Recovering Bodies

Wisconsin Studies in American Autobiography

William L. Andrews
General Editor

Recovering Bodies

Illness, Disability, and Life Writing

G. THOMAS COUSER

With a Foreword
by Nancy Mairs

The University of Wisconsin Press

The University of Wisconsin Press
2537 Daniels Street
Madison, Wisconsin 53718

3 Henrietta Street
London WC2E 8LU, England

Library of Congress Cataloging-in-Publication Data
Couser, G. Thomas.
   Recovering bodies: illness, disability, and life-writing /
G. Thomas Couser.
   334 pp.   cm.—(Wisconsin studies in American autobiography)
   Includes bibliographical references and index.
   ISBN 0-299-15560-9 (cloth: alk. paper).   ISBN 0-299-15564-1 (paper: alk. paper)
   1. Sick—United States—Biography—History and criticism.
2. Physically handicapped—United States—Biography—History and criticism.
3. Sick—United States—Psychology.   4. Physically handicapped—United States—
Psychology.   5. Autobiography.   6. Biography as a literary form.
   I. Title   II. Series.
   R726.5.C73   1997
   616'.001'9—dc21   97-11952

In memory of my cousin
Sara Jane Couser Johnson
1946–1990

Contents

Foreword

Nancy Mairs

You sit in a tiny room, probably white, probably without windows, the walls decked with posters showing parts of your anatomy you might rather not contemplate. With luck, you've got your clothes back on; otherwise, you're wearing a scanty smock that bares anatomical parts you'd definitely prefer no one else to contemplate. If you're wise, you've brought with you a parent, child, spouse, or sibling. Voices from the surrounding rooms leak through the walls, but the two of you eye the posters in silence. No matter how fluently you communicated this morning over the breakfast table, nothing seems worth saying in the fluorescent glare of this cubicle.

Something is amiss, you know, or else you wouldn't be here; unless you're a doctor or a hypochondriac, you have no idea what the problem is, but you're inclined to believe that the wonders of modern medicine will soon make it go away. Then the doctor raps once, slips through the door, and speaks your doom. In my case, it was multiple sclerosis; in my husband's, melanoma. Suddenly, you feel lopped off from the social body, shut up here in this bright little box, unutterably alone. Being a rational creature, you know you're not the only person to have heard these words; statistically, people all over the world are hearing something like them at this moment. Such knowledge doesn't matter. Each of us experiences the self as a singularity, and you've just been sucked into a black hole.

Fortunately, this histrionic state tends not to last. You set about doing whatever has to be done: buy a cane, go to physical or occupational therapy, schedule surgery, join a support group, revise your will. Being a social creature as well, you soon long for the guidance and companionship of other sufferers and, as you begin to get the hang of your situation, to serve as a guide and companion yourself. Then, if you're a writer, you start to scribble.

In a note at the opening of *A Whole New Life* (1995), Reynolds Price offers his account of surviving a malignant spinal cord tumor "to others in physical or psychic trials of their own, to their families and other helpers and then to the curious reader who waits for his or her own devastation." "In my worst times," he goes on a few sentences later, "I'd have given a lot to hear from veterans of the kind of ordeal I was trapped in," although he doesn't relate any efforts he might have made to seek these out. Wilfrid Sheed, in the introduction to *In Love with Daylight*, the 1995 book in which he recounts his surviving polio, addiction-depression, and cancer of the tongue, speaks more explicitly about both the price he'd have been willing to pay and the futility of his search:

I would have sold my soul cheerfully (if I could have done anything cheerfully) just to hear from someone else who had passed this way and could tell me what was actually happening to me and what to expect next. But among all the thousands of inspirational and pseudoscientific words I could find . . . not one came close either to describing what I was going through, or suggesting anything useful to do about it. . . . So I've had to write it myself, scene for scene—all the things I would like to have read back then.

All writers, it occurs to me, my be driven to their desks less by creative genius than by the desire to produce the book they would most like to read. Margaret Mitchell was probably just dying to curl up with a romantic epic set in the Civil War. Edward Gibbon couldn't for the life of him find a satisfactory account of the decline and fall of the Roman Empire. *Nobody's done a decent job with this material*, the writer laments. *I'll simply have to do it myself*. When the work relies on personal history, instead of or in addition to research, the impetus becomes even stronger; although human experience may not vary widely from one person to another, individual perceptions of it do, leaving each person convinced that her story is unique and must be told by her alone.

Writers of what I've come to call the literature of personal disaster or the memoir of mischance—works about illness, disability, and death—are being a little disingenuous, then, when they claim to wish that they'd had the book they've just written back when they needed it most. In their heart of hearts they're glad such a book didn't exist, because then they felt compelled to write it. What they mean is that—lucky you!—you now hold in your hands the information and advice they so sorely lacked (though, if you're anything like the rest, this won't quite satisfy, and you'll have to write a book of your own).

In truth, personal narratives about illness and injury abound, and they're not all as sorry as Sheed suggests, although altogether too many of them are. The would-be reader can hardly be faulted for failing to search them out, however. "Disability studies" is a fairly recent coinage, and because most bookstores and libraries don't catalogue works under this rubric, they may be scattered in a variety of categories: biography, autobiography, memoir, or journalism; belles lettres or essays; health or medicine. Because they are grounded in feminist theory, mine are generally classified under women's studies, and I once found one in the philosophy section of a Los Angeles bookstore and gave myself airs for some hours thereafter.

Though a practitioner of the form myself, I became aware of illness narratives as a distinct subgenre of autobiographical writing only gradually. Several years ago I began to discern a pattern to the books for which I was asked to write reviews or endorsements. Despite general similarities, the situations revealed in these works were far from uniform. Many entailed loss, for example, but this might be of a parent, child, spouse, limb, or mind. Ages varied widely, although, not surprisingly, socioeconomic level generally did not. The narrator might be afflicted herself or might be caring for another. I use the generic feminine here, but in fact I began to perceive that more women than men write, and write more intimately, about physical and emotional distress.

Some writers stated explicit purposes for their undertakings, but most did not; in fact, they often seemed unaware that they were producing a "book" and not merely a log or daybook. Nevertheless, they were obviously people who relied heavily on language (rather than, or in addition to, alcohol and sleeping potions) to get them through an ordeal. Some underlying motives might be to aestheticize pain, memorialize the beloved, rage against fate or the system (these two are often conflated), order chaotic experience, or merely hold hands with an imagined reader in similar distress.

Most of these works have an accidental basis: one simply does not set out to have melanoma as one sets out to earn a college degree. In both cases, the ends are fixed (the former perhaps more inexorably than the latter), but one course is as disorderly as the other is methodical. For this reason many writers, especially those without literary background, are apt to keep a journal; essays and memoirs are also common. On the whole, the closest rhetorical analogy may lie in the letters and diaries of early explorers. The terrain is similarly unknown and fraught with peril.

We're not talking a handful of books here. Dozens have poured forth from publishers large and small in the United Kingdom as well as the States. My shelves groan under their weight. Until a few years ago, when I met Tom Couser at a conference on autobiography hosted by Hofstra University, I wasn't sure that anybody else had observed this proliferation. But indeed Tom had noticed and was already well into the project that would become this welcome book.

When a genre emerges, it does so without either fanfare or operating instructions. As a result, even highly literate people like Price and Sheed may not know that what they want exists, and practitioners and readers alike may not recognize the rules whereby it is successfully written and evaluated. Rules there must always be, as chaos theorists have demonstrated. These may be internally generated, although in the case of literature a good many conventions carry over from one genre to another. What Tom has done so valuably in *Recovering Bodies* is to call attention to the autobiography of illness and disability and to define some of the conventions peculiar to it. Only with such solid grounding can a truly intelligent reading of these works be done.

Wisely, I think, Tom has limited the scope of his study to books dealing with HIV/AIDS, breast cancer, paralysis, and deafness. He couldn't have covered every physical catastrophe that has occasioned a memoir, and these are good choices for representing the variety of issues associated with illness or disability, which are not necessarily synonymous. HIV/AIDS has stricken gay men in disproportionate numbers, whereas in all but a few hundred cases breast cancer occurs in women; generally speaking, paralysis and deafness don't show any particular gender bias, though the responses to them often do. Whereas AIDS appears to be, at this time, inevitably fatal, as is breast cancer all too often, paralysis may or may not be, depending on its cause, and deafness, in and of itself, virtually never. *Stigma,* in sociologist Erving Goffman's sense of the word, attaches to every abnormality, but the rationale for social exclusion varies. Because their condition is associated with homosexuality and intravenous drug use, people with HIV/AIDS are apt to be isolated by moral disapproval; deaf people, linguistically; those in wheelchairs, by physical barriers; victims of breast cancer, by pity and horror. Such variables make it possible for Tom to analyze literary production under a wide range of circumstances.

Though fully realized in its own terms, *Recovering Bodies* remains in some sense preliminary. That is, because some conditions not considered here—mental disabilities like Down syndrome, autism, and bipolar illness, say, or the limitations imposed by aging—have inspired works that may augment or modify the conventions Tom has identified, ample room remains for further investigation. Genres other than autobiography, both in literature and in the other arts, might yield fruitful insights into strategies for representing illness and disability. Approaches from different disciplinary standpoints—theological, psychoanalytic, and the like—could enrich our understanding of the experiences that inspire narratives of distress and the purposes they fulfill.

Nevertheless, Tom has made a brave beginning—and I use the word advisedly. On the whole, critical attitudes toward art produced by people in mental or physical anguish have been condescending at best and often downright dismissive. In a *New Yorker* article a couple of years ago dance critic Arlene Croce labeled it, with an all but audible sneer, "victim art" (1994). Refusing even to see a production by an HIV-positive choreographer that dealt with AIDS, she demurred, "I can't review someone I feel sorry for or hopeless about," a stance that denigrates and, if inadvertently, mystifies suffering in a way that is helpful neither to those afflicted with some mental or physical disorder nor to those who will become so afflicted, as all who live long enough, including Croce, will do. In the critical community Croce's presence is "magisterial," in the words of one of her colleagues (Jowitt 1995). A scholar, recognizing the merits of a neglected body of work, requires some courage to ignore the disdain of the éminences grises and set about studying it with the dignity, insight, and wit Tom displays here.

References

Croce, Arlene. "Discussing the Undiscussable." *The New Yorker,* December 26, 1994, and January 2, 1995: 54–60.

Goffman, Erving. *Stigma: Notes on the Management of Spoiled Identity.* New York: Simon & Schuster, 1963.

Jowitt, Deborah. "Critic as Victim." *Village Voice* January 10, 1995: 67, 69.

Price, Reynolds. *A Whole New Life: An Illness and a Healing.* New York: Plume, 1995.

Sheed, Wilfrid. *In Love with Daylight: A Memoir of Recovery.* New York: Simon & Schuster, 1995.

Preface

Because of my sense of the broad interest in the growing literatures of illness and disability, I have made a conscious effort to make this book accessible to "lay" readers—that is, nonacademics. To that end I have tried to minimize discussion of methodology and the use of academic jargon. Also, because many readers may be primarily, if not exclusively, interested in the literature of one of the four major conditions whose literature I discuss—breast cancer, HIV/AIDS, paralysis, and hearing impairment—I have tried to make these chapters independent of one another.

Because the books I survey are relatively recent and generally not well known, I have also departed from the academic convention of assuming readers' familiarity with the texts under discussion. I have tried to supply enough information about each—without resorting to plot summary—to give readers a sense of the life into which illness or disability intrudes. I hope that my book will serve as a guide to reading the primary sources as well as an introduction to the issues raised by narratives of illness and disability.

This book has been (too) long in preparation. Indeed, it would still be in progress if not for a timely grant from the National Endowment for the Humanities. With additional generous support from Hofstra University I was able to take an extended leave from teaching during which I completed the manuscript. Dean Robert Vogt and Associate Dean Bernard Firestone of Hofstra College deserve special thanks for arranging for my leave of absence. I also benefited from other support that is less tangible but no less valuable. Colleagues took precious time away from their work to read and comment on mine. I am grateful for the generosity of Timothy Dow Adams, Kay Cook, Susanna Egan, and Rosemarie Garland Thomson, who read parts of the manuscript, and to Paul John Eakin and Nancy Mairs, who read all of it. I am grateful too to William Andrews for his interest in the project and to the University of Wisconsin Press for its expeditious review process. Polly Kummel's alert copyediting improved the book in subtle but significant ways. And I am grateful to the editors of *a/b: Auto/Biography Studies* for permission to adapt material from my contributions to a special issue on illness, disability, and life writing (vol. 6, no. 1, spring 1991), and to Willard Spiegelman for permission to use material previously published in *Southwest Review* (summer 1996).

My sister, Jane Barton, provided encouragement and clippings of relevant book reviews. My wife, Barbara Zabel, has lived with the book as long as I have and knows better than anyone what it means to me.

Recovering Bodies

1

Introduction

Human Conditions—Illness, Disability, and Life Writing

> What happens to my body happens to my life.
> —Arthur W. Frank, *At the Will of the Body*, 1991, p. 13.

> For illness is a real loss of control that results in our becoming the Other whom
> we have feared, whom we have projected onto the world.
> —Sander Gilman, *Disease and Representation*, 1988, p. 2.

Over the several years I spent on this book, when friends and colleagues would ask what it was about, most seemed nonplussed when I replied, "Personal narratives of illness and disability." Some would express mild interest; others, commiseration: "Gee, that sounds depressing."[1] But the most common response was, "How did you get interested in *that*?" I took this to indicate that, even in an age when cultural studies legitimates almost anything as an object of academic inquiry, people considered my topic eccentric, perhaps even unnatural or morbid. The question also seemed to anticipate and invite an autobiographical answer: on some level it was an inquiry about my health or my history. People seemed to find it odd that a healthy-looking individual who is not disabled would be interested in illness and disability. In part, this reflects an all-too-common cultural denial of bodily dysfunction. In part, it reflects the influence of identity politics. For the idea that one's identity and politics are, or ought to be, based in some shared attribute—such as race, ethnicity, or gender—has recently been extended to illness and disability. One unfortunate consequence of identity politics has been a tendency to reify or reinforce differences between groups so defined. In the academy this has meant all too often that like studies or teaches like—in my view not an ideal manifestation of multiculturalism. Thus

3

the practice, if not the theory, of multiculturalism can discourage interest in identities other than one's own. For various reasons, even though illness and disability represent forms of marginalization to which we are all vulnerable, they remain truly marginalized topics within the academy.

Although the deaths of my mother (in her midsixties) and a cousin (in her early forties) of cancer and the deaths of friends and colleagues of AIDS have had an undeniable effect on my awareness of illness, the sources of my interest are not primarily biographical—at least on the conscious level. (Admittedly, the advent of middle age, with its intimations of mortality, is a contributing influence.) My interest in narratives of illness and disability is less a function of personal history than an extension of a long-term concern with autobiography and other "life writing" genres, and in particular with issues of authority—who (or what) controls or shapes life narratives.

Like other scholars in the field, I have been attracted to life-writing genres (which include autobiography, biography, memoir, and diary) partly because of a sense that, located on the borders of the literary, they are particularly accessible to marginalized individuals. I am wont to quote William Dean Howells to the effect that autobiography is the most democratic province of the republic of letters (1909, 798): in theory, anyone in a modern democratic society can write an autobiography. In practice, life-writing genres have hardly been equal opportunity employers; various constraints have made autobiography, especially, a male-dominated genre. Indeed, a prominent concern in much recent work on life writing has been who gets a life and who doesn't: whose stories get told, why, by whom, and how.

As it happens, those who produce narratives of illness and disability are not diverse in terms of race and class. They tend to be white and upper middle class. Before they became ill or impaired, many were already professional writers or worked in professions where writing was part of the job. When such people experience serious illness or disability, it jeopardizes an already valorized individuality; writing, already a valuable professional skill, bids to be an agent of recovery as well as self-expression. Nevertheless, by definition the subgenre does represent marginalized individuals—especially in the case of stigmatic diseases like AIDS. Indeed, in recent decades the flourishing of narratives of illness or disability poses a significant challenge to the stigmatization of illness and disability and to the general valorization of mind over body in Western culture, the tendency to deny the body's mediation in intellectual and spiritual life.

It is obvious upon reflection (though most of us rarely reflect upon it) that we have our being in the world, and act upon it, through our bodies. Yet, although our selves and our lives are fundamentally somatic, the body has not until recently figured prominently in life writing. Traditional biographers usually treat illness as an interruption of the life that is their proper concern, except when it threatens life or ends it. And although autobiographers are better situated than biographers to report on the somatic lives of their subjects, traditionally they too have seemed disinclined to do so.

In the last several decades, however, illness narratives have been written and published in unprecedented numbers. According to Anne Hunsaker Hawkins, "As a genre, pathography is remarkable in that it seems to have emerged *ex nihilo*; book-length personal accounts of illness are uncommon before 1950 and rarely found before 1900" (3).[2] Unnoticed by most scholars doing textual and cultural studies, a new form of life writing has flourished in the post-World War II era, gaining momentum in the era of civil rights and other liberation movements.

The relation between bodily dysfunction and personal narrative is a complex one; the former may both impel and impede the latter. Bodily dysfunction may stimulate what I call *autopathography*—autobiographical narrative of illness or disability—by heightening one's awareness of one's mortality, threatening one's sense of identity, and disrupting the apparent plot of one's life. Whatever form it takes, bodily dysfunction tends to heighten consciousness of self and of contingency. As Arthur W. Frank puts it, "Illness takes away parts of your life but in doing so it gives you the opportunity to choose the life you will lead, as opposed to living out the one you have simply accumulated over the years" (*Will* 1). If introspection is conducive to autobiography, illness and disability would seem to be apt preconditions for writing one's life.

Although bodily dysfunction may be conducive to autobiography, only a fraction of those who are ill and disabled actually write, let alone publish, narratives. One reason is that the conditions that may stimulate autobiographical reflection may also obstruct its expression. After all, many of the sick and disabled are simply too ill—too debilitated or traumatized by their condition—to imagine writing about it. Crucial events or periods may be unavailable to the autobiographical *I* because of literal unconsciousness resulting from coma or anaesthetic. More important, and more generally, illness or disability may turn people so far inward that they become virtual black holes, absorbing energy rather than emitting illumination. Moreover, those with chronic disability or illness may have difficulty reconciling their experience of illness with the comic plot expected of autobiography; in many cases the culturally validated narrative of triumph over adversity may simply not be available. And for some disease annihilates selfhood, or ends life, before they can undertake a narrative—what distinguishes the autobiographical subject may also extinguish it. Conversely, if the illness or disability is acute and not chronic, temporary and not terminal, it may seem, retrospectively, an interruption of life rather than an integral part of it. Those whose dysfunction is temporary have the luxury of denying their physical vulnerability and bodily contingency.

Personal narratives of sickness and disability may, of course, take forms other than autobiographical accounts. Broadly considered, the category would include journals, essays, and full-life narratives (*illness narrative* refers to writing about the episode of one's illness, whereas *full-life narrative* refers to a comprehensive account of one's life, including the illness). (Indeed, although I limit myself to published book-length personal narratives here, representation of illness and disability may also take the form of self-portraiture, as do the paintings of Frida Kahlo, and audio or video recording.) Although illness and disability do seem to single out individuals, these conditions inevitably also affect those close to those individuals, especially their families; as a result, illness has also been a stimulant to relational, as well as autobiographical, narratives. In the case of narratives by family or friends—illness memoirs, as opposed to autobiographies—some of the obstacles I have cited do not pertain.[3] Although memoirs cannot render the subjective experience of illness, they can represent conditions (and outcomes) unavailable to autobiography. To a lesser extent so can the diary (or journal), precisely because it does not await the resolution—whether in recovery from or accommodation to dysfunction—that seems to license most retrospective autobiographical accounts of illness and disability.

For various reasons bodily dysfunction has recently been precipitating into print lives that would not otherwise have been written. Yet, like members of other marginalized groups, individuals who are ill or disabled do not always control the representation of their lives even in personal narratives. Some groups of individuals also find powerful cultural obstacles to life writing. For example, Deaf people (deaf individuals who use American Sign Language, value Deaf culture, and who identify with other such people) are unlikely to produce written personal narrative; the Deaf community does not offer much cultural sanction for autobiography, and literacy in English tends to be low. Even when others write the lives of Deaf people, the verbal medium may misrepresent them and their lives in significant ways. For reasons particular to HIV/AIDS, narratives related to this disease far more often take the form of memoir than of autobiography. Issues of authority are especially complicated in the case of memoirs of illness, in which the person who is ill or disabled is not the narrator; such narratives may be unconsciously patronizing. For various reasons, then, illness and disability may at once stimulate the production of written lives and inhibit authoritative self-representation.

Perhaps the major stimulus to my interest in personal narratives of illness and disability has been the writing itself, which has flourished remarkably in the last several decades. Dysfunction may remain in the background, as when serious illness or disability stimulates reassessment of a whole life, but usually it is squarely in the foreground, as when the narrative is coextensive with the condition. Recent trends have favored such "single-experience" autobiographies. Indeed, as Peter Kramer, the author of *Listening to Prozac*, remarked in the *New York Times Book Review* in 1996, "Ours is the era of autopathography. Bookstore shelves groan with memoirs of heart disease and asthma. No mental disorder, from alcoholism and autism to schizophrenia, is without its confessions. Obviously, these titles represent niche book selling, a guide for every challenge" (27).

The tepid interest of most of my literary colleagues in narratives of illness reflects a sense that such niche books must necessarily be sub- or extraliterary—too narrow in focus, too confined in theme, too conventional in form to be of much interest or lasting significance. And although I have been drawn to the subject by some splendid books published in the last few years, I find it hard to name many titles that most colleagues would recognize. Yet the lack of acknowledged classics may have less to do with the inherent qualities of these books than with a system of values that marginalizes narratives about illness and disability as it does people with those conditions. Furthermore, although the field is maturing quickly, it is still relatively young.

Several related phenomena seem to be coinciding. One is that writers already established in other, more literary genres, such as poetry and fiction, have been turning to autopathography; for them bodily dysfunction has provided an occasion for an experiment with life writing. Works in this category would include William Styron's *Darkness Visible* (which deals with depression), John Updike's *Self-Consciousness* (psoriasis, stuttering, asthma), *No Laughing Matter* by Joseph Heller and Speed Vogel (Guillain-Barré syndrome), Audre Lorde's *The Cancer Journals* (breast cancer), Reynolds Price's *A Whole New Life* (spinal cancer and paraplegia), Richard Selzer's *Raising the Dead* (Legionnaire's disease), Paul West's *A Stroke of Genius*, and Paul Monette's *Borrowed Time: An AIDS Memoir*. Closely related to these books are nonliterary celebrities' narratives of illness (often collaborative in authorship)—books like Arthur Ashe's *Days of Grace* (AIDS) and Gilda Radner's *It's Always Something* (ovarian cancer). In both sets of examples the fame of the authors guarantees their books an audience; the narratives are published by well-known presses and often widely and prominently reviewed. Bookstores shelve them under *nonfiction* or *biography*.

Less prominent but perhaps just as significant is a complementary groundswell, the publication of illness narratives by less well-known individuals. These people would likely never have written books, certainly not personal narratives, if they or someone close to them had not become ill or impaired; indeed, their books are likely to be the only ones they ever write. Sometimes naive in their approach, they tend to be published by small presses and are not usually widely or prominently reviewed. Bookstores shelve them under *health*, according to the condition they describe.

The same factors stimulate both trends. One is the destigmatization of illness and disability, which such narratives at once reflect and seek to advance. Another is the extension of identity politics to illness—especially in the case of diseases specific to particular groups, such as breast cancer. Further, those illnesses that are especially threatening—either because they are common or because they are particularly fraught with cultural significance—tend to provoke relatively large numbers of narratives. (Thus narratives of tuberculosis were fairly numerous in the nineteenth century. In the period immediately following World War II polio narratives proliferated.)

Life writing about illness and disability demands attention at this moment for a number of reasons. First is AIDS, a disease that has become uniquely and powerfully stigmatic, irrationally (and rationally) feared, widely (sometimes cruelly) publicized, and highly politicized. Such a contemporary calamity is AIDS—first, but not only, for the gay community—that, like the Holocaust (to which it is often and inevitably compared), it has given rise to a literature of its own. Although the best-known works about AIDS are plays and novels, it has also been the subject of many illness narratives. Because AIDS carries such a burden of myth and metaphor (which quite literally adds insult to injury), these narratives often involve an extraordinarily complex negotiation between private experience and public expression and a delicate balancing of literary, moral, and political considerations. AIDS, then, simultaneously generates and complicates life writing about illness. Other dreaded diseases, such as breast cancer, have also given rise to literatures of their own in recent decades. Indeed, Susan Sontag's breast cancer was one of the stimuli for her 1978 *Illness as Metaphor*, which initiated a critique of the representation of disease that has been given further urgency by the stigmatization of AIDS.

But the rise of interest in life writing about disease has to do with larger cultural forces than the ravages of such diseases, for people also are writing narratives about relatively rare illnesses and about conditions that have no particular currency. Since the early 1980s people have published narratives devoted to a large range of illnesses: asthma (Brookes), chronic fatigue syndrome (Duff), heart disease (Greene), prostate cancer (Broyard), diabetes (Pray), lupus (Chester), and even, improbably, Alzheimer's disease (McGowin).[4] In the background is the tenor of contemporary American mainstream culture, which is at once both health and disease conscious. Thus even as narratives of illness and disability proliferate, so do magazines about health and fitness. (This counterpoint is perhaps most intense in gay culture, which simultaneously affords us images of the most assiduously cultivated and the most disease-ravaged male physiques.)

The concerns with health and illness are not contradictory; rather, both are expressions of a powerful cultural mandate that individuals control their bodies. Indeed, according to one increasingly influential "alternative" way of thinking about health—exemplified in the "wellness movement"—"sick persons are understood to be responsible for incurring their illness, usually by their life-style, stress, or feelings of unresolved anger and depression, and they are also responsible for getting well again" (Hawkins 129). (This paradigm would tend to encourage confessional forms of autopathography.) As late twentieth-century Americans (of the middle- and upper-income brackets, at least) come to take for granted increased longevity, as many work at fitness and health, and as governments, employers, and insurance companies encourage people to take greater responsibility for their health, instances of illness and disability seem all the more remarkable—and all the more sinister. Thus the backdrop against which we need to regard the flowering of illness narrative is a historical era in which certain groups of people may take health for granted. When illness and disability are seen not so much as inevitable natural phenomena but as unexpected and perhaps disastrous events, they become noteworthy and (potentially) narratable. Bodily dysfunction is perhaps the most common threat to the appealing belief that one controls one's destiny. Perhaps, then, narratives of disability and illness serve to expose and dramatize what we would prefer to ignore most of the time, to arouse and (ideally) assuage our anxiety about our somatic selves. As Sander Gilman has observed, "The fixed structures of art provide us with a sort of carnival during which we fantasize about our potential loss of control, perhaps even revel in the fear it generates within us, but we always believe that this fear exists separate from us" (2).

According to Hawkins, "It is surely no accident that the appearance of pathography coincides with the triumph of scientific technological medicine" (xii). Herein lies an irony, if not a paradox: as the efficacy of U.S. medicine has increased, public confidence in the medical establishment has decreased. The nature of the biomedical paradigm is to promise more than it can deliver—a quick fix for every bodily ill. Even when it does cure, it too often alienates us from our bodies. The same phenomena that have made contemporary diagnosis and treatment so sophisticated have, ironically, diverted doctors' attention toward disease and away from illness, toward the laboratory and away from the bedside, toward curing and away from healing. Modern medicine has enabled many people to survive illnesses and conditions that once would have killed them; many, however, are not fully cured and become members of what Frank calls the "remission society." Medicine may give them continued life, but it cannot give that life meaning. Indeed, medical practices, regimes, and discourse threaten to diminish or distort its significance. Thus even when medical treatment may be objectively successful, patients may feel that they have been poorly treated (Shorter 21–23). They often express anger at depersonalizing treatment and sometimes advocate alternative modalities (Hawkins 5).

The treatment of illness or disability typically, and necessarily, involves a sort of narrative collaboration between doctor and patient— the creation of a new "life text." Diagnosis often relies at least in part on a medical history; the patient offers up testimony that the doctor interprets according to codes and conventions generally unavailable to the patient. In order to be treated, then, patients generally must have their medical history "taken." In diagnosis doctors provide patients with an interpretation of their lives—an act that, regardless of what follows, may at least make sense of a baffling past. Diagnosis leads in turn to prescription, treatment, and prognosis, all of which extend physicians' authority over patients' lives. Thus doctors may both reinterpret patients' pasts and literally pre-script their futures. The process is collaborative but one sided; patients submit their bodies to tests, their life histories to scrutiny, while doctors retain the authority to interpret these data. By means of this process (interrogation and interpretation) the physician reconfigures the sick person's illness as the patient's disease.

Of course, this is what most sick people expect, and perhaps even desire, from doctors, and this process is not inherently malign. Yet the process involves relinquishing control over one's body, and one's story, in a way that may seem objectifying and objectionable to many people. The narrative thus "collaboratively" produced may serve the physician's needs more fully than it serves the patient's.[5] Thus, just as patients wish to vanquish the illness that alters their lives, they may also wish to regain control of their life narratives, which they have yielded up to "objective" medical authority.

Increasingly, patients are resisting or challenging medical authority or seeking to share it. One manifestation of this trend has been the patients' rights movement. Well before the onset of AIDS and the activism it engendered, the women's movement played a key role in the reconception of the relationship between patients and doctors; the problematic—intimate yet objectifying—relationship between gynecologist and patient has been the site of a reexamination of the politics of medicine as a whole. Thus contemporary patients are more likely to seek second opinions, assert more control of their treatment, second-guess—and sue—their doctors. A related phenomenon is that, in the wake of the civil rights advances of the 1960s and 1970s, people with disabilities have claimed their right to greater participation in public life.

According to Frank, the postmodern experience of illness is distinguished by the impulse of patients to reclaim their bodies and their stories from medical discourse; the postmodern era is also, then, postcolonial (*Wounded* 10).

> Post-colonialism in its most generalized form is the demand to speak rather than being spoken for and to represent oneself rather than being represented or, in the worst cases, rather than being effaced entirely. But . . . the post-colonial impulse is acted out less in the clinic than in stories that members of the remission society tell each other about their illnesses.
>
> The post-colonial stance of these stories resides not in the content of what they say about medicine. Rather the new feel of these stories begins in how often medicine and physicians do *not* enter their stories. Postmodern illness stories are told so that people can place themselves outside "the unifying general view." For people to move their stories outside the professional purview involves a profound assumption of personal responsibility. In [Talcott] Parsons' [classic sociological analysis of the] sick role the ill person as patient was responsible only for getting well; in the remission society, the post-colonial ill person takes responsibility for what illness means in his life. (13)

As we shall see in Chapter 2, this resistance to medical discourse has important implications for medical practice, for doctor-patient relations in all their subtle political ramifications. But it also has interesting implications for life writing, especially autobiography. As patients seize, or at least claim, more authority over their treatment, they may also be more inclined to narrate their stories, to take their lives literally into their own hands in part to reestablish their subjectivity in the face of objectifying treatment. As Frank notes, personal narrative enables patients, whom the biomedical paradigm assigns a passive care-receiving role, to be active agents, providing care through their narrative to others (*Wounded* xi). Frank's schema of illness narratives suggests that most reflect neither best-case "restitution stories" (a quick, complete, and uncomplicated restoration of health) nor worst-case "chaos stories" (dysfunction that cannot be ameliorated) but "quest stories":

Quest stories meet suffering head on; they accept illness and seek to *use* it. Illness is the occasion of a journey that becomes a quest. What is quested for may never be wholly clear, but the quest is defined by the ill person's belief that something is to be gained through the experience.

The quest narrative affords the ill person a voice as teller of her own story, because only in quest stories does the *teller* have a story to tell. In the restitution narrative the active player is the remedy: either the drug itself . . . or the physician. Restitution stories are about the triumph of medicine; they are self-stories only by default. Chaos stories remain the sufferer's own story, but the suffering is too great for a self to be told. The voice of the teller has been lost as a result of the chaos, and this loss then perpetuates that chaos. Though both restitution and chaos remain background voices when the quest is foregrounded, the quest narrative speaks from the ill person's perspective and holds chaos at bay. (*Wounded* 115)

It may be, then, that prolonged, serious, or chronic illnesses and disabilities may ultimately yield more complex and multidimensional narratives than acute illnesses; because lasting dysfunction has to be lived with for some time, rather than survived as a mere episode, it may lead to quest stories rather than to restitution stories—in literary terms, autobiography rather than autopathography.

Thus illness by itself does not lead to autobiography; autobiographers also must have some cultural authorization, some sense that their story is valid and valuable; the more public the form of expression, perhaps, the stronger the social sanction required. And until recently, such cultural authorization has been lacking. Increasingly, then, narratives of somatic dysfunctions explore the ways in which culture constructs illness and disability, whatever their proximate causes, according to its anonymous and seemingly arbitrary dictates. One common purpose is to invalidate dominant cultural narratives of invalidism.

More generally, however, life writing about illness and disability promises to illuminate the relations among body, mind, and soul; indeed, it is significant not just because it represents a relatively new category of life stories but also because it promises to foreground somatic experience in a new way by treating the body's form and function (apart from race or gender) as fundamental constituents of identity. The effects of disease on identity and self-perception may be most fundamental and troubling in the case of mental illness. However, some physical ailments may radically undermine a patient's sense of self. The neurologist Oliver Sacks has made a literary form of case studies of patients with physiologically altered egos. But perhaps our conventional notions of bodily integrity, individuality, and mortality are most profoundly challenged when surgeons successfully transplant vital organs—including that most metaphorically and symbolically charged of all such organs, the human heart. Such operations, once the stuff of science fiction, have interesting, and unsettling, implications for life writing, because they threaten the boundaries of self and life that autobiography usually assumes. When illness and disability foreground the body in this way, life writing has a new opportunity to explore the ways in which the body mediates identity or personality.

Whether the works in question put illness in the foreground or the background, whether they are autobiographical or biographical, private or public in conception, writing of this nature occurs at the intersection of culture and what Adalaide Morris has called "that most insistent and intimate locus of materialization, the living human body" (571). With the current turning away from the most cerebral of literary theories, such as deconstruction, to approaches more attentive to social and historical contexts, from a sense of language as an impersonal and autonomous system to a sense of writing as a concretely situated personal appropriation of a public instrument, narratives acknowledging and exploring the embodiment of the self have much to say to us today.

The irony is that when the study of marginalization in the form of race, gender, class, and sexual orientation has moved to the center of literary and cultural studies, few have studied the most widespread forms of marginalization—illness and disability. Indeed, Arthur W. Frank has referred to the first-person narrative of illness as "an orphan genre"— by analogy with "orphan diseases," which occur so rarely that they do not seem worthwhile subjects for research ("Reclaiming" 2). Since I began the inquiry that resulted in this book, however, the situation has changed dramatically; two other scholars in particular have moved to adopt the orphan genre. Anne Hunsaker Hawkins's groundbreaking work in this area culminated in her *Reconstructing Illness: Studies in Pathography* (1993), which provides an indispensable overview of the field. More recently, Frank's 1995 book, *The Wounded Storyteller*, theorized about illness narratives (including unpublished ones) in a broad cultural perspective.

A medical sociologist by training, Frank is especially interested in the ethical significance of patient testimony—in relation to, though not contained by, medical practice. Hawkins, who was trained as a literary scholar, approaches illness narratives largely in terms of the myths they use to ascribe meaning to illness. In distinction from my two precursors I am more interested in the relation of illness narratives to other forms of life writing and to the discourses of illness and disability. Thus perhaps my inquiry can best be distinguished by saying that I accent the poetics and politics of illness narrative as both separate and related aspects of the literature. By *poetics* I mean the questions the books raise as narratives. Most fundamentally, how do illness and disability—which in extreme cases might obstruct or defy narration—get written at all? How does one make a (coherent) story out of bodily dysfunction? What particular challenges do illness and disability pose for personal narrative? (To look ahead I see a particular challenge in the little-appreciated but quite powerful life-writing convention of the comic plot. The challenge for autobiographical narrative is to achieve closure of any sort, but especially comic resolution, with regard to conditions that are chronic, systemic, or degenerative.) What genres, conventions, points of view, and formulas do stories of illness use? How do they draw on, revise, or expand the existing repertoire of life-writing conventions in order to represent previously unrepresented conditions?

I am interested too in how and when illness narrative becomes life writing more generally. Under what circumstances does the story of a bodily dysfunction come to represent an entire life? The distinction is troublesome, because it can be both a matter of kind (or intention) and one of degree (or quality). Thus some books feature illness as their primary, even sole, focus, whereas others may use illness as a pretext for exploring broader issues. Generally, however, narratives that confine themselves to a chronological clinical account of illness do not get published (outside of medical discourse). Most books discussed here at least gesture in the direction of life writing. To put it somewhat schematically writers may integrate illness narrative into a larger life narrative chronologically, by linear extension, or simultaneously, by conflation of other issues with the somatic. The first strategy involves embedding a somatic crisis in a full-life narrative (as a phase or "chapter"); the second explores the full existential implications of an illness or disability. Although it may seem counterintuitive, narratives of somatic dysfunction tend to become life writing to the degree that the writer identifies the self with the body. Thus pure illness narrative tends to disengage the body from the self in the way that medical discourse often tends to do. Full life-writing is facilitated, authorized, or even required when one assumes that what happens to one's body happens to one's life (to paraphrase this chapter's first epigraph). I do not claim to have laid out a systematic poetics of illness narrative, but I hope that I have taken an important step in the direction of understanding illness narrative as a significant and relatively new form of life writing.

In *politics* I comprehend at least two dimensions, internal and external. By internal politics I mean the distribution of power between those who are ill or disabled and those who represent (or misrepresent) them in narrative. To what extent do the narratives involve self-representation? Are some conditions more conducive to autobiography than to memoir? (For reasons to be explored later breast cancer and paralysis

annotations specify the illness in question, the myth(s) used to organize the narrative, and other attributes that will assist focused research or reading.

5. In *The Illness Narratives* (1988) Arthur Kleinman explores the role of oral testimony in medical care and makes a case that truly therapeutic medicine requires careful and empathic attention to the testimony of the ill. Similarly, Cheryl Mattingly has observed how, in the rehabilitation of people with disabilities, collaborative "therapeutic emplotment" can shape recovery (1994).

6. Another obviously stigmatizing condition would be mental illness. Although my omission of any such disorder risks reifying what is increasingly seen as a false dichotomy between physical and mental illness, it is based on two considerations. One is that the literature of mental illness—of which depression seems to be the contemporary paradigm—is developing so fast that I could not keep up. Another is that, despite my sense that *mental illness* is in large part a misnomer, dysfunctions like schizophrenia and depression raise complex and largely independent issues—such as the representation of altered consciousness—that I was ill equipped to address. (For some pioneering work in this area see Sidonie Smith's 1996 essay on autism.)

2

Medical Discourse
and Subjectivity

"Patients," people whose illnesses or disabilities require medical care or other therapies, are usually objectified in the process to the extent that they perceive their bodies as literally belonging to someone else.
—Barbara Hillyer, *Feminism and Disability,* 1993, p. 170.

As I was lying there, trying not to move as the machine registered its images, it occurred to me that the individuality we pride ourselves upon, our personhood, rests almost entirely on intangible qualities of character and efforts of mind, all of which are completely invisible to medical technology.
—Musa Mayer, *Examining Myself,* 1993, pp. 24–25.

Medicine, I think, needs to be seen as a meeting between patient and physician, on equal footing, in the real world, with the aim of promoting self-understanding.
—Tim Brookes, *Catching My Breath,* 1995, p. 283.

The considerable power of the medical profession today depends on the medicalization of society and the concomitant granting of a virtual monopoly on diagnosis and treatment of illness to trained specialists. Thus, as Eliot Freidson puts it,

In matters of health the opinions of laymen are very likely to be subordinated to the opinions of professional experts. This subordination is based on the assumption that a professional has such special esoteric knowledge and humanitarian intent that he and he alone should be allowed to decide what is good for the layman. This assumption forms the ideological foundation of health and other highly professionalized human services. (ix)

The claim to "special esoteric knowledge" is not merely a professional requisite; it also plays a functional role in the healing process in two ways: modern Western medicine is effective not just because its treatments are empirically based in "special knowledge" of physiology and biochemistry but also because patients believe that "doctor knows best." In its reliance on the patient's trust in the healer's superior knowledge modern Western medicine is like most other systems of healing; it differs in that its authority depends on the deployment of a specialized scientific vocabulary rather than, say, esoteric rituals (although one could argue that it has its share of those as well). As Kathryn Montgomery Hunter has said, "Medicine's claim to science, like the white coat that manifests that claim, is a part of its magic and serves as its rational, disinterested ideal" (25).

Increasingly, people—inside as well as outside the medical establishment—are acknowledging that medical discourse, ostensibly and ideally the language of healing, may be at times counterproductive—that it may contribute to patients' suffering even as it purports to ease it.[1] Recent studies of the medical profession make clear that its discourse may obstruct rather than enhance empathy; autobiographical accounts of medical training and personal narratives of illness reveal how medical discourse may alienate doctors from patients and patients from their bodies and bodily experience. These various perspectives—sociological and historical accounts of institutional practices, personal accounts of medical education, and personal narratives of illness—expose the unequal distribution of power between doctor and patient in medical discourse and its implications for treatment.

As Eliot Freidson has pointed out, modern Western medicine bases its authority on its presumed expertise and humanitarian intent. Collectively and individually, physicians (like academics) establish, exercise, and perpetuate their power by means of the development and deployment of specialized languages ("expert-ese"). Furthermore, although physicians usually rely to some extent on information provided by patients, they assume total responsibility for diagnosis (the identification and description of illness), prognosis (the prediction, or pre-scription, of its course), and therapy (the course of treatment). After a patient presents his or her case to the physician, the role of the patient in conventional medical discourse is to attend to, and to comply with, "doctor's orders." The politics of medical discourse thus favors the professional; doctors exercise their medical authority through their privileged place in a specialized discourse.

That this is true not just in general terms but in the actual face-to-face interactions of doctors and patients is confirmed by Candace West's *Routine Complications: Troubles with Talk Between Doctors and Patients* (1984), an empirical analysis of such dialogue:

Male physicians interrupted their patients (especially their Black patients) far more often than the reverse, and they appeared to use interruptions to exercise control in their interactions with patients. However, there was no evidence which indicated that this pattern of physician-initiated interruption was beneficial for patients' health. If anything, the exercise of this form of control seemed likely to hinder doctors' efforts at healing, through the loss of valuable information pertaining to patient treatment. (150)

The major deviation she noted from Talcott Parsons's asymmetrical model of the physician-patient relationship was that "patients interrupted their female physicians as much or more than their doctors interrupted them" (150). West's analysis suggests that the asymmetrical power distribution of the physician-patient relationship reflects gender and racial hierarchies as well as professional authority. Until recently, the gender and race of physicians reinforced their status as professionals; the domination of the profession by white men intensified the privileging of the professional and the objectification of the patient.[2]

Despite its theoretical basis in expertise and intent, in practice the basis of medical authority is incumbency. The presumed expertise of physicians endows them with authority that in effect inheres in office, because most patients are laypeople neither able nor eager to assess their doctors' academic and professional credentials. And, like any other professional behavior, medical practice involves role-playing, the presentation of a professional image according to conventions that are in part discursive. Further, as medical historians and sociologists have seen, one manifestation of medical authority is the control of information, keeping it from nonprofessional competitors and patients alike. According to Freidson, a physician may be "jealous of his prerogative to diagnose and forecast illness, holding it tightly to himself. But while he does not want anyone else to give information to the patient, neither is he himself inclined to do so" (142). (The rationales for withholding information have to do with the presumed inability of patients to understand or use it—precisely because they are nonprofessionals and because as patients they lack "objectivity" in regard to their conditions.) Similarly, Paul Starr has noted that professionalism involves a code of "ethics" that strictly controls how, when, and from whom patients should receive information regarding their illnesses. (This may at times be in patients' "best interests," but it also helps to avert open conflicts over diagnosis and treatment; this code of medical ethics ensures that professionals' competence will rarely be questioned—and never in front of a patient [Starr 94].) Thus discourse between patient and doctor occurs in a way that may be at odds with the root meaning of *communication*, the making common of information; professionalism shapes it to serve physicians' needs more than those of patients.

In fact, the dual bases of medical-professional authority, esoteric knowledge and humanitarian intent, are sometimes at odds. Indeed, the crux of the problem of medical discourse may lie in the nature of its relation to the discourse of science: the claim to expertise rests on the prestige of science, but the scientific tendency to objectify and quantify human experience may obstruct the profession's humanitarian intent. One need not want to undermine the authority of physicians to be uneasy with many aspects of medical discourse, such as its tendency to infantilize patients, reify illness, and medicalize experience.

To turn from a synchronic to a diachronic view of modern medical professionalism is to confirm our sense of the paradoxical role of medical discourse, which helps to create the authority on which healing may depend but may also unnecessarily alienate physician from patient, healer from supplicant. According to Michel Foucault, the "birth of the clinic" around 1800 involved a shift in the site and the paradigm of medical practice; accompanying this shift was the development of a powerful new medical discourse, the function of which was to monitor and regulate the health of the body politic. With the consolidation in the clinic of medical education and medical treatment came a new kind of observation of patients; the medical academy focused the gaze of its newly credentialed observers on symptoms that only the trained eye could interpret as signs of disease (and that autopsy would eventually confirm). Even before the invention of the x-ray, then, new techniques like percussion and listening projected the doctor's "vision" into the body (Cousins and Hussain 141–65).

In *Medicine and the Reign of Technology* (1978) Stanley Joel Reiser offers a detailed, comprehensive, and skeptical account of the powerful role of technology in the new paradigm and its sometimes negative effects on the physician-patient relationship—one of which is to discount patient testimony. In the seventeenth century the testimony of the patient, in the form of a narrative elicited by the physician, was the main basis for diagnosis (1). But since then a whole array of diagnostic tools—the laryngoscope, ophthalmoscope, microscope, fluoroscope, endoscope, x-ray, the medical laboratory, and various electronic scanning devices—have offered increasingly detailed and "objective" evidence of the body's internal workings. The effect has been to extend the range and domain of the medical gaze and to efface the skin as an obstacle to vision and thus to diagnosis. (The common suffix *scope* is symptomatic of the privileging of vision as the preeminent sense for diagnosis. Significantly, the term *stethoscope* refers to a tool for listening as though it were a device for seeing: its root meaning is 'I see the chest'.)

The physician's and the patient's relation to the body diverged dramatically; increasingly, physicians had sensory experience unavailable to patients. These devices tended to supplant or simply bypass the patient's testimony; indeed, new devices have often been recommended on the ground that they circumvent unreliable or distorted patient testimony [Reiser 31]. As a result, "many modern physicians . . . [regard] facts obtained through complex scientific procedures . . . as more accurate and germane to diagnosis than facts they detect with their own senses, which, in turn, they value more than facts disclosed by the patient's statement" (170–71). Since the birth of the clinic, diagnosis has depended less and less on face-to-face dialogue between patient and physician; physicians can and do make their diagnoses in consultation with specialists on the basis of evidence supplied by their patients' bodies—in the absence of patients themselves.

The scientific understanding and efficient treatment of disease achieved undeniable gains at the expense of loss of sight of the whole patient, of the personal, social, moral, and spiritual significance of illness. More and more, doctors saw disease "in terms of discrete, picturable lesions, as a disturbance of one part of the body more than of the person himself" (Reiser 55). The development of diagnostic devices does not represent the autonomous march of technological progress but a shift in attitude toward disease and toward the patient's body that licensed the physician to take greater and greater liberties with patients' bodies and to ascribe less and less credence to their testimony. As a result, medical discourse has become more alien, and potentially alienating, to patients; the gap between the language in which patients "confess" their symptoms and that in which physicians diagnose illness has widened.

Although medical schools continued to teach history taking and physicians continued to practice it, a new objectivism may have worked against the empathy-inducing effect and therapeutic function of the patient's narrative:

With the start of the twentieth century, it became increasingly routine for students and hospital physicians to take histories and do physical examinations by following an outline. This approach represented an effort to prevent distortion of the information from the patient by collecting answers to a standardized set of questions. It also helped deter the patient from attempting to reveal to the doctor irrelevant experiences. Such a medical history was patterned after the conduct of a physical examination on a passive patient; it was far from the two-person interchange of dialogue in which both participants probed deep into the nature of the issue at hand. In the outline method, the human relation between doctor and patient during history-taking, while perhaps more personal than when the doctor was listening to the heart or feeling the abdomen, was minimal. (Reiser 180)

The advent of psychoanalysis provided some potential for amelioration of the depersonalization of the patient, because it privileged testimony over physical examination, focusing on the patient as a person and establishing the physician-patient relationship as central to therapy. But for obvious reasons such emphasis on patient testimony remained marginal, even suspect, in the medical establishment as a whole (181). As yet another medical specialty, psychoanalysis may have the effect of reinforcing the split between mind and body. And today, with the rise of psychopharmacology, the talking cure faces a new challenge to its legitimacy and efficacy.

Edward Shorter's *Bedside Manners* (1985) confirms Reiser's account; with advances in medical technology after World War II the emphasis in diagnosis shifted away from the history toward the empirical test, away from the personal interview to the check sheet administered by a nurse or other surrogate and the laboratory examination of samples drawn directly from the body. As Shorter notes, "The price paid for this intensification of testing is the downplaying of history-taking and the physical exam, steps of the consultation that can have therapeutic power in and of themselves" (200). Whatever the other effects of this shift, it has tended to deny patients the "cathartic benefit" of telling their story (200). Their role in discourse has shifted profoundly; no longer the sources of invaluable testimony to their symptoms and suffering, patients are subjected to oral interrogation or technological screening or scanning. Patients have moved from a position of unique and privileged subjectivity to one of quantified objectivity, from the source of personal testimony to the source of bodily specimens.[3] However impressive the technologies of detection, diagnosis, and treatment developed by modern clinical medicine, they have been accompanied by shifts in discourse and in the position of the patient in that discourse, such that medical "care" has sometimes been purchased at the cost of the silencing or disenfranchisement of the patient.

These changes in professional attitudes toward patients over many generations can also be traced biographically in the development of professionals within a generation. Ontogeny recapitulates phylogeny: in becoming doctors medical students retrace developments in the profession as a whole. For example, Coombs notices how medical students, who at first tend to identify strongly with patients, learn to adopt "a detached scientific attitude. . . . Thus, students focus on the technical aspects of

their work rather than on individuals per se. Losing oneself in the pathological details—thinking about diseased tissue—is less personally involving than pondering about the patient as a suffering human being.
In this way, patients can become medical entities, objects of scientific interest" (239). In particular Coombs notes that "to help themselves
through awkward encounters [with the families of deceased patients],
students develop communication skills that serve as a coping mechanism. One is the frequent use of technical language in referring to
death. These terms tend to insulate and isolate death by classifying it as
a medical event" (132).

Not only disinterested or skeptical analysts of the profession—such
as historians and sociologists—but also physicians have noted these
changes. One subgenre of modern Western autobiography is the narrative of initiation into a profession, and the medical profession has provided one of the most grueling of such initiations. Recent survivors of
this process have remarked on how it depersonalizes the physician-
patient relationship. Professional authority and legitimation come at
the cost of sharply constrained subjectivity. Because one constraint on
doctors is discursive, testimony critical of the initiation process is rare;
it amounts to a kind of counterconversion narrative in which physicians speak out against—and outside of—medical discourse.

Melvin Konner's *Becoming a Doctor: A Journey of Initiation in Medical
School* (1987) testifies to the subtle but unmistakable desensitization
that accompanied his empowerment as a physician:

It is obvious from what I have written that the stress of clinical training alienates the doctor from the patient, that in a real sense the patient becomes the
enemy. . . . At first I believed that this was an inadvertent and unfortunate concomitant of medical training, but I now think that it is intrinsic. Not only stress
and sleeplessness but the sense of the patient as the cause of one's distress contributes to the doctor's detachment. . . . In the end, we all—doctors, patients,
hospital staff—have a sense that the doctors are doctors, and can be allowed to
do what they do, *because of* the rigors of the training. Because we view it as
painful, stressful, life-distorting, and terribly long, we allow it to justify the remarkable power we give the doctor over us. The doctor has paid for the power
with suffering. (373)

One interesting feature of this passage is movement back and forth between first- and third-person pronouns and the slippage in the referent
of the first-person plural pronoun. At times Konner speaks as a physician, at times on behalf of patients. This shift does not reflect or effect a
broadening of perspective; on the contrary, it implies, or presumes, that
patients consent to this process of legitimation. In Konner's account it
is as though the point of medical training were to authorize doctors to

overcome inhibitions, psychological or moral, against assuming too much power over another person. Konner seems to affirm not only the empowerment of physicians but also the way in which a grueling, depersonalizing initiation seems to justify that power. The price of professional empowerment is detachment, loss of empathy. (Of course, this cost is passed on to the consumer; ultimately, the patient pays the price of the physician's training.)

At first Konner seems surprised and disappointed by some effects of medical training, but in the end he seems to accept these as the unavoidable costs of an efficient modern medicine. His metaphors for doctoring reinforce the modes of domination and indifference to others' subjectivity into which he has been all too successfully initiated. Thus he characterizes the first two years of medical school as a kind of foreplay, preceding physical contact with patients; he thus identifies such contact with intercourse, with the physician in the superior (i.e., male) position. It is perhaps not surprising, then, that he describes his first surgery as being like sexual penetration: "[My] fingers had been inside another person's body, not just in the mouth or the vagina or the rectum, but beneath the protective surface of the skin, the inviolable film set up by millions of years of evolution, the envelope of ultimate individuality" (38). His constructs his professional initiation as a reenactment of sexual initiation, achieved by the penetration of a submissive (unconscious) other. So even as he appears to criticize the depersonalization of professional training, he implicitly (and unwittingly) accedes to it. Although he finally chose to pursue medical anthropology rather than to practice medicine, Konner to some extent reinforces the mystification he set out to expose.

In her book, *A Not Entirely Benign Procedure* (1987), the pediatrician Perri Klass is more successful at analyzing and resisting the insidious effects of medical training. Her ability to withstand medical socialization may have had something to do with her having been pregnant in medical school. In addition to being a woman in a male-dominated institution, she was a patient; as an incipient mother, she found the lessons of her birthing classes to be in sharp contrast to those of her medical studies, where pregnancy was viewed as a "perilous, if not pathological, condition" (42). Despite her partial insulation from the process of socialization, she acknowledges that, in rewriting essays published while she was still in medical school, she had to strive to preserve (that is, to simulate) a point of view she no longer held and a voice that was no longer hers—that of the novice: "I have found that in order to write about my training so that people outside the medical profession can understand what I am talking about I have had to preserve a certain level of naïveté for myself"(16).[4]

Among the subjects of her book is the most disturbing kind of medical discourse, physicians' backstage talk about patients. Klass notes, for example, a telling grammatical idiom: "You never say that a patient's blood pressure fell or that his cardiac enzymes rose. Instead, the patient is always the subject of the verb: 'He dropped his pressure.' 'He bumped his enzymes.' . . . When chemotherapy fails to cure Mrs. Bacon's cancer, what we say is, 'Mrs. Bacon failed her chemotherapy'" (73–74). Clearly, making the patients the subject of these verbs in no way acknowledges their personhood or their power; indeed, the grammar of these assertions assigns the patient responsibility for *in*voluntary processes— without involving them as competent parties in their healing. This idiom doesn't empower anyone; rather, it insulates doctors from the sickness they (over)see. It reflects—or effects—a lack of empathy.

A similar idiom is the use of a peculiar kind of depersonalizing synecdoche, the reference to patients as particular (malfunctioning) organs: for example, "the liver in 201." Such tropes are entirely reductive; by reducing the whole patient to one crucially afflicted part, they suggest that the organ is all that matters and all that is being treated. This professional trope not only recalls but in some sense enacts the old medical joke—"the operation was a success, but the patient died"—for in this synecdoche the vital organ survives, bloodlessly severed from the patient, whereas the patient "dies," his or her subjectivity completely annihilated.

Like Konner, Klass is tempted to adopt a pragmatic perspective: "The more extreme forms aside, one most important function of medical jargon is to help doctors maintain some distance from their patients. By reformulating a patient's pain and problems into a language that the patient doesn't even speak, I suppose we are in some sense taking those pains and problems under our jurisdiction and also reducing their emotional impact" (76). The jargon separates the syndrome, the disease, from the patient, brings it into a system of discourse in which it is manageable without reference to a patient's idiosyncrasies. The opacity and impersonality of this language may provide necessary distance for the patient as well as the doctor, though its purpose is apparently to ease the physician's, rather than the patient's, suffering.

In her next chapter, however, Klass grapples with another troublesome idiom of medical discourse, the pervasive trope of treatment as aggression, even war:

If we are at war, then who is the enemy? Rightly the enemy is the disease, and even if that is not your favorite metaphor, it is a rather common way to think of medicine: we are combating these deadly processes for the bodies of our patients. They become battlefields, lying there passively in bed while the evil armies of pathology and the resplendent forces of modern medicine fight it out. Still, there are very good doctors who seem to think that way, who take disease as a personal enemy and battle it with fury and dedication. The real problem arises because all too often the patient comes to personify the disease, and somehow the patient becomes the enemy. (81)

In this metaphorical matrix patients may slip from the privileged role of innocent civilians invaded or taken hostage by enemy forces to that of collaborators or traitors—after all, they "host" and sometimes conceal the enemy. So what should be empowering for both patient and doctor can subtly erode or disrupt empathy. The parties who ought to be seen as allied may be characterized instead as opposed—a graphic illustration of the potentially counterproductive effects of medical discourse.

The effects of medical discourse also appear in personal narratives of illness, or autopathographies, a form of counterdiscourse in which patients "address and sometimes seek to avenge the damage done by medical care to their bodies, care that took no care of them" (Hunter 154). One particularly illuminating text is Samuel Sanes's *A Physician Faces Cancer in Himself* (1979), which recounts the author's battle with terminal cancer. A retired pathologist and medical school professor, Sanes shared his experience of illness in a series of articles in the *Buffalo Physician*; after his death his widow edited and published them as a book. For most lay readers the striking thing about the book is the highly technical language in which Sanes describes his illness. For example, his description of his initial discovery of a lump shifts into medical jargon as his consciousness registers what may lurk below the surface of his body: "I had found the first small lump, about the size of a lima bean, while bathing. It was on the left side of my chest, posterior to the left axilla. Nervously I palpated the rest of my body. I found a smaller lump in the mid-pubic region, and another in the postero-lateral aspect of the upper part of the right arm" (2). This language can be explained, or justified, in a number of ways. First, it would have been in some sense appropriate to the original audience; to the readers of the *Buffalo Physician* such language would have seemed neither opaque nor remarkable. Second, when the patient is a doctor, as is the case here, medical jargon may accurately express the experience of the patient, who cannot suppress his professional knowledge. It may, then, reflect his subjective point of view, the terms in which he naturally constructs his bodily experience; it may thus be authentic discourse, the language with which he is most comfortable.

In his account Sanes characteristically retreats from the vulnerable position of the patient to the privileged one of the medical school lecturer who addresses a professional audience over the body of a patient—or slides of the body (the book is illustrated with snapshots of its author in various stages of treatment)—in this case, himself. Indeed, he organized the book less as a running account of his illness than as a series of lectures on various related topics, as the chapter titles suggest: "Discovery and Early Reactions," "Responses of Lay Persons and Physicians to Patients with Cancer," "Responses of Professional Colleagues and Co-workers to a Physician with Cancer," and so on. Still, his authority here is not so much professional—his specialty is pathology, not oncology—as autobiographical; he speaks with the authority of experience, as one who has seen illness from both sides. And his explicit intention is to sensitize his audience to the subjective reality of cancer, to help physicians empathize with their patients.

Given this aim, his antiseptic jargon is at best only partially successful; at worst it is self-defeating. Considered as autobiographical discourse, the language creates an eerie effect in part because it suggests such profound alienation from self. Indeed, the book suggests that, if medical discourse can come between patient and doctor in normal circumstances, when a doctor falls ill, expert-ese may split the self in two; the perspective of the ailing doctor may vacillate between the objective position of physician and the subjective one of patient, between professional and lay discourse. In his account of his discovery of his lump the phrase "nervously palpated" nicely represents this dichotomy: the verb is a fairly technical term, consistent with the language he uses to locate the lump on his body; his subjectivity as a patient intrudes only in the adverb. His action is professional, his manner is emphatically not.

The book is full of such vacillation between two modes of self-perception and self-representation. One can see that medical jargon in this instance may have served subjective needs; it may have insulated Sanes from his dire prognosis, and it may have offered him a seeming linguistic mastery of his uncontrollable and finally fatal tumor. Yet the depersonalization and reification inherent in medical discourse become especially ironic when the physician is a patient. Sanes's expertise seems to be an affliction that exacerbates his experience of his illness: "Someone has said that cancer is a lonely disease. It is especially so if the victim is a physician, above all if he is a pathologist whose outlook is influenced by the destructive and fatal results of the disease as he has seen them at autopsy" (3–4). It is hard to tell whether Sanes is helplessly trapped within professional discourse or whether he half-consciously takes refuge in it. Although it may protect him from anxiety, his language distances him from the lay audience reached by the posthumous publication of his articles. The overall effect is that of a subject immured in medical discourse. Ultimately, despite its transparency to his original audience of physicians, his language undermines most of his advice to that audience about the value of empathy and sensitivity (28–29), about the value for medical students of "general literature . . . by and about chronic 'incurable' patients" (39), and about how to communicate openly, with rapport and concern, using "simple, understandable English, not medical terminology or jargon" (190).

Sanes's book offers a good illustration of the potential effect of a lifelong immersion in the role of doctor, even on a humane practitioner-teacher, for Sanes cannot quite bring himself to drop the sterilized verbal gloves with which he palpates his bodily self; as a result, his account remains antiseptic, unable to touch us directly. His book thus illustrates how medical discourse, though empowering for doctors, may be disabling for ill people, even when doctor and patient inhabit one body. Medical discourse in this instance appears to be part of the problem, not the solution. Itself pathological, the language of pathology gives new meaning to the phrase "communicating disease."

Personal narrative is an increasingly popular way of resisting or reversing the process of depersonalization that often accompanies illness—the expropriation of experience by an alien and alienating discourse. Jean Cameron's narrative of her fatal cancer, *For All That Has Been: Time to Live and Time to Die* (1982), politely but powerfully counters the subjection of patients to institutional discourse—including, ironically, the supposedly empathy-enhancing paradigm of Elisabeth Kübler-Ross's "stages of dying." Like Sanes, Cameron was a health-care provider who succumbed to cancer, but as a hospice worker rather than a physician (and thus not as invested as Sanes in the biomedical paradigm) Cameron was more attuned to the depersonalization of medical discourse, especially regarding the terminally ill. As her illness worsened and her role shifted from that of colleague to that of patient, she suffered a social death that cruelly anticipated her physical death. Despite her conviction that her illness increased her empathy and authority as a caregiver, her colleagues thought that her cancer disqualified her, because it compromised her objectivity:

There are helpers and there are patients; one apparently cannot be both. I felt in a kind of no-man's land for a while, and then I crossed the line. I understood, but the experience was frustrating. It came at a time when, having experienced first-hand so many of the feelings and symptoms that patients described, I felt that I had more to offer now, not less. Moreover, I was beginning to feel a small sense of urgency. . . . It was hard to be so close and yet not allowed to act.

When someone has been bereaved it is generally suggested that he or she should wait a year before attempting to help others in similar circumstances. I have always thought that this was sound advice. . . . But you can't wait until you have actually died before you help the dying. There is no coming back. I think standards have to be a little different. (57)

Though in life she acquiesced to her forced retirement, in her book she does, in a way, "come back," speaking from the grave to change, or at least challenge, the standards that excluded her.

While a patient, Cameron became an unknowing subject in an experiment that involved the secret substitution of an unknown substance for her usual anodyne, the Brompton mixture. Detecting a difference in taste and effect despite a misleading label, her suspicions were confirmed by a series of calls inquiring as to the intensity of her pain—an extreme example of apparently empathetic discourse disguising a cruelly manipulative (and presumably unethical) experiment. Eventually, after she penetrated the masquerade, sympathetic doctors offered her usual medicine, but she chose to continue to participate in the experiment: "Knowing that I could always change my mind, I decided to continue and experience the whole experiment as all the others must who lacked my opportunity. But I would keep a record of events and my reactions; maybe someday someone would care to know just how a patient felt" (50). Informed consent made all the difference. But Cameron did not simply consent retroactively to be an experimental subject: she converted the experiment to her own uses, collecting and analyzing her own data. Indeed, this chapter is the publication of her findings, one of which is that the young medical student who made the phone calls was intensely troubled by his assignment. He too had been conscripted into a discursive relationship in which professional authority was exercised at the expense of empathy. Cameron's experiment puts her treatment on trial in a different sense as well; her narrative encourages other patients to challenge the authority conveyed through medical discourse.

The limits of medical discourse are most evident with terminally ill patients. The terminal stage of an illness puts a patient beyond the reach of discourse that is bent to the vanquishing of disease. In recent years, however, a specialized discourse has been developed for understanding and easing the predicament of the terminally ill. One of its authors is Kübler-Ross, whose theory of the stages of adjustment to terminal illness has been highly influential in dealing with the doomed. Yet Cameron found the Kübler-Ross model problematic; by predicting the nature and sequence of the emotional stages of dying, the paradigm tends paradoxically to disempower patients: "If each time one is angry it is called part of the 'normal' state of dying, it doesn't really have to be dealt with. It doesn't matter whether the anger is justified. It can be labelled 'displaced'" (77).

The whole schema of stages can be patronizing if it is not sensitively interpreted and sensibly applied. Despite Kübler-Ross's empathetic premises and goals, the effect of the theory of preordained stages can be to minimize or devalue individual variations and needs. The medical establishment responds to the paradigm, not the patient—the syndrome, not the subject. Thus, although some people began to distance themselves from Cameron as soon as they knew her diagnosis, others gave up on her later because she didn't die on schedule (97). She outlived their empathy, which was based on a prescripted and presumptive narrative of terminal illness. Cameron's life and death, then, were overdetermined; in addition to the injury of having her death caused by cancer, she suffered the insult of having her emotional responses dictated by a supposedly therapeutic paradigm. Her book is a modest attempt to fight back, not against brain cancer, which she knew would finally render her non compos mentis, but against the theory of dying, which rendered her voice inaudible.[5]

The prospects for the future appear mixed. On the one hand, as Julia Epstein notes, "instead of moving toward a more unified understanding of *psyche* and *soma*—mind/self and material body as an aggregate economy of the human—the superspecialized organization of medical professionals works in the opposite direction. The growth subspecialties that carry the most prestige and highest earning capacities are those that most anatomize and resect the human body" (4–5).

On the other hand, there are signs that the medical establishment is beginning to respond to the issues raised here. One such sign is Arthur Kleinman's *The Illness Narratives* (1988), which thoughtfully takes up the problem of the depersonalizing effects of medical discourse. He concedes that an

unintended outcome of the modern transformation of the medical care system is that it does just about everything to drive the practitioner's attention away from the experience of illness. The system thereby contributes importantly to the alienation of the chronically ill from their professional care givers and, paradoxically, to the relinquishment by the practitioner of that aspect of the healer's art that is most ancient, most powerful, and most existentially rewarding. (xiii–xiv)

Yet he remains convinced, and tries to convince his colleagues, that

the interpretation of narratives of illness experience . . . is a core task in the work of doctoring. . . . Moreover, an interpretation of illness is something that patients, families, and practitioners need to undertake together. For there is a dialectic at the heart of healing that brings the care giver into the uncertain, fearful world of pain and disability and that reciprocally introduces patient and family into the equally uncertain world of therapeutic actions. That dialectic both enhances the therapy and makes of it and the illness a rare opportunity for moral education. (xiii–ix)

Kleinman's book describes and attempts to exemplify a more humane doctor-patient discourse, truly dialectical or dialogical. But Kleinman is a psychiatrist, and his book is concerned exclusively with the chronically ill—for whom the biomedical model may seem inadequate or irrelevant—which suggests the limits of his leverage on a profession geared to high-tech intervention and curing rather than prevention and caring.

Kathryn Montgomery Hunter argues in *Doctors' Stories: The Narrative Structure of Medical Knowledge* (1991) that narrative is at the heart of contemporary medical diagnosis and treatment. She traces the transformation by physicians of patients' narratives into case reports, anecdotes, charts, and other professional genres. Although most of these revised narratives are alien, and some are completely unavailable, to patients, Hunter argues that the transformation of their stories is not only necessary but therapeutic; the translation of subjective reports into medical terminology makes patients' experience available to diagnosis and treatment and may serve, not incidentally, to validate their experience. To a degree, then, in her view objectification in medical discourse is not only inevitable but literally healthy.

Hunter recognizes, however, that these institutional narratives may go beyond objectification to dehumanization, and she addresses the potential of medical narratives to hurt as well as to heal. Under treatment by a physician ailing people become patients; their narratives becomes cases: "Such metonymic imperialism is a hazard of the act of representing another person in a narrative of one's own construction, and it contributes to the professional shortsightedness that sees maladies rather than people as the objects of medical attention" (Hunter 61). In Hunter's view the lay and professional narratives are finally "incommensurable," but that is no excuse for the lack of genuine dialogue between patients and physicians. The incommensurability can be worked around, if physicians acknowledge it, "first, in their attention to the patient's story during the interview that begins the encounter and, then, in their careful return of the story—not only in understandable terms but with the acknowledgment that it, like the life it relates, belongs to the patient" (xxii–xxiii).

Returning the patient's story is a tricky and problematic endeavor:

This transformed account of illness must be reintegrated as an interpretation of events into the patient's ongoing life story—whether that story is one of health, illness, successful treatment, physical limitation, or approaching death. This is not always easy since in its medical translation the patient's account of the experience of illness is distorted and flattened, almost obliterated. Returned to the patient in this alien form (as occasionally it is by a physician who either has forgotten the common language of illness or ignores the need to use it), the medical narrative is all but unrecognizable as a version of the patient's story—and all but useless as an explanation of the patient's experience. A silent tug-of-war over the possession of the story of illness is frequently at the heart of the tension between doctors and patients, for that tension is in part a struggle over who is to be its author and in what language, a struggle for the interpretation of life (and death) events. (13)

Hunter is clearer on what doctors should do than on how they should do it, but perhaps a process that must take shape within an intersubjective relationship cannot be prescribed. The acknowledgment that physicians need to return patients' stories to them in comprehensible terms, however, is certainly encouraging.

As it happens, a good deal of recent work in the field of "medical humanities" has been devoted to the role of narrative in making meaning of illness and in therapy. An exemplary article is Howard Brody's "My Story Is Broken: Can You Help Me Fix It? Medical Ethics and the Joint Construction of Narrative." Like other recent theorists in this area, Brody advocates the collaborative authorship by patient and physician of a meaningful, individualized, and therefore therapeutic, narrative of the patient's illness. One distinctive feature of his piece is that it cites empirical evidence that "patients will be more inclined to get better when they are provided with satisfactory explanations for what bothers them, sense care and concern among those around them, and are helped to achieve a sense of mastery or control over their illness and its symptoms" (80).[6]

Nevertheless, acknowledging the ethical and therapeutic value of respecting the priority and authority of patients' stories and allowing them a fuller role in medical discourse is not enough, for medical discourse is heavily implicated in larger historical phenomena (for example, the reliance of medical authority on the prestige of science). Medical discourse does not change independently of the larger culture in which it is embedded. Indeed, in the view of Howard Waitzkin, one effect or function of medical discourse, as exemplified in medical encounters, is to preserve the status quo by minimizing or ignoring social and cultural factors contributing to illness. Even as physicians may profess frustration with their lack of ability to affect the roots of the illness and impairment incurred by their patients, physicians' discourse with patients tends to detach health problems from the social context. By what they do not say as much as by what they do say, physicians tend to reinforce dominant ideology and social control. Indeed, one pattern in interruptions of patients by physicians during history taking is that of the doctor steering patients' testimony away from political and economic factors as contributors to individual distress. Waitzkin argues that, regardless of their political leanings as individuals, health-care professionals tend to "subtly direct patients' actions to conform with society's dominant expectations about appropriate behavior" (8).

However, some evidence exists of large-scale cultural changes that will allow or effect significant changes in medical discourse. As we have seen, the notions of treating the whole person and of genuine dialogue between physician and patient are getting more attention these days. The medical establishment is beginning to acknowledge that it does not have all the answers for all patients. Doctors are paying more than lip service to the goal of generating more humane and empathetic medical care. One example would be the founding of the C. Everett Koop Institute at the Dartmouth Medical School, one purpose of which is to encourage future doctors to be more sensitive in dealing with patients. Indeed, the majority of accredited medical schools require students to study physician-patient relationships; from the admissions process onward some schools are emphasizing humanistic dimensions of medical care, such as ethical questions and the need for good communication with patients.

Demographic changes and changes in gender roles are relevant here too. The admission of more women to medical school probably both reflects and advances the reconception of professional medical care (Angier). Certainly, the women's movement, with its emphasis on control of one's body, and the empowerment of ill and disabled people by analogy with other civil rights movements, have made it possible, or necessary, to imagine a new discursive relationship between patients and doctors. As I hope I made clear in Chapter 1, personal narratives—especially autobiographical ones—have been one way in which laypeople have responded to the dehumanizing tendencies of medical discourse. Changes in medical care of the sort advocated by Kleinman and Brody may ameliorate some tendencies that have provoked narratives of illness—especially the angrier ones. No matter how meaningful and egalitarian in authorship the narratives jointly created in patient-physician encounters, however, they will never be adequate to fully express the experience of the ill person; they may serve the relatively narrow purposes of Western medicine, but they will not exhaust the meaning of serious illness from the patient's point of view. As we have begun to see, the impulse toward illness narrative often addresses precisely those factors that medical discourse—even at its most enlightened and humane—may be impotent to challenge.

As Hunter and other authorities on medical discourse and education recognize, medical discourse is beginning to change in response to various counterdiscourses and the countercultures that give rise to them. People who are ill or disabled often also have to contend with more pervasive cultural discourses. The dominant culture assigns some degree of stigma to all the conditions we will discuss. As we shall see, illness narrative then often involves reclaiming one's body from more than just medical discourse.

Notes

1. *Medical discourse* is a broad term encompassing a variety of genres and rhetorical situations. I am concerned here mainly with medical discourse as it bears most directly on patients: as it is used to describe or refer to them and as it is used in dialogue with them.

2. An abundant literature testifies to the way in which the gender differential often reinforces the power differential between doctor and patient. See, for example, John M. Smith, *Women and Doctors* (1992), and Helen Roberts, *The Patient Patients* (1985).

3. In Foucault's account the clinic was born when doctors began to correlate symptoms with autopsy results; significantly, the literal meaning of the term *autopsy*, which has nothing to do with death, is 'seeing for oneself'. Invasive modern medical tests may be considered, then, a kind of antemortem—and, ideally, antimortem—autopsy.

4. She also had to overcome an ugly attempt to silence her; an anonymous enemy accused her of plagiarism and even went to great lengths to fabricate evidence to incriminate her.

5. Cameron does not attack the Kübler-Ross theory by name; indeed, she alludes favorably to Kübler-Ross in her acknowledgments. The book has a foreword by Kübler-Ross as well as one by the head of the hospice in which Cameron worked. Presumably, then, Cameron faults not the paradigm so much as its mindless application. Still, it is a curious feature of the book that it is published under the imprimatur of the medical establishment that it politely attacks. The two medical authorities who introduce her book do so in a slightly, and presumably unconsciously, patronizing way. The book thus acts out posthumously the same sort of asymmetrical physician-patient dynamics that it critiques.

6. See also works listed in the references by Charon, Churchill and Churchill, Donnelly, Mattingly, and McCullogh.

3

Self-Reconstruction

Personal Narratives of Breast Cancer

> My self, my existence as a solid person in the world, starts from my chest, from which I feel myself rise and radiate.
> —Iris Marion Young, "Breasted Experience," 1990, p. 189.

> Breast cancer . . . is more than a disease of the body, far more than the sum of errant cells run wild. Like any life-threatening illness, cancer invades the entire context of a life, disturbing its balance, heightening its struggles.
> —Musa Mayer, *Examining Myself*, 1993, p. 6.

Examining Breast Cancer

Breast cancer is probably the disease most feared by contemporary American women, for good reasons. Although lung cancer kills more women overall, breast cancer kills more women aged forty to forty-nine than any other cause ("Mammograms"). Although it is treatable and survivable, it is often not definitively curable; thus, once diagnosed with it, most women live thereafter in fear of recurrence. As Juliet Wittman puts it, "Throughout my life, I'd always confronted crises with the sure knowledge that eventually they would be over. . . . But this crisis of cancer would never be over, and it could mean the end of the world, at least for me. I would be in danger for the rest of my life" (173). Moreover, the incidence of breast cancer appears to be increasing, particularly among younger women.[1] In addition to breast cancer's threat to life, its striking an organ distinctive of women makes it a potential threat to a woman's identity.[2] Cancer—and the usual surgical "treatments," lumpectomy and mastectomy—can literally and symbolically disfigure a woman. (And some suspect the silicone implants once routinely used in surgical reconstruction carry their own risks to health.)

Less obvious reasons for women's dread of breast cancer lie in non-surgical treatments like radiation and chemotherapy, which are at best tedious and unpleasant, at worst torturous. One of the less well-known potential side-effects of chemotherapy is the early onset of menopause; thus the eradication of cancer may end a woman's fertility. In addition to denying a woman with cancer further children, this premature change in life phase may be disorienting and traumatic. For all these reasons breast cancer can radically alter a woman's life narrative. Moreover, because of the stigma attached to it, women often suffer the disease in silence; the secrecy imposed on them is itself punishment, a kind of solitary confinement.

All these factors help to shape narratives of breast cancer, which have been published with increasing frequency since the mid-1970s. Although conditioned by the physical manifestations of the disease and the medical protocols of treatment, women's responses to the disease, individually and collectively, ultimately script such narratives. Regardless of their explicit politics, then, all the narratives may be viewed as doing important cultural work; whether announced or not, one common purpose of these narratives is to expose to public view a deadly disease that warrants individual wariness, public concern, and aggressive research into causes, prevention, and treatment. Although the authors are inevitably and appropriately self-concerned during their illnesses, in the act of writing they seek to enhance others' chances of survival and to support them by sharing their experiences.

More than the narratives of many other diseases, then, narratives of breast cancer generally have a public mission, an agenda that is in some sense political. Indeed, as an autobiographical subgenre they have some affinity with slave narratives, which were also written in the hope of abolishing a threatening condition that their narrators were fortunate enough to escape. Thus survivors of breast cancer, aware that their individual escape may be temporary, wish to focus public attention and resources on their disease in the hope of minimizing its potency. And, just as white abolitionists sometimes authorized slave narratives in introductions or forewords, medical professionals sometimes validate breast cancer narratives. But whereas slave narratives primarily addressed an audience not subject to enslavement—Northern whites—breast cancer narratives are written primarily for an audience at risk, especially perhaps for women struggling to comprehend and cope with their diagnoses.

Thus two focuses emerge: the personal (addressing the illness as an individual concern) and the political (addressing the disease as a women's health issue). Some books end with supplements recommending various resources to the ill, and the autobiographical narrative may appear as an exhibit in a self-help book. Some end with calls to action—

for fund-raising or lobbying for research money, for greater concern about environmental carcinogens, and so on. But the two strategies are positions on a continuum rather than mutually exclusive options; motives and strategies are generally mixed. Curiously, the narrative that ends with the most explicit call for mobilization is one of those least informed by feminist insights. Joyce Wadler's *My Breast* (1992) is distinguished largely by its attempts at humor, yet it appends an afterword by the renowned breast cancer specialist Dr. Susan Love, whose urgency is reminiscent of the militancy with which abolitionists presented slave narratives: "We have been good little girls for too long. It is time for us to start yelling and screaming and being obnoxious. . . . We can't let this disease pass on to another generation. Our lives depend on it" (179). By definition slave narrators, as escaped slaves, write from a position of greater safety than breast cancer survivors; because, unlike slavery, cancer is not susceptible to legislative abolition, the appeal to politics in the cancer narratives has a compensatory dimension. Unsure of their fate, women with breast cancer exert what rhetorical and moral leverage they can to ensure the health of subsequent generations.

Breast cancer does discriminate: it is more common among some ethnic, racial, and socioeconomic groups than among others. For reasons that are not clear its incidence in the 1990s is higher among Caucasian women of higher socioeconomic status (Love 184). On the other hand (and less surprisingly), although mortality rates for breast cancer overall have held steady, the mortality rate is higher among poor women, and in the 1990s is rising among African-American women (Altman 34–36). Those who narrate their illnesses are generally white women of the middle- and upper-middle classes who have the literacy, leisure, and inclination to write their stories—and the contacts to get them published. (The authors of most narratives surveyed here are professionals; many were already writers.) Their privileged status also means that they generally got prompt high-quality medical treatment; moreover, medical professionals treated them with considerable respect.[3] Finally, all these women have supportive families and/or friends; no published narrative, to my knowledge, tells of a woman suffering in isolation, as many women must. These patterns reflect general trends in illness narratives. Autobiographical accounts of illness tend to inscribe best-case scenarios; with breast cancer the ill woman has an unusual array of resources—emotional, social, and financial—and her case usually turns out well.

Although breast cancer is not a new disease, published narratives of it are clustered in the recent past.[4] Essentially, the breast cancer narrative, as an autobiographical or autopathographical subgenre, developed in the 1970s and 1980s, when various forces—especially the women's movement—transformed breast cancer from a private, even shameful, ordeal into a publicly narratable personal crisis. Perhaps the watershed event was the publication in 1970 of *Women and Their Bodies* (better known by the title it carried in later editions, *Our Bodies, Our Selves*) by the Boston Women's Health Collective. As its title suggests, the book identified women with their bodies in order to assert their right and their responsibility to understand, control, and enjoy those bodies. In the seventies and eighties the perception of illness, cancer, and women's bodies changed significantly. An index of this shift was the acknowledgment by various celebrities across the political spectrum—from Gloria Steinem to Betty Ford and Nancy Reagan—of their having breast cancer. A range of national and local presses (depending more on the preexisting visibility of their authors than on the quality and significance of the books) has published narratives of breast cancer. Thus Little, Brown brought out the narrative of the movie star Jill Ireland, whereas the relatively obscure Spinsters Ink published Audre Lorde's *Cancer Journals*. The variety of writers and publishers involved is a testament to a profound shift in the perception of illness, cancer, and women's bodies in contemporary America. That breast cancer narratives are almost all autobiographical accounts is significant; as we shall see, narratives of HIV/AIDS and of deafness are far more likely to take the form of memoir.[5] In its form (point of view) as much as its content the breast cancer narrative asserts women's control of their bodies.

Closure in Breast Cancer Narratives

By definition women who write narratives of their breast cancer experience are survivors; they narrate their stories only when they are emotionally and physically well enough to undertake a sustained project— typically, after successful treatment of an initial incidence of breast cancer. That they recover sufficiently to compose a coherent conclusive narrative means that they are not necessarily representative of women with the disease; their narratives offer encouraging scenarios. Although some of these women subsequently suffered recurrences, and some have died of their cancer, their narratives tend to end with recovery of some tentative assurance of health and vitality. The master plot, then, of the breast cancer narrative, like that of autobiography generally, is a comic one; it ends "happily," with some significant recovery; the narrators are healed, if not cured. Without exception, then, the narrators are, or claim to be, better off at the end than at the beginning.

For obvious reasons the resolution provided by these narratives appeals to writers, editors, and readers; few people want to read (and no one wants to write) an autopathography with a tragic plot. One power-ful motive in going to the considerable effort of composing a book-length narrative of one's illness must be precisely to achieve closure, emotional as well as narrative. For other women diagnosed with can-cer such positive resolution provides hope; for readers who are at risk the master plot rehearses a desirable scenario and may thus psycholog-ically neutralize a nightmare. Reading such narratives may serve as a kind of therapy—a way of averting or controlling fear by vicariously undergoing a life-threatening experience.

The timing of the composition with regard to the experience of illness follows a significant pattern. Some begin as journals during the illness. (This is a way of keeping a personal chart: plotting their own case ap-peals to some patients.) But most seem to begin only after the writer has reached some equilibrium; few women are evidently willing to invest in the act of narrating their illness until and unless they sense that the out-come will be favorable. The narratives are generally composed, then, in the immediate aftermath of recovery from treatment. As a result, they are typically published about five years after initial diagnosis. Thus they often appear at about the five-year mark—a milestone of sur-vival—as a kind of celebration of their authors' survival and recovery.

Built into the first-person retrospective accounts of the disease, then, may be a misrepresentation of the disease. Although a narrative must stop autobiographical time in order to conclude, historical time goes on. Because of the inevitable lag between the creation and the reception of a book narrative closure is always out of date: the condition of the author is not necessarily the same as that of the narrator, who typically "re-covers" at the end of the story. The time lapse between the composition and the consumption of these narratives is a breach through which un-certainty leaks; the lag between the reader's sense of the narrator's con-dition and the author's actual health mimics the inherent lag between the status of the author's cancer and her awareness of it. This funda-mental extratextual consideration complicates the dynamics of reading these narratives. Inherently comic in their plots, and sometimes extrav-agantly affirmative in the tone of their endings, these narratives never-theless communicate to all but the most naive readers an implicit un-dercurrent of anxiety.

Comic closure may be particularly misleading in the case of breast cancer, now considered a systemic rather than a localized disease. (This is one reason behind the trend away from radical mastectomy and to-ward more aggressive chemotherapy [Love 263–71].) Despite their often explicit awareness of this, the temptation, and the tendency, for narra-tors is to treat their breast cancer experience as over—an episode in, or an interruption of, a normal healthy life that the author eventually resumes (though this is never narrated).[6] What distinguishes some of the more satisfying narratives—those of Gayle Feldman, Elizabeth Gee, Dorothea Lynch, Musa Mayer, Juliet Wittman, and Christina Middlebrook—is the way in which they balance the need for closure with the demands of truth and vigilance. A subtle but significant difference lies between claiming definitive closure, which implies that the story of illness (as well as the written narrative) is over, and achieving composure, which implies readiness for whatever is in store. The latter seems more appropriate—healthier in every sense—in narratives of an illness like breast cancer.

Because breast cancer is rarely considered cured—because having "had" cancer almost always means being susceptible to recurrence, being constantly vigilant—the retrospective closed-end autobiographical narrative is always somehow false to the experience. So autopathography has its inherent limits. The desire of the breast cancer patient as a mortal individual may be to wrap up the story, encapsulating the malignancy and preventing it from infiltrating the entire life, whereas her best interest is served by maintaining a wary watchfulness without succumbing to despair or panic. This difference is dramatically enacted in Joyce Wadler's *My Breast: One Woman's Cancer Story* (1992), which puts a great deal of energy into achieving closure. Her case requires extra exertion in this regard because Wadler's relatively favorable initial diagnosis was later reversed: "That was where my cancer story was going to end. Then, nearly a year after the lump has been removed from my breast, an extraordinary thing happens: my greatest-little-cancer-in-the-world diagnosis changes, and I discover that not all of the slides of my original biopsy had been sent from Roosevelt to Sloan-Kettering" (149).

After undergoing a newly prescribed regimen of chemotherapy, Wadler again declares victory over her cancer: "So that is it—That is the story of my breasts and me and our cancer. Score: Joyce, One; Cancer, Zero" (163). (In a nervy gesture she asks to be awake during her lumpectomy, and she inspects her tumor immediately after its extraction, as if she could stare down her now exposed enemy.[7]) Much of her work as a narrator, however, is tactfully undermined, if not undone, by Dr. Susan Love's afterword, which reminds the reader how little is known about why particular women get cancer and about how to treat it, much less to prevent it. This is unsettling enough, but Love's most emphatic gesture is to call into question the closure Wadler has struggled to attain:

Joyce Wadler ends her story here, with her treatment nearly completed. But this is where the story for most women really begins. The adjustment to living with what could be a life-threatening diagnosis is enormous, not only for the woman herself but for her family, her children, her significant other. Learning to live with uncertainty is very difficult. Learning to trust your body again when it has betrayed you is very hard. . . . The hardest time psychologically is after the treatments are completed. (179)

Here the physician says what the patient does not yet know or cannot yet acknowledge; Love speaks over the patient's head (and body) to the potential patients in her audience, questioning the confident closure of Wadler's narrative and projecting the narrative line into an indefinite future.

Generic Conventions

Breast cancer is one of a few diseases sufficiently common and of sufficiently wide public interest that it has generated a distinctive autopathographical subgenre, the breast cancer narrative—an autobiographical literature of growing significance. At least two dozen book-length narratives have been published since the mid-1970s. One thing one learns from these narratives, if one doesn't know it already, is that breast cancer is not a single phenomenon; indeed, one refinement of cancer treatment involves carefully distinguishing between different tumors and devising different therapies for each.

And yet, despite the variety in the actual tumors and the options for treatment, not to mention the individual reactions to the illness, certain features do appear repeatedly in the narratives. Read serially, they yield some common elements, in addition to the use of a comic plot. A number of topics or scenes appear in nearly every narrative, generally in the same order: discovery by the author of a suspicious lump in her breast; diagnosis of cancer; the assessment of treatment options; some form of surgical treatment, lumpectomy or mastectomy; some form of adjuvant treatment—radiation, chemotherapy, hormone therapy, or a combination of these; recovery and resolution in the form of favorable reports and restoration of (relative) peace of mind.[8] Thus medical protocols—not the "progress" of the disease so much as the way in which it is detected, diagnosed, and treated—would seem to dictate the basic constituents of the master plot.

In addition to virtually obligatory medical scenes, the narratives have a number of other recurring topics and motifs. Those who have mastectomies discuss whether to undergo reconstructive surgery, wear a prosthesis, or neither. Shopping for a prosthesis and/or a wig to hide chemotherapy-induced baldness is a common scene. When one shops not to adorn a healthy body but to simulate a missing part, a conventional female pastime becomes uncharacteristically fraught. Feminism, which has helped to empower women to relate their breast cancer experiences, complicates this aspect of recovery. Many women experience the decision about reconstruction or prosthesis as a double bind. Patriarchal culture fetishizes women's breasts and thus puts a premium on at least the appearance of intactness; nevertheless, it may condemn reconstructive surgery as vain. (Defining reconstruction as 'cosmetic' justifies the view of others, including insurance companies, that it is not essential and indeed is frivolous.) Moreover, some feminists criticize any attempt to reconstruct or simulate a two-breasted body as submission to the male gaze. It is worth pointing out here that the act of recounting one's breast surgery is itself a courageous acknowledgment that one's body is no longer intact. Despite their differing approaches to the problems of body image, all the autobiographers under consideration chose not to try to pass as "full-bodied"—by virtue of the publication of their stories.

In addition, many authors have sought out alternative supplemental therapies, including support groups, massage or acupuncture, herbal treatments, and the use of crystals. A motif in some books, then, is discussion of the worth and purpose of such therapies; these women are inquisitive enough to investigate all approaches, anxious enough to try almost anything, skeptical enough to have reservations about some of what they try, and sensible enough not to claim too much for any of the alternative therapies.

Breast cancer narratives, then, often involve both a kind of master plot and a series of recurrent scenes and topics. Despite these shared features, the illness does not write the narratives, and physicians do not script them. Indeed, several narrators remark on the extent to which choices of treatment are left up to them. As Juliet Wittman points out, this may be less a function of the empowerment of patients than of the relatively primitive state of knowledge about the disease. Were one treatment indubitably superior to others, physicians would universally recommend it and perhaps patients would universally adopt it. As it stands, however, survival rates do not differ significantly between alternatives, so women are often free to customize their treatments. This is cold comfort, but it too makes the illness more susceptible to autobiography, because the choice of treatment reflects personal values and circumstances rather than medical mandate. It also invests the narratives with an undercurrent of anxiety; because doctors routinely disagree about the best course of treatment, and because no treatment can be guaranteed to work, patients often live in fear that they have chosen incorrectly.

As with any (sub)genre, the generic plot provides both a convenient narrative armature for the author and a source of predictable gratification for the reader (who is generally assured of the narrator's recovery). But autopathography becomes autobiography by means of two related processes. One is the integration of illness by individual authors into distinctive ongoing life narratives: the author's making her illness her own by exploring the issues it raises in her case helps illness narrative to transcend its ready-made formulas. The story of an illness becomes the story of a life. The other is the enrichment of the genre by successive writers who defy, complicate, or refine its conventions. Later writers can profit from the familiarity of the genre's conventions; as we shall see, the growing familiarity of certain scenes makes it possible for later narratives to convey their meaning through compression or even omission. The formula's familiarity enables them to minimize the obligatory illness scenes and treat their illness as an occasion for probing other issues.

Tropics of Cancer

Though the nature of the disease and the medical protocols of diagnosis and treatment undoubtedly are powerful shapers of the genre, they are not the only or primary ones. Disease is always culturally constructed, and people write autopathographies as much in response to discourse about disease as to the diseases themselves. With conditions such as breast cancer (and HIV/AIDS, deafness, and paralysis) the most threatening discourse is not medical discourse; it is the general cultural discourse that ascribes stigma to a bodily dysfunction. Susan Sontag has incisively delineated the problems posed by the cultural discourse of cancer. Cancer, she argues, is a "tropical" disease, one seen through particular—and particularly insidious—metaphors; the prevailing tropes of cancer add insult to the injury inherent in the disease, imposing a heavy penalty on the ill. Sontag's counterdiscursive response to her breast cancer was not to try to tell her story—indeed, in *Illness as Metaphor* (1978) she did not explicitly acknowledge her illness—but rather to analyze and attempt to reform cancer discourse itself:

My subject is not physical illness itself but the uses of illness as a figure or metaphor. My point is that illness is *not* a metaphor, and that the most truthful way of regarding illness—and the healthiest way of being ill—is one most purified of, most resistant to, metaphoric thinking. Yet it is hardly possible to take up one's residence in the kingdom of the ill unprejudiced by the lurid metaphors with which it has been landscaped. It is toward an elucidation of those metaphors, and a liberation from them, that I dedicate this inquiry. (3–4)

As a deadly disease of unknown or poorly understood causes, cancer, like tuberculosis in the nineteenth century, has been imagined in terms of extravagant and toxic tropes. Sontag notes that

the controlling metaphors in descriptions of cancer are, in fact, drawn . . . from the language of warfare: every physician and every attentive patient is familiar with, if perhaps inured to, this military terminology. Thus, cancer cells do not simply multiply; they are "invasive." . . .

Treatment also has a military flavor. Radiotherapy uses the metaphors of aerial warfare; patients are "bombarded" with toxic rays. And chemotherapy is chemical warfare, using poisons. (64–65)

Because we think with such metaphors, they seem natural, inevitable, transparent—not figurative at all. But as Sontag is at pains to point out, such metaphors conscript patients into wars fought over, on, and in their bodies; among other things, such tropes may encourage the use of "heroic" measures of questionable effectiveness that may cause unnecessary suffering. Moreover, when doctors approach cancer using military metaphors, they sometimes identify patients with the enemy through a kind of conceptual slippage:

Punitive notions of disease have a long history, and such notions are particularly active with cancer. There is the "fight" or "crusade" against cancer; cancer is the "killer" disease; people who have cancer are "cancer victims." Ostensibly, the illness is the culprit. But it is also the cancer patient who is made culpable. Widely believed psychological theories of disease assign to the luckless ill the ultimate responsibility both for falling ill and for getting well. And conventions of treating cancer as no mere disease but a demonic enemy make cancer not just a lethal disease but a shameful one. (Sontag 57)

Sontag points to another cancer trope that is perhaps more pernicious: "The disease is often experienced as a form of demonic possession—tumors are 'malignant' or 'benign,' like forces—and many terrified cancer patients are disposed to seek out faith healers, to be exorcised" (69). Sontag has brilliantly illustrated how cancer discourse has tended to stigmatize and marginalize the ill, condemning them in two senses—simultaneously censuring and sentencing them. (As we shall see, this is perhaps even more the case with HIV/AIDS.)

Although Sontag has pointed out the ill-logic of the cancer metaphors we live (and die) by, singlehandedly changing cancer discourse is difficult for individuals, no matter how powerful of intellect: such discourse is anonymously created and communally perpetuated. Unfortunately, much of the discourse that Sontag condemned continues to plague us. Sontag's influence is, however, apparent in breast cancer narratives. Several narrators mention her work; some make manifest efforts to avoid detrimental tropes.[9] Although Sontag, who had breast cancer, does not remark on the discourse specific to it, Deborah Kahane, a social worker who survived breast cancer in her thirties, has summarized an insidious stereotype of the woman with breast cancer:

She was deformed, less sexually attractive, less feminine, and therefore had less worth as an individual. . . . She would be rejected by future suitors or abandoned by her partner, and somehow was "less a woman." This stereotype evolved from our culture's linking of a woman's identity to her attractiveness and worth, and of her femininity to her breasts and body. A woman's value also has been defined in relation to men: How could a woman who is considered "damaged goods" ever attract a man? (1990, 10)

Such negative gender stereotypes make an inherently threatening disease all the more to be dreaded: even if it doesn't take a woman's life, it may destroy her womanliness.

Malignancy, Motherhood, and Mental Illness: Betty Isaac, *A Breast for Life* (1974)

The power of breast cancer as a threat to womanliness is illustrated by what is (as far as I can determine) the first published book-length narrative of a breast cancer experience, Betty Isaac's *A Breast for Life*. At least, her book shows what can happen when a woman takes too literally the association between her breasts and her womanliness (in her case her maternal role). Hers is a disturbing narrative because of the extremity of her response to the loss of her breast. Upon diagnosis she is so averse to sacrificing her breast that, even though she is told mastectomy is the only way to save her life, she refuses to accede to it until a second physician forcefully supports the view of her doctor and her husband.

Isaac's postmastectomy pain was both physical and mental. After her operation she experienced an anomalous symptom, a painful urge to nurse, and she deeply resented medical advice that she forego having any more children (she already had five daughters) for fear that the additional estrogen during pregnancy would encourage further tumors. For Isaac more devastating than the amputation of her breast—which she acknowledges did not permanently impair her as a mother—was the realization of her dispensability when she returned from the hospital to a tidy home: "Mommy wasn't *always* indispensable! Sometimes, Daddy *was*! I couldn't have felt more secure and loved as I did just then, but something beyond my control was creeping stealthily over me" (80). If Mother wasn't indispensable, maybe her breast wasn't either, and perhaps her lifelong association of womanliness, motherhood, and breastedness was invalid. Upon returning home after her surgery, rather than recovering physically and emotionally, Isaac suffered a nervous breakdown that required hospitalization and repeated electroshock treatments to cure.[10]

The sequence of the two illnesses—one physical, one mental—is so compressed as to imply that the first caused the second—indeed, that they were a single mind/body crisis. So invested was Isaac in her role as mother, so much did she identify her maternal identity with a two-breasted body, that mastectomy threatened her core sense of being: her ego apparently could not survive the loss of a breast. Oddly, neither she nor her therapists explores this line of thinking about her predicament. But—in the absence of other explanations, and the narrative is not particularly introspective or confessional—it seems to explain why mastectomy was so calamitous for her. Unique among the published accounts of breast cancer, hers narrates a subsequent (and apparently consequent) psychic collapse. It is as though she could imagine only two roles for a woman—mother and daughter; when she is temporarily disqualified from running her household, she regresses to a kind of infantile dependency. "Curing" her involves returning her to the original role, still unexamined, of mother-woman. It is probably significant that her narrative is distinctive from the others in supplying almost no autobiographical context; it gives little insight into her life before cancer and little context beyond her immediate domestic circle. She seems to have little sense of her value outside her role as provider of life and care to her family, and when breast cancer removes her temporarily from that role—and seems to compromise it symbolically—her hitherto solid world dissolves.

Eventually, Isaac recovers, and the narrative ends with her resuming her maternal role in her family. She does not claim, like the typical illness narrator, that she has grown or changed as a result of her illness. Rather, the implication is that, after all, she is only physically different; otherwise, she is the mother-woman she was before her cancer. The plot is thus circular rather than truly comic; the protagonist restores her equilibrium but learns little in the process. Her lack of insight into her psychological collapse and recovery makes hers an unsatisfying, though unusual and revealing, narrative. The narrative cries out for analysis— particularly feminist analysis—because the author's devastated reaction to her plight seems disproportionate to what she describes. However, given the dearth, at the time of her diagnosis, of available accounts of breast cancer, perhaps her reaction is not so exaggerated. Although the narrative falls far short of becoming autobiography, and although its readership has apparently not been wide, it sounds a cry for help— for a politics and a worldview according to which the loss of a breast need not be such a calamity.

Collected Narratives and Counterdiscourse

The book that most programmatically addresses the need for counterdiscourse on breast cancer is Deborah Kahane's *No Less a Woman: Ten Women Shatter the Myths About Breast Cancer* (1990). Kahane's book presents a group of narratives as explicit counterexamples to the cruel and

misogynist stereotype of the woman with breast cancer. As its title suggests, the book has a thesis: for psychologically healthy women breast
cancer is a survivable crisis; indeed, women can come through it with
their lives not merely restored but enhanced.

Kahane does not deny that breast cancer can be a threat to a woman's
self-esteem as well as to her existence, but she counters this truth in two
ways: by arguing that the threat to self-esteem is rooted in patriarchal
ideology and by supplying ten first-person narratives she elicited from
women who were not devastated by the disease. Among the virtues of
this approach is the variety of cases Kahane has assembled. Although
these women are generally middle income, they are not all as privileged
as those who have written full-length narratives of their illnesses. Thus
they represent a larger range of ages, races, and ethnicities and religious,
occupational, and socioeconomic backgrounds than the authors of such
narratives. Individual voices do come through; refreshing colloquiality
and candor emerge from the process of eliciting, transcribing, and editing oral interviews. In response to Kahane's stimulus each woman begins by discussing her childhood and her life before cancer and ends
with an assessment of the overall influence of breast cancer on her life;
this approach avoids the convention of beginning with diagnosis and
helps to minimize the powerful impulse to end by closing off the illness
plot. Generally, then, their experience of breast cancer is, unlike Isaac's,
contained in a larger narrative frame.

The accounts are less varied than they might be, however, because of
the way they were, in effect, coauthored by Kahane. At Kahane's
prompting the ten witnesses explicitly address the issue of their self-
image and self-esteem after breast cancer, and their answers are uniformly and predictably affirmative. (Kahane is quite open about her
criteria for selecting subjects; she chose them as exemplars rather than
typical representatives.) Kahane's method of asking all the women to
address the same issues in the same order provides its own formula and
reduces individual differences. These collaboratively produced narratives are thus analogous to those slave narratives that abolitionists
elicited to serve as antislavery propaganda. Most would not have been
spontaneously created, and they are shaped in service of a single thesis
rather than reflective of personal circumstance. The attempt to produce
forceful counterdiscourse results in a deadening uniformity.

Kahane devotes the latter half of the book to her generalizations about
the women; she distills from their individual experiences the shared attributes that may account for their successful adaptation to their illness.
She divides her chapters into short sections, each headed by a specific
generalization supported by evidence from the narratives. Some of her
generalizations seem purely descriptive—such as "Lumpectomy Pa-

tients Had the Least Difficulty Integrating the Changes," "Mastectomy Patients Chose a Variety of Means to Recreate Their Sense of Physical Wholeness"—but the vast majority are implicitly prescriptive: "They Chose to Survive," "They Did Not Relinquish Their Power," "They Participated in Their Treatment Decisions," "They Reached Out for Support," "They Laughed," "They Made Plans for the Future," "They Owned Their Illnesses."

Although I do not question the validity of her generalizations nor Kahane's motives in glossing the individual narratives in this way, I think the ultimate effect of this section may be counterproductive. The operative pronoun is now the third-person plural rather than first-person singular; the women who emerged as distinct and lively individuals in their narratives are now collapsed into a composite Superwoman. To her credit Kahane tries to distinguish between successful adjustment and survival (being "healed" and being "cured"); she even notes that one subject died before the book was published, so the book acknowledges that long-term survival is not the only scenario. However, the composite heroine appears to survive breast cancer as a result of her initiative—her decision and her ability to take charge of her life. Thus the book implicitly characterizes illness as a test of character—indeed, of true womanliness: "each woman eventually was able to turn her breast cancer crisis into an opportunity for growth and change. . . . They emerged as self-directed, more autonomous women, who were proud of their accomplishments and had a newfound self-respect" (243). Although such positive models are no doubt intended to inspire, they may well intimidate some women with cancer. Such examples and such conclusions may be dispiriting for those who have trouble merely coping. Kahane's insistent didacticism may undermine the cultural work that the narratives do more effectively. Like too many so-called self-help books, this one sometimes resorts to a rather facile formula for recovery; in doing so it makes implicit (and finally irresponsible) claims for the power of mind over malignancy.

Another possible drawback to Kahane's approach is that it may give more weight to the stereotype than it deserves. Talking back to negative stereotypes may be preferable to ignoring them. But the women who have written full-length narratives of breast cancer generally do not express much defensive concern about their womanliness[11]; certainly, loss of a breast is not their primary concern. Indeed, rather than finding themselves abandoned by husbands or lovers repulsed by their altered bodies, several decided to terminate relationships that they no longer found satisfying. Illuminated by a sudden brush with mortality, relationships, like all aspects of one's life, are subject to healthy reassessment. The indifference of these narrators to the stereotype of the

mutilated and discarded woman may be a function of the self-assur-
ance that empowers them to write their narratives, but their narratives
answer the stereotype in their quietly effective way.

Perhaps the most affirmative version of a scene repeated in virtually
all narratives involving mastectomy—the patient's first viewing of her
scar—is that in Gayle Feldman's *You Don't Have to Be Your Mother* (1994):
"It was all so neat, no lumps, no bumps, no breast. As I looked down, I
felt my spirits lift, I felt curiously unfettered, happy almost. . . . I was so
glad simply to be alive. The loss of the breast didn't seem to matter that
much" (155). (Feldman had just given birth to her first child, reassuring bodily evidence of her womanliness.) Given the high probability of
a primary cancer in the remaining breast, Feldman underwent a second, prophylactic mastectomy. Although she found the second mastectomy far less traumatic than the first, she acknowledges that "the inexpressible, innate sense of femininity that comes from having breasts
was gone." Nevertheless, "the emotion that surged above the sadness,
gave sense to it all, was the overwhelming sense of relief. I had sacrificed healthy tissue to keep me healthy, had done all I could to help myself and my boy. I would not, now, develop a new primary breast cancer. It was the right decision. I had no regrets" (248). Although she had
worn a prosthesis after her first mastectomy for the sake of symmetry,
she abandoned it after her second, accepting her body's new shape. Her
physicians predict that she will eventually elect reconstruction, but she
asserts that she has had enough body-altering surgery. Such individual
responses, fully contextualized in life circumstances, may be more
powerful counterdiscourse than edited collected testimony that is to
some extent homogenized.

The Politics of Prosthesis: Audre Lorde, *The Cancer Journals* (1980)

If the problem with Isaac's book is that she seems no wiser at the end
than at the beginning, in part because she seems so isolated from other
women, the problem with Kahane's is that in deconstructing and
rewriting the cultural script of breast cancer she obscures individuals'
accommodations to their illnesses. If Isaac severs the personal from the
political, Kahane subsumes the personal too completely into the political. Breast cancer narratives are most powerful—and perhaps most autobiographical—when they avoid these two extremes.

The most aggressively deconstructive account of breast cancer—and
also a compelling personal account—is Audre Lorde's *The Cancer Journals*. Despite its title, it is not a diary but a series of essays derived from
and illustrated by journal entries expressing her immediate responses
to her illness. The book shifts back and forth between the proximate

and the distant, between the emotional and the intellectual, as Lorde struggles to bring all her resources to bear on a new and frightening challenge. The strength of the book is in its inclusion of both her private responses—cries of pain and outrage—and her political analysis—seasoned, reasoned discourse. Her explicit politics makes her book powerful counterdiscourse. Already quadruply marginalized—a female, black, lesbian poet—Lorde is particularly sensitive to the marginalizing effect of illness—especially a "woman's" illness. The marginalization that deprived her of specific role models may have helped to free her: "This is it, Audre. You're on your own" (28–29).

Because of her race and sexual orientation she is acutely aware of the hypocrisy of passing for what one is not. Thus she focuses on the process by which women are pressured into buying and wearing prostheses. She points out that although most prostheses are designed to compensate for the lack of function of a missing body part, breast prostheses serve only to compensate for its absence, providing a cosmetic facade that hides the surgery. This seemingly benign gesture—of enabling women to appear as they once were, two-breasted, full-bodied—in fact erases not only the effects of surgery but the presence of their illness in society (16). It enables others to ignore the disease, and it prevents women with breast cancer from recognizing each other and working together against both the illness and the patriarchalism that defines women as objects to be adorned and consumed. Wearing a prosthesis alienates women from their bodies because of the disjunction between the public and private images of their bodies: outwardly, they appear as they were; inwardly, they know they are different. Thus it denies them their grief and encourages living in the past (57).

It also "encourages a woman to focus her energies upon the mastectomy as a cosmetic occurrence, to the exclusion of other factors in a constellation that could include her own death. . . . It encourages her to ignore the necessity for nutritional vigilance and psychic armament that can help prevent recurrence" (57). Lorde points out the gendered double standard that makes a male's surgical scar heroic and thus displayable in public, whereas a woman's mastectomy scar is shameful and stigmatic. She recalls trying on a prosthesis offered to her in the hospital by the Reach for Recovery Program:

I came around my bed and stood in front of the mirror in my room, and stuffed the thing into the wrinkled folds of the right side of my bra where my right breast should have been. It perched on my chest askew, awkwardly inert and lifeless, and having nothing to do with any me I could possibly conceive of. Besides, it was the wrong color, and looked grotesquely pale through the cloth of my bra. Without it, I looked strange and uneven and peculiar to myself, but somehow, ever so much more myself, and therefore so much more acceptable, than I looked with that thing stuck inside my clothes. (44)

The prosthesis is not merely dead but deadening, not merely false but falsifying: "The emphasis upon wearing a prosthesis is a way of avoiding having women come to terms with their own pain and loss, and thereby, with their own strength" (49).

Unlike Sontag, who saw cancer metaphors, and the war metaphor in particular, as the patient's enemies, Lorde embraces the trope of war; she takes pride in identifying her one-breasted self as an Amazon warrior, and she chooses to define her scar as a badge of honor:

Well, women with breast cancer are warriors, also. I have been to war, and still am [at war]. . . . For me, my scars are an honorable reminder that I may be a casualty in the cosmic war against radiation, animal fat, air pollution, McDonald's hamburgers and Red Dye No. 2, but the fight is still going on, and I am still a part of it. I refuse to have my scars hidden or trivialized behind lambswool or silicone gel. I refuse to be reduced in my own eyes or in the eyes of others from warrior to mere victim. . . . I refuse to hide my body simply because it might make a woman-phobic world more comfortable. . . . I realized that the attitude towards prosthesis after breast cancer is an index of this society's attitude towards women in general as decoration and externally defined sex object. (60)

She becomes a warrior against what she sees as the forces that cost her the breast.[12]

In an interesting twist on the theory that repression causes cancer, she raises the possibility that oppression may have caused her cancer: "And if a lifetime of furies is the cause of this death in my right breast, there is still nothing I've never been able to accept before that I would accept now in order to keep my breast" (34). In implying that hegemonic culture may be responsible for her illness, she characterizes herself as a martyr to causes long espoused. She imagines, and hopes by her example to recruit, an army of Amazons to take on cancer and patriarchy—related threats to women's health. She incisively reveals how much the treatment of breast cancer is determined by mainstream cultural values rather than by purely medical concerns and how it works to keep women powerless and isolated from one another. Clearly her object in writing these journals is not so much individual recovery as generativity—the creation of solidarity among women and the encouragement of social critique and transgressive behavior. By expressing her loss she hopes to support others in theirs and to challenge a system that construes that loss in a way that makes it unduly traumatic.

Her literary form is significant in this endeavor, beginning with the slightly misleading title. In a way, Lorde does what Kahane did: she edits a personal account of cancer and distills certain lessons from it. Lorde's book differs both because her lessons are far more radical in their implications—less about women's self-esteem as individuals and more about their collective lot,and because it is entirely hers. Moreover, her fusion of essay and journal writing affirms both the intimate experience of the female body and self-assertion through force of intellect. She does not use her journals as a hidden source for her essays; rather, she embeds the relatively raw entries in essays that reflect upon and analyze her initial responses to her illness. Her literary form thus draws on and affirms the tradition of women's private writing while making her journals emphatically and aggressively public. Further, her decision to quote selectively from her journals, rather than to recreate a single retrospective time line, helps to liberate her from the master plot of illness narrative with its personal focus, obligatory scenes, and its emphasis on outcome. (One notable feature of Lorde's book is an eloquent silence: she devotes minimal space to scenes involving physicians and medical discourse.)

The result simultaneously models both the theory and practice of breast cancer testimony. Declining to wear a prosthesis and scorning reconstructive surgery—refusing to closet her postsurgical body—Lorde performs elective reconstructive surgery on her self—not her body— using her pen: "Any amputation is a physical and psychic reality that must be integrated into a new sense of self" (16). Her writing, retracing and reweaving the threads of her life, recreates her personal integrity and at the same time seeks to stitch her experience together with that of other women. Rereading her journal entries involved resubmitting herself to her earlier crisis and perhaps preparing for a dreaded recurrence; the act is therapeutic, demystifying both past and future. (And indeed in her later book, *A Burst of Light* [1988], she handled recurrence and metastasis with great aplomb.) Giving her pain private articulation served her immediate needs; the reshaping of her earlier responses into a public political manifesto aims to reconstruct society as well, to adjust culture to her body and self rather than vice versa.

Narrative Time, Mortality, and Immortality: Elizabeth Gee, *The Light Around the Dark* (1992)

In a retrospective autobiographical account of an illness such as breast cancer the narrator knows more than her readers do: what's coming. At the same time, however, the reader can presume a more or less positive outcome to the experience of illness. The form guarantees that the subject survived to tell the tale and implies a comic resolution (though not cure). So a kind of double insulation is inherent in retrospective autopathography; the reader can relax to some extent in the hands of a narrator who knows the future and who is assured of having one. When we turn from retrospective to concurrent (serially composed) accounts of breast cancer, however, our relation to the narrator shifts decisively. With a diary we have no guarantee of positive resolution; the master plot is not necessarily comic. (Indeed, diaries need not have plots at all, though we tend to impose plots on them as we read.) Moreover, assuming that the author has not revised the entries, the narrator knows little more than the reader. Reader and writer proceed together into the unknown—and perhaps foreshortened—future. At any moment may come a turn for the worse that will lead away from the positive resolution that both reader and writer desire. Thus the experience of reading the two forms is quite different. The diary is inherently tentative, far more fraught with anxiety than the retrospective narration.

In some instances readers may know of the subsequent death of the author from the illness recounted. Whether the book is a retrospective or a concurrent narrative, such knowledge indubitably affects our reading, drastically changing the general account of the reader-writer relationship given earlier. In both forms it supplies a dramatic irony; the readers now know what the author did not: the end of the story. But this works differently in the two forms. The irony of our knowledge of the author's death is less corrosive in the case of the diary, which typically does not attempt or claim the same sort of closure as the retrospective narrative. Although it has recently been fashionable in the academy to treat the individual as a cultural and linguistic "construction," and autobiography as "fictive," reading accounts of illness where life is literally at stake exposes a crucial divide between fiction and nonfiction. Fiction may evoke a wide range of genuine emotions in readers, but nonfiction can evoke emotional responses of a different order. Certainly, fictional characters, no matter how autobiographical, have a different relation to their authors than their autobiographical counterparts.

The authors of the first cancer diaries to be discussed here—Elizabeth D. Gee's *The Light Around the Dark* (1992) and Dorothea Lynch's *Exploding into Life* (1986)—died before their books were published. Reading a diary of an author known to have died of her illness tends to be a particularly uneasy experience. If we assume that the narrative will trail off and end as hope wanes and the author resigns herself to her fate, the temporal process of reading acquires a troubling dimension. The gradual shifting of pages from the right hand to the left becomes a kind of tangible index of time running out on the diarist; as the reader approaches the end of the narrative, the diarist approaches the terminus of life. Some impulse—not suspense exactly (in a sense one already knows the outcome) but the powerful demand for resolution—impels one to finish the narrative, but this means in some sense finishing off the narrator. Insofar as one equates the remaining pages, consciously or not, with the subject's remaining lifetime, one may feel complicit in the shortening of the narrator's life as one reads, for the reader controls the rate of the consumption of the written life.

Part of what impels us, however, is not the urge for resolution for its sake but curiosity about the end that awaits us all—and which some are condemned, or privileged, to see in advance. Thus one motive to keep turning pages is the hope that the narrative will tell us what it's like to die—or, because that is the one experience no autobiographical account can retrospectively narrate, what it's like to see death approaching. Diaries of deceased authors seem to hold out the promise of answers. However much we want the story to turn out well, the narrator to recover her health, some part of us may be drawn to narratives that foresee death. Thus, although retrospective narratives tend to be written from a more or less secure vantage point and tend to close off the threat of recurrence, diaries are more open-ended and may finally admit death as a looming prospect.

One reads Gee's diary knowing of her subsequent death; her narrative is framed by various documents written by others—friends, colleagues, her daughter—that give away its ending. In addition, the text of the diary acknowledges its author's death in various ways. Among these is its morbidity; cancer pervades her consciousness even as it does her body: "I'm amazed at how quickly cancer has staked out a wide territory in my ordinary thoughts and daydreams" (27). Thus the entries—especially the early ones—are full of nightmares of dying, and they have a pervasive (but sober rather than panicky) sense of doom. Such morbidity is actually quite unusual in cancer narratives, and it is particularly noteworthy here because it is not a function of actual foreknowledge at this point that her cancer would prove fatal. (More likely, her family history of cancer made her pessimistic.)

Another way in which Gee's narrative acknowledges the possibility of her death is its narration of the death of an aunt. Gee inscribes in her diary excerpts from her grandmother's retrospective account of nursing her daughter in her final illness, which Gee did not witness. Perhaps Gee finds solace in her grandmother's explicit and confident references to an afterlife. By including her foremother's death from breast cancer, she bravely rehearses and confronts her own, supplying a surrogate for a scene that defies literal inclusion in any autopathography. Moreover, by importing into her narrative her grandmother's grieving but griefeasing account of her daughter's death, Gee finds a cathartic outlet for her repressed fears and proleptic grief.

Its frank and deep spirituality also distinguishes this narrative. It illustrates, in fact, that autopathography can take the form—and serve some functions—of a now somewhat unfashionable and neglected form of autobiography, spiritual autobiography.[13] This is no deathbed or crisis conversion narrative, however: a lifelong Mormon, Gee was evidently a believer whose faith never wavered. She is unabashedly, though not dogmatically, religious, as concerned with the state of her soul as with the condition of her body. Thus, although her narrative proper ends with a suspicious lesion proving benign, she bases the narrative resolution and closure not on diagnostic reassurance—which we know will prove premature—but rather on a mystical sense of peace that pervaded her before the test.

In an epilogue dated a year after the last diary entry Gee announces that she has found another suspicious lump. After initial panic, "the fear started to surrender to that peaceful reassurance, and it is with me now, a sense that I am in touch with something higher than myself, or something higher within myself" (142). The narrative ends at this point, with the status of the lump undetermined but the narrator composing herself through reference to God and immersion in nature. The narrative gives the firm impression that she can weather any test result; tapping the deep well of her faith, she achieves a kind of composure that may falter but will not fail. Gee's is a sober and sobering book in its acute recognition of mortality and in its sense of impending doom, but at the same time it is reassuring in its representation of the process by which the mind and spirit can—and must—constantly renegotiate their relationship with a mortal body.

Collaborative Narrative

An Eye with an I: Dorothea Lynch and Eugene Richards, *Exploding into Life* (1986)

Another cancer diary, Dorothea Lynch and Eugene Richards's *Exploding into Life*, makes a special contribution to the literature of breast cancer for two reasons. First, it carries the narrative of a fatal cancer further than most. If Lynch began her diary not knowing how her story would come out, she seems to have known when she ended it that her cancer was going to kill her. The diary ends when she feels she has told as much of the story as she is able to tell. Second, the book is collaborative; Eugene Richards, her domestic partner, edited the text from Lynch's diary (with help from a professional) and supplemented it with photographs he took during her illness. One subplot is the solidifying of the sometimes shaky relationship between Lynch, the writer, and Richards, the photographer. It is not just a matter of the relationship's surviving the shared ordeal of her cancer, however; rather, the two agreed to pool their talents to record and publicize the experience of other cancer patients. Their taking on a joint project gave another, more public, dimension to their domestic partnership.

The collaboration that produced Lynch's diary was initially intended to publicize the plight of other patients. For various reasons, however (including increasing resistance from physicians and hospital authorities), Lynch and Richards never finished the planned book. Still, partly because of its origins *Exploding into Life* is more than a simple diary focused on Lynch. Indeed, during and after her recovery from the initial cancer Lynch's diary entries and Richards's photos concern other patients suffering from other cancers. Thus this narrative has a broader focus than most illness narratives.

Still, the photos of Lynch provide the most powerful testimony. Confronted with the possibility of a mastectomy, she is frustrated not to be able to obtain photos—rather than sanitized sketches—of the results. She quickly intuits that she has found a cultural blind spot, and one prime motive of her book is to illuminate this dark place—to let other patients see, if they wish to, what their bodies will look like after surgery; thus her words and Richards's pictures are part of an ambitious and successful attempt to demystify cancer. When breast cancer narratives include photos, they are usually family snapshots supplementing the written narrative; they serve less to record physical changes in the patient than to represent moments of relative health and normality—to embed the ill person in a larger context. I am aware of no other American breast cancer narrative that actually pictures a mastectomy scar.[14] The Lynch and Richards book is unique in using the camera as a witness to so many stages of illness and treatment. The pictures are uncaptioned, which creates some ambiguity about what they represent. Words and images are thus truly interdependent and synergistic; fully to comprehend either, one must consult the other.

It might seem that the use of pictures would exacerbate the voyeuristic potential of an illness narrative, but that does not seem to be so here for a couple of reasons. According to the diary, Richards took the photos of Lynch at her insistence—indeed, against his initial inclination—and she evidently was not opposed to their posthumous publication. Thus she authorized them—Richards did not take them against her will or without her knowledge; she was a willing, even eager, subject—at least at first. They represent not an invasion but, like any autobiographical gesture, a sharing of her privacy.

The issue of privacy also is foregrounded in Gee's *The Light Around the Dark*, when she records her dismay and discomfiture with her radiation therapy, during which someone projected an image of her, naked to the waist, on a video monitor in the hall adjoining the lab. "Here am

I, someone with supposed expertise in bioethics, in moral principles of 'patient autonomy' and 'respecting persons,' and I am submitting to these indignities" (47). She protested through her powerful husband, then president of the University of Colorado, to little effect. But clearly a motive in her journal was to take back her body and her privacy. The publication of her private record, far from reenacting her exposure, is a reassertion of control, for in it *she* determines how much of herself to reveal to the world. The same is true of the photos of Lynch.

Aesthetically, these photos mediate between the intimate portrait and the objective documentary. The images are often grainy or shadowy, like documentary photos, but the photographer's access to vulnerable moments and the subject's apparent ease with that access give them a redeeming intimacy. Several photos are truly shocking without being sensational. One is the first image of Lynch after chemotherapy has rendered her totally bald. Many breast cancer narratives deal with the issue of hair loss; this one alone startles the reader with the sudden radical transformation of the patient's appearance. However shocking this image is to an eye accustomed to the previous images of Lynch's face framed by black hair, it is far from repellent. The absence of hair (and glasses) permits her facial features to emerge, and because it is a close-up in which she gazes directly into the camera, the image is disarming rather than grotesque.

The most disturbing photograph is an image of Lynch's torso soon after her mastectomy. Seeing it, one understands why women have been discouraged or prevented from seeing postoperative photos: the sutured scar that diagonally bisects Lynch's left chest is still raw and painful looking. Her swollen left arm is lifted, obscuring her face, which is turned toward the physician who examines her. One might be inclined to read this as an image of pain and mutilation, of disfiguration. On the opposite page, however, Lynch records her reaction to first seeing the result of the surgery:

Deep breath. I look down at the purple black line, an eight-inch-long, puckered and black-stitched cut. There is a drainage tube stuck in a hole in my side. It is kept from falling inside my body by a safety pin. The breast remaining is a surprise, its nipple as pink as a girl's pout. Where I had expected a gaping hole and raw flesh, there is a little skin remaining—their attempt to leave as much as possible. Clean, necessary. (32)

The juxtaposition of words and image makes the photo less voyeuristic and less grisly; the photo is not literally from her point of view, but, by depicting for readers what she sees, it enables them to appreciate her perspective on her wound, which is remarkably matter-of-fact—resigned to its necessity, gratified by its neatness.

At other times the photos fill gaps in the narrative, depicting experiences that elude verbal representation. For example, intentionally or not, breast cancer narratives tend to minimize the long periods of discomfort and nausea some women suffer from chemotherapy. Richards's single photo of Lynch, sitting on the bathroom floor next to the toilet—looking dazed and miserable with nausea—is probably the most candid record we have of the unpleasant side-effects of this treatment. This photo does seem intrusive, and she records her ambivalence about it: "'Aren't you going to take a picture of this, too?' I snarl at him, as if I were the camera's victim instead of the director" (91).

At times one senses that, contrary to his initial objection to photographing her on the ground that the camera "would be in the way" (21), Richards may have sought refuge in the distance the camera put between him and Lynch. Still, the photos are highly affecting, never arty. They manage not to objectify her—in part because she has her own medium through which to express her subjectivity, in part because Richards observes a certain decorum. There are scenes he will not shoot, images he will not publish. For example, the photos do not, as they might, carry the narrative further than her words do. A possibility here—one used in some AIDS documentaries and narratives—would have been for her point of view to give way to the survivor's, with Richards photographing her in late stages of illness, even in death. What happens instead is that images and words commence and cease simultaneously. Except for a brief epilogue by Richards that informs the reader that Lynch died (and when), she has the last word. She acknowledges the likely course of her illness without quite acceding to it:

The garden out back of our house sprouts one-half-inch here, an inch there, and I am changing too; cancer plods on from node to node, remarkable and yet not remarkable at all, like summer itself. Just another growing season after all. Is this resignation? I hope not. I do not intend to give up without a struggle, but more and more I see myself as a thread in a huge and royal tapestry—important to the central design but having an end, a place, a physical destination. (161)

Her last testament, then, combines personal resistance with philosophical resignation.

The last series of photos is of Lynch being prepared for high-tech treatment of her metastases. In the first set she appears supine, with her head strapped to a table. In the first image she is photographed close up; her eyes and lips glisten, her face is composed, her expression serene. If not for the context, she would seem to be the picture of health. In the next one we see the same scene from a different angle on a TV monitor; the image is washed out, grainier, and a shadow slashes across her face. One senses here the ominous reason for her distance from the photographer, who presumably needed to be shielded from the radiation. The next, and penultimate, image is of Lynch, again supine, hands clasped over her head, lips closed, looking somberly up through her thick glasses at a radiation machine overhead. The room is dark, but the machine casts a square grid of light on her chest. Her mastectomy scar, though visible, is quite well healed; we know, however, that this procedure is designed to destroy a deeper invisible cancer—beyond the reach of surgery, conventional photography, and quite possibly radiation.

The final image is a detail of this one; cropped to exclude the machine, it pictures her from the top of her head to midchest. Although merely a segment of the previous image, its effect is stunning. Most brightly lit is the area of her chest where her cancer had first been discovered; her face, on the flanking page, is in half-light, but because her face is in better focus and because that is where we look for signs of emotion, it is very much the center of interest. It has little expression—not surprisingly, because she is facing an inanimate, though potentially life-saving, machine. The image hints at inner life but provides no access to it. The repetition of images functions like a freeze-frame in a motion picture; on one level it suggests resolution, stasis—and thus the cessation of life. And in context, as the narrative's final picture, this close-up functions as a kind of death mask. Like the narrative as a whole, the movement from full shot to close-up draws the viewer deeper into the patient's life and closer to the brink of death. The collaborative diary—words and images—ends here.

An *I* with an *I*: Sandra Butler and Barbara Rosenblum, *Cancer in Two Voices* (1991)

The last cancer diary discussed here is the perhaps the most daunting, because it narrates a case of advanced breast cancer up to and beyond the death of the woman with cancer. It achieves this by means of its collaborative authorship; it is the story of Barbara Rosenblum—whose story was one of the ten short narratives in Kahane's *No Less a Woman* and to whose memory that volume is dedicated—and her partner Sandra Butler. Rosenblum's was a worst-case scenario in many respects; her tumor was initially misdiagnosed, and by the time it was correctly diagnosed, it was quite advanced. (From a blue-collar background, she faults class deference for preventing her from seeking a second opinion.) Within a couple of years she suffered metastases to other organs that required repeated, then more or less constant, chemotherapy; she died a mere three years after her initial diagnosis in 1985—less time even than the initial prognosis of five to eight years.

She was, however, blessed in having a strong and steady partner, and a malpractice settlement made it possible for her to travel in her last years. (Although she won her suit, the legal process was triply objecti-fying. Transforming her medical case into a legal one involved under-going nontherapeutic tests, surrendering her story to an advocate who argued the worst-case scenario, and putting a price on her suffering.) What most offsets the sadness of the rapid decline of her health is her avid appetite for life and the energy and insight with which she wrote about her final years. As San Francisco Bay area lesbians with many gay friends, Rosenblum and Butler approached the illness as more than an individual crisis; they mobilized friends to support them in practical ways and in periodic rituals. More important, they conceived of them-selves as pioneers and models; their writing, they hoped, would help ease the journey for any who might follow. In addition, they wrote to make their experience fully legible to themselves: "We wanted to tell our story, finally, because this writing made us visible to ourselves as we were living it" (i). Their collaborative writing, then, is not merely a record of this period in the two women's lives; rather, it is a way of truly living through it.

From the outset both women were committed to the project of the narrative, parts of which they published during the illness, the whole of which Butler edited after Rosenblum's death. The book is made up largely of a series of journal entries alternating between the two women, interrupted occasionally by longer, more focused pieces and Rosen-blum's periodic letters to friends updating them on her condition. Their writing is a means of simultaneous engagement with and retreat from each other: one major pattern of the narrative is a cycle of separation and reunion. The collaborative composition has the advantage, then, of always providing two perspectives and uniquely illuminating the dif-ficult predicament of the ill person's partner, typically overshadowed by the needs of the sick person. (Indeed, Butler worries openly about the danger of having her life sucked into the vortex of Rosenblum's can-cer, of having their schedules determined entirely by Rosenblum's needs.)

Collaborative composition also means that the narrative can achieve firm closure with Rosenblum's death and Butler's grieving. Books that point to their author's death are difficult to read, for reasons I have sug-gested. This is certainly true of this narrative, but the sadness of tracing Rosenblum's decline is somewhat compensated for by access to a griev-ing consciousness. Although people suffering from fatal illnesses can to a degree work through their grief, it is difficult for them to communi-cate that in autopathography; here, with one author/partner surviving, the narrative can enact, rather than just initiate or hint at, this process.

The completeness and closure of the narrative may be suggested by one scene unique to it among these breast cancer narratives—the composition of a will. Rosenblum sees that the legal testament will serve, like her collaborative narrative, as an inscription of the sort of person she was; the challenge is to ensure the posthumous enactment of her values by translating them into legal discourse. Although Butler respects Rosenblum's autonomy in this matter, she finds herself resenting that she will not be the prime beneficiary. (Rosenblum had aging parents and a young nephew to take into consideration.) The once-married Butler finds herself expecting the sort of protective legacy that a widow might expect; after all, she has played the caregiver to her ailing partner, and the couple had held a ceremony of commitment early in the illness. At the same time she fears that the insurance settlement will make Rosenblum the dominant partner insofar as money determines power. Under pressure of a quite literal deadline the two find themselves in conflict over the documents and rituals that will give public and permanent expression to their unconventional relationship. In the end Butler defers to her partner's needs: "Cancer is my work. . . . Cancer swallows up the air of my life and insinuates its presence everywhere. Nothing remains untouched, inviolate. So I am excused. I don't want to be separate now. . . . I will be separate soon enough. . . . I excuse myself from autonomy. I need now to yield, to allow the dependence on this woman who has become my life" (48). The book is not incidentally a record of a lesbian couple's life, making visible its particular stresses and satisfactions. That the book constructs a bulwark against the cancer that tears them apart, before and after the Rosenblum's death, suggests the resilience of the couple's response to illness. The book is counterdiscursive less in its content, which is far less political or feminist than Lorde's testimony, for example, than in its egalitarian collaboration, which enacts the mutuality of the same-sex union without embarrassment or apology.

From Autopathography to Autobiography: Juliet Wittman, *Breast Cancer Journal: A Century of Petals* (1993)

A few recent retrospective accounts of breast cancer transcend the limits of the subgenre, moving beyond autopathography toward full autobiography. This achievement is possible in part because, although relatively new, the breast cancer narrative is old enough to have matured remarkably as a genre. Enough narratives have now been published that new ones can take for granted and either "rewrite" or build on earlier ones. Driven or justified by motives of advocacy, early narratives sometimes coupled short personal narratives with compendiums of information and resources intended to empower women in their quest for effective and humane treatment. This is certainly the case with Rose Kushner's *Breast Cancer*; published originally in 1975 (not long after

Isaac's *A Breast for Life*), it was updated in 1982 as *Why Me?* and again in 1985 as *Alternatives: New Developments in the War on Breast Cancer*. (Significantly, Kushner renamed her book in response to reports that the bluntness of the original title was off-putting; concerned that women would avoid her useful book, she gave the second version a discreet title that would not intimidate potential purchasers or readers.) The modest title belies Kushner's approach. Kushner was an activist patient, and hers is the original narrative of (self-)empowerment; from the inception of her illness she researched her options carefully and shopped aggressively for treatments and physicians she believed in.

Though many later narratives also list resources in appendixes, most do not attempt to be exhaustive or current in this regard; rather, they focus on the experience of illness—offering support and validation more than advice. Thus the genre has moved away from one of its initial impulses, which was more utilitarian than autobiographical. Now, as examples of the genre proliferate, breast cancer narrators can assume some familiarity with the typical scenario; scenes repeated so often in early narratives as to seem obligatory cease to be so. Recent narrators are free to expand their focus from the single, sometimes all-consuming, experience of cancer to the way in which illness assumed meaning in the larger patterns of their lives. The founding of a tradition involves the establishment of generic conventions; the same process, however, makes possible innovation. Intertextuality, which begins as repetition, continues as variation and deviation.

Juliet Wittman's *Breast Cancer Journal* clearly profits from work that has come before and builds on it. On one level her book continues the self-help tradition of women with cancer initiating and advising others with the same illness. The introduction to her narrative is by the founder a support group for cancer patients that she found helpful, and she addresses two appendixes to women at risk. The first addresses larger political concerns—causes of breast cancer that may have been overlooked, such as birth control pills—and the need for universal health care. The second—"What I Wish I'd Known When I Was First Diagnosed"—addresses itself specifically to the recently diagnosed; as if to accommodate women who lack the time to read the whole narrative, Wittman distills some practical lessons from her experience. Aside from these framing texts, however, her autopathography has a density of detail, a maturity of reflection, and quality of prose that make it autobiography.

Without asserting that mind controls matter—indeed, she rejects the idea of the cancer personality—she recognizes that cancer is as much an existential crisis as a physical one. With a disease such as breast cancer much of one's initial suffering is mental anguish (uncertainty, anxiety, and fear), and much of that arises from disruption of one's internal auto-biography in progress. Self-consciousness, which constantly writes and rewrites this account, suddenly has its authority challenged by the uncertainty of illness—as by any major life crisis. Thus at one point Wittman finds herself "wondering whether the nightmare was really re-ceding, or whether I was just enjoying a brief respite, a kind of floating trough between tumultuous waves. Was this the beginning of a normal life, or would the cancer return to engulf me again?" (148). The signifi-cance of the episode will depend on what it proves to be, but having to wait for retrospective assessment is itself traumatic, especially for those whose projected lifespan may appear to have suddenly shortened.

Cancer diagnosis radically alters autobiographical perspective; every aspect of life narrative—past, present, and future—looks different. Di-agnosis is inevitably followed by the frantic trying out of various scenar-ios, the trying on of various roles. Wittman incisively isolates the alienat-ing qualities of diagnostic and prognostic discourse: abstraction and sterility. (She also remarks on one problem of communication between physicians and patients with life-threatening diseases: the information communicated has such emotional force that patients have trouble as-similating it, at least at the moment it is first conveyed.) For instance, she can't connect the antiseptic diagrams of a mastectomy with the reality of "severing a body part . . . cutting my warm familiar breast from my body, turning it into something bloody and alien and disposing of it . . . how? . . . My imagination faltered and stopped" (15). What at first seems to frustrate imagination, however, in the end stimulates it; herein lies one powerful source of illness narrative. Part of successful adjust-ment—the management of one's emotional response to the illness—is the process of sorting out these scenarios, rejecting the less likely, and working to convert statistical prognoses into flesh-and-blood stories.

Wittman's narrative gives exceptionally frank and vivid accounts of her terror and her sense of fragility: "any wisdom or resignation or un-derstanding I'd acquired, my proud ability to lead a normal life in the face of cancer—all these things were only a thin skin. . . . The yawning chasm that opened within me, was always there" (251). For Wittman, however, writing her story was instrumental in weaving the sudden eruption of cancer in her body into ongoing narrative lines and themes. (Already a professional journalist and a budding fiction writer, she found that her illness gave her a compelling topic for her first book.) Al-though her illness is always in the foreground, the fundamental cause and subject of the narrative, she embeds that experience within a full account of her life—indeed, within her family history. Her suddenly sharpened sense of her mortality enables, perhaps emboldens, her to revisit her mother's final illness; similarly, Wittman's great fear of abandoning her daughter helps her imagine how intensely her father, who died when Wittman was four, must have wanted not to abandon her by dying. Her illness also gives greater reality and poignancy to her sense of how the Holocaust wiped out members of her family: "few of my relatives, Jews in Central Europe, had been given the chance to die of disease" (9). At times her cancer turns her in on herself, but she gains from it a self-understanding that she translates into fuller imagination of the meaning of family, generativity, and history.

One distinction of Wittman's narrative is its self-consciousness about the built-in limits of the genre—such as the comic master plot. Although she cannot completely escape them, her acute awareness of generic constraints endows her with greater autonomy than most narrators. For example, although her story ends happily, she acknowledges more fully than most retrospective narrators the possibility of her death—in several ways. One way is by narrating her mother's final illness, which may foreshadow her own. Another, paradoxically, is to acknowledge her need to maintain a psychological barrier between herself and those with advanced cancers: "a cancer patient erects the same kind of barrier between herself and someone with metastasis that most of the world erects between itself and her" (244). With her acknowledgment of this psychological defense Wittman exposes the extent to which the typical cancer narrative represses the knowledge of mortality that it claims—by relegating the threat to the past, implying that the author *had* cancer. Cancer narratives often explicitly criticize the denial of death in American culture, but many are to some degree complicit in it. (Perhaps because of the high mortality rate of AIDS, and because of the rarity of autobiographical testimony, HIV/AIDS narratives are more candid in this regard; people healthy enough to write about their cancer generally express confidence in their survival.)

Wittman devotes her last chapter to an unusual means of advancing her healing—by observing, at the suggestion of her physician, another woman's mastectomy. One odd thing about much autopathography is that some of the most crucial, defining events occur when the narrator/subject is literally unconscious and entirely passive—being operated upon. Because Wittman's surgeries consisted of a biopsy-lumpectomy and a diagnostic removal of lymph nodes rather than a mastectomy, her account of another's mastectomy does not precisely fill the gap in her story caused by anaesthesia. It does, however, add a crucial scene to the repertoire of breast cancer narrative—the scene of mastectomy itself.[15] Within her narrative its role is somewhat ambiguous. It may stand for the operation she underwent or for an operation she may yet have to undergo. Either way, what is reassuring to her about this vicarious experience is the care she observes being administered to the unconscious

patient and the subtle art of the surgery; the operation is far more delicate than she had imagined. The significance of this episode is layered;
her observation of the operation is motivated by her status as a patient,
but it also reaffirms her status as a journalist whose professional training presumably affords her the requisite detachment to witness the
surgery. Her vision is at once passionate and dispassionate, and the
episode points both backward and forward in her narrative.

It is gestures like these that achieve what I call composure rather than
the sometimes facile, premature, and misleading closure of less satisfying narratives. In her coda, set in her garden, the resolution Wittman affirms is appropriately modest: "I thought about the blind worms pushing through the clumps of soil and the reaching filaments of root. And
I thought about the last year—the old flashes of pure joy, the constant
fear that underlay my daily living and became acute with every freckle,
cough, headache or misspoken word. And I thought, I am alive. *Alive.*
Can anyone, anywhere, with any assurance, say more?" (271)

Malignancy and Menopause: Musa Mayer, *Examining Myself: One Woman's Story of Breast Cancer Treatment and Recovery* (1993)

Three aspects of *Examining Myself* warrant singling it out for discussion. The first is the way in which it illustrates the tendency of illness
narrative to transcend itself by means of grafting another story onto the
plot of bodily malady. This tendency is perhaps especially strong with
a disease, like breast cancer, that is not susceptible to easy resolution and
definitive closure on its terms. Here Mayer's ordeal of breast cancer,
chemotherapy, and breast reconstruction—precisely because it *doesn't*
yield the desired closure—gives rise to a more comprehensive account
of her life. To use her metaphor her illness provides an armature on
which she sculpts a new self. In Mayer's case, however, her breast cancer is not complemented by a single additional plot; rather, her illness,
with its aging effects and its powerful intimations of mortality, causes
her to reassess her life. Self-examination and reconstruction involve her
whole being, then, not just her breasts. Although the book's temporal
scope is fairly restricted, it is autobiography in the sense that it documents a process of benign growth that offsets her malignancy—which,
even when excised, remains a threat in her consciousness. One of her
treatments, chemotherapy, induces menopause prematurely, and Mayer
comes to realize that the loss of her breast represents a change of life beyond the expertise of her physicians and even the understanding of her
husband or her friends. Ultimately, then, Mayer's account finds its subject as much in the midlife passage of menopause as in the more acute
and frightening episode of breast cancer.

Breast cancer radically challenges her sense of herself as a mature and self-assured woman. On the one hand, she undergoes menopause early, aging before her contemporaries. On the other, one of her reactions to the crisis of her illness is to regress psychologically. Thus, even as her treatment accelerates the process of aging, Mayer's illness threatens to reverse the process of maturing. She suddenly has to contend with selves both younger and older than her chronological age; her body is out of step with her psyche. The experience is at times utterly disorienting.

One coping strategy is to accept her illness as a major challenge to her identity rather than a mere medical condition that she can put quickly and completely behind her. Seeing her illness as more than a physical crisis paradoxically makes it more manageable; rather than "suffering" cancer passively, she seeks to make it a chapter in a larger life. Privileged with the leisure and the resources to permit this response to her illness, she addresses herself to finding meaning in, as well as treatment for, her cancer. Among the resources she explores are some New Age remedies for what ails the soul—various alternative and holistic therapies, including religious retreats and a trek in Tibet—but Mayer remains skeptical of facile attempts to ascribe meaning to illness (such as theories of cancer-prone personalities); she is open-minded without being gullible or desperate. In the end she sees that the meaning of her illness is not to be found "out there"—ready-made, prescribed—but to be created by her out of the fabric of her life.

The emphasis on significance means that the book is at times less narrative than expository; individual chapters are not chronological units so much as accounts of different aspects of her illness. Among these is the long multisurgery process of breast reconstruction, a good example of how a crisis for the body raises much deeper issues and of how illness narrative tends toward full autobiography. In the end, although she is satisfied with the result of her reconstruction, she acknowledges that it does not bring her the gratification or resolution she sought. It gives her, at best, only the appearance of wholeness. Her dissatisfaction with it is not a function of feminist qualms about prosthesis; she respectfully disagrees with Audre Lorde on this and insists that no single feminist position exists. Rather, she finds that her reconstruction does not resolve but accentuates the disparity between her outer and her inner self.

She comes to realize that the loss of her breast had become a metonym for a loss of womanliness that the reconstruction of the breast could not by itself recover: "my own inner sense of femaleness had changed profoundly . . . through an accretion of related concerns, each of which had some bearing on this basic issue of sexual body image. Infertility, hysterectomy, weight gain, aging, menopause—all of these factored into the equation" (120–21). If the loss of a breast was an outward sign of an inner deficit, the correction of the external deficit did not repair the internal one. Instead, the restoration of her womanliness was accomplished by the more arduous process that the book as a whole recounts.

The second facet of Mayer's book that warrants discussion here is the way in which it stretches the first-person point of view to include others. Mayer discovers that the sheer length of her ordeal exhausts even her most sensitive and well-intentioned friends. Finding her friends not always capable of bearing witness, she joins a support group. There she finds solace, succor, and solidarity, antidotes to the "invisibility, isolation, and uncertainty [that] are hallmarks of this disease" (147). Indeed, at times Mayer's narrative moves toward a first-person plural point of view. (At a crucial point in her story, when she is about to announce the result of an annual check-up, she interrupts her story with those of others in her group.) But Mayer is quite candid about the complex emotional dynamics of support groups, the way in which the cancer that unites the members also divides them, dealing out different fates to different members. The resulting narratives sometimes threaten the unity and integrity of the group, which has to learn to survive its losses. Only by looking beyond her support group and identifying with all women can Mayer locate herself in an unambiguously comic plot—a teleological narrative of the conquest of cancer: "We stand on the edge of a new era of early prevention, diagnosis and treatment of breast cancer. Women are mobilized now, and won't rest until this leading killer of women is eradicated or at least controlled. Dr. Love believes this will happen in her lifetime" (170). If her breast cancer forces her to look beyond her mate for solace, moments like this are the antidote to the image of lonely insomnia with which the narrative opened.

The third distinguishing feature of *Examining Myself* is its handling of the issue of narrative closure. As is perhaps appropriate for someone attuned to Eastern philosophy, Mayer achieves narrative closure in part through the acknowledgment of its unavailability. The "resolution" of her crisis is her resolve to go on without definitive assurance of continued good health. This is partly a function of her sense that cancer cures are not to be trusted. In her case, when she is told by her oncologist two years after diagnosis to put cancer behind her, she suspects that this is a generic message not indicative of her particular chances (155–56). She consciously and conscientiously declines to label herself a survivor, both because such a claim may prove premature and because in her view it is an invidious term that implies disloyalty to her less fortunate sisters (166–67). Rather than boasting of her survival, or seeking full closure, Mayer prefers to insist on the chronicity of her illness. But the unattainability of closure, she reminds her readers, is not peculiar to

people with cancer or to narrators of illness narratives; closure in autobiography is always fictive, arbitrary, premature.

Malignancy and Maternity: Gayle Feldman, *You Don't Have to Be Your Mother* (1994)

Like Mayer's narrative, Gayle Feldman's is forthright about the lack of
closure available to her. That is, she acknowledges that her case will not
admit of definitive resolution: whatever narrative closure she achieves
cannot be assumed to stand for complete physical recovery. This is particularly noteworthy because hers was the lucky case in which her
physicians declared her cured soon after her surgery rather than waiting for her tumor-free survival for a period of years. Her refusal to confirm or accept their verdict is partly a function of superstition rooted in
her intimidating family history, which can never be completely erased
from consciousness: "My mother had once listened to a doctor who had
told her nothing needed to be done. She had died five years after that"
(178). Far from being relieved, Feldman is frustrated by her doctors' decision that no further treatment is necessary; though aware that this represents a best-case scenario, she yearns for the reassurance that decisive
action might bring. Her fear of cancer, then, proves more invasive, more
difficult to eradicate, than any tumor.

In the absence of strong narrative closure—that is, a sense of her secure recovery—she turns to confession as a distancing device; that is,
she finds that public *dis*closure provides a measure of emotional closure.
Although she had already impulsively begun to write the account of her
illness that she eventually published, she found the prospect of confid-
ing in her editorial colleagues daunting. Only after considerable vacillation, then, did Feldman decide to reveal to them the true reason for her
long leave of absence: "I didn't just have a baby, I had cancer as well"
(225). The "simple" act of divulging her illness helped to seal off the experience (as the verb tense implies), and it brings its own gratification
and relief: "I was glad I had chosen to speak about the cancer, to be a
kind of witness, a simple advocate, to tell the truth" (226). As her reference to witnessing suggests, the completion of her written account provided further detachment from her illness by putting it into a larger biographical and historical perspective.

Two elements unrepresented in other accounts of breast cancer distinguish, provoke, and justify Feldman's book. The first is the coincidence of breast cancer with pregnancy. (Induced labor and the birth of
her son are followed almost immediately by procedures more typical of
cancer narratives, a biopsy and a mastectomy.) Feldman probably
would not have written about her pregnancy had it not been compli-

cated by the discovery of a malignant lump in her breast, nor would she likely have written about her cancer had she not been simultaneously pregnant. But the coincidence of two such antithetical experiences gave her a clear claim to a story worth writing. (Indeed, it is symptomatic of the maturing of the breast cancer narrative that new ones evince the need for a new angle; once the genre has been established, the experience of cancer is not necessarily sufficient to justify a narrative.)

The second unusual element, alluded to in her title (a slogan appropriated from an ad for athletic shoes), is a family history of breast cancer. The defining gesture of the narrative, then, is to locate Feldman in relation to two generations—between her son, whom she desperately wants to live to nurture, and her mother, whose fatal illness coincided with Feldman's adolescence (she died at forty-seven, when Feldman was fifteen). The resulting book, rather than being exclusively an "illness" narrative, is an account of a relatively short period of her life when Feldman experienced in quick succession a number of radical changes in her self-image and life narrative. By causing her to reflect on larger patterns of family history and of women's history—as well as the immediate issue of her survival—these coinciding challenges opened up her narrative.

Feldman defines herself and her story relationally to an unusual degree:

> I am the daughter of a woman who died of breast cancer in her forties, the age I am now.
>
> I am the granddaughter of a woman whom I never knew as a living person, my mother's mother . . . [who] died of lung cancer in her fifties without ever having smoked a cigarette. . . .
>
> I am the wife of an Englishman whose younger brother married [a woman who] died of breast cancer in her mid-thirties.
>
> And I am a woman who, at age forty, while in the eighth month of a first, much-desired, and difficult-to-achieve pregnancy, discovered that I had breast cancer and had to face not simply the imminent possibility of my own demise and the awful uncertainty engulfing the unborn child within me, but the knowledge that, should we both survive the passage to birth and beyond, everything would be different, changed irrevocably, the ghosts of cancers past intimate companions forevermore.
>
> It seems to me that like some second, malevolently tangled DNA, cancer has twisted through my cells, providing a defining thread to my life as surely as the genetic skein that has given me large eyes, small bones, brown-black hair. As I grew from age eleven through fifteen and watched my mother die, my own chaotic teen years served as an outward mirror to the uncontrolled growth taking place within her body. Already, even then, I knew that my mother's death would be the formative experience of my life, and the paths I have taken and not taken to this day wind back to that crossroads so many years before. (11–12)

Just as Feldman reached puberty, she had impressed upon her a powerful and frightening association of womanhood (and especially motherhood) with breast cancer—indeed, with death. From puberty on Feldman had lived in fear that her destiny was inscribed upon her body, encrypted in her genes. She was haunted by a terrifying "family plot": "in those memories, motherhood and death appear as intimates, intricately intertwined, bound together by cancer. . . . Being a mother and dying of cancer: the two went together, and I did not want that for myself. The simplest way to avoid it was not to become a mother at all" (52). She thus deferred getting pregnant, so long that it compromised her fertility.

At one point Feldman makes the startling confession that in the late stages of her mother's illness she had feared contamination from her mother's soiled bedclothes, as if she could catch her mother's cancer (207). After her mother's death Feldman evidently suffered from a less melodramatic form of the same fear. But although the narrative suggests the Gothic possibilities of illness narrative, it does not, like Betty Isaac's, realize them. Feldman overcomes her fear, paradoxically, when she is diagnosed with cancer and sees that the course of her illness is not necessarily going to repeat that of her mother; her fate is not preordained. Ultimately, then, she is able to incorporate the tragic narratives of her sister-in-law and her mother into her narrative without projecting them onto it; at appropriate moments she folds them into the chronicle of her illness from diagnosis to cure. She is finally able, then, to honor their stories. By distinguishing carefully between their cases and hers, she exorcises their ghosts and demystifies their stories. Ultimately, then, she is able to return her mother's gift of life, reviving her mother in narrative, even as she gives birth to a son in the flesh.

In part because of her family history of cancer Feldman's narrative foregrounds the power of scripts. On the one hand, scripts may be imposed on people—by nature (in the form of heredity), individual memory (in the form of superstition), or culture (in the form of widely shared beliefs about illness). Early in her illness she, like many patients, was plagued by the sense that her life story was no longer in her control: "We felt as though our lives were becoming public property. And we knew that they were being orchestrated elsewhere, that we were playing by the doctors' score now" (35–36). On the other hand, stories can also be liberatory narratives shared with others. One simple but valuable resource of which Feldman makes use in her crisis is the confidences of survivors, who spill out their stories upon learning of her condition; their narratives help to offset the stories of the women closer to her—those related by blood or marriage: "I needed to see, in the flesh, that you could do battle with cancer and survive. I needed it especially since I had seen cancer up close, and nobody . . . had made it through" (61). A sense of membership in a larger sisterhood, most of whom survive cancer, helps to dilute the threat of cancer without weakening her ties to her relatives. The writing of her story can be viewed as a more formal and public way of providing precisely this sort of comfort to others, the literary equivalent of the everyday sharing of oral autobiographies.

She puts further distance between her and her mother's haunting example by putting both their cancers in historical perspective, reassuring herself that even if her cancer should mimic her mother's, her chances of survival would be better. Feldman would not be subjected to the "one-step" procedure that rendered patients like her mother completely passive in their treatment. Moreover, Feldman's situation would be different, thanks in part to the efforts of intervening women:

> The "one-step" procedure they called it, doing the biopsy under general anesthesia, rushing the tissue for analysis, removing the breast while the patient waited, insensible. . . . So much easier, doing it that way, all at once, convenient, straightforward.
>
> Until, that is, a few pushy, questioning women, in the free-for-all of the late 1960s, began to challenge the doctors, read the fine print, demand that the biopsy be done separately, as a thing in itself. They also began to question the terrible, disfiguring surgery. Did it have to be so radical, to leave them so caved in?
>
> I was the beneficiary of their struggle. By the early 1970s, the medical philosophy had begun to change and the "two-step" procedure gradually became the norm. Not only that, but the Halsted radical gave way to the modified radical mastectomy, which left the major chest muscle intact and the woman flat, rather than just ribs and skin. Thinking had even gone beyond that now, with lumpectomy and radiation often an alternative to taking the whole breast. (75–76)

Feldman's brief account of changes in medical treatment—emphatically *her*story—emphasizes progress without minimizing residual risk. Her narrative makes her a beneficiary of a trend toward more responsive and responsible procedures and toward more respect for female patients as individuals and agents. Indeed, she makes her rather unusual case a chapter in a larger narrative in which women collaborate to change the script(s) of breast cancer. One pertinent difference between her and her mother—not perhaps as important as advances in treatment but nevertheless of some comfort—is the availability to Feldman's generation of published accounts of breast cancer: "[in her] case, there was so little to go on, so much was hidden. Betty Rollin, Rose Kushner, Jill Ireland, Betty Ford . . . the women who would speak and write publicly about their breast cancer hadn't done so yet" (38).

Even in a subgenre whose master plot is comic, this story is a notably positive account of breast cancer—though cautiously and responsibly so. This is partly because her cancer was relatively nonaggressive; lumpectomy was considered to have removed the threat of her first cancer; prophylactic mastectomy, that of any further breast cancer. She is that all-too-rare patient whose doctors pronounced her cured: "The doctors all count me among that happy band—those who've had cancer and can consider themselves cured" (249). In addition to this affirmative aspect of her case is the narrative of her pregnancy, which provides its own happy outcome—the birth of a healthy child (who, being male, would be minimally vulnerable to breast cancer). The narrative is positive not just in the narrow sense that Feldman does not relive her mother's sad history but also in the broader sense that it emphasizes the ways in which women today are in many ways better off than their mothers in relation to breast cancer. They are better off not only in medical terms—surgeries are less radical, reconstructive techniques more advanced—but also in cultural terms—their condition is less stigmatic, others' stories are more accessible.

"Advanced" Breast Cancer Narratives: Christina Middlebrook, *Seeing the Crab: A Memoir of Dying* (1996); Terry Tempest Williams, *Refuge: An Unnatural History of Family and Place* (1991)

Seeing the Crab and *Refuge* are "advanced" narratives of breast cancer in different senses. Both are advanced in the sense of being particularly original and innovative accounts of illness. But *Seeing the Crab* is advanced in a more literal sense: it is an autobiographical account of a cancer so advanced (Stage IV—metastatic—when first diagnosed) as to warrant the seemingly oxymoronic subtitle: "A Memoir of Dying." Like Williams, Middlebrook is a sufficiently skilled and confident writer to depart significantly from established formulas and conventions. Because her cancer is so advanced—an unfortunate term—Middlebrook skips over many of the obligatory scenes of preceding narratives. Thus she dispenses with her initial discovery of a lump, diagnosis, surgery, and chemotherapy in a single sentence (32), beginning to narrate in detail only with her autologous bone marrow transplant—a last-ditch and controversial treatment. The result of this procedure was to put her cancer in remission, but she insists that she has merely bought additional time, not a reprieve: "Cancer will kill me. It will sneak up on me, make microscopic but lethal invasions into tiny parts of my body without my even knowing it. And while it happens, I will be looking healthy" (99).

Indeed, so pressed is Middlebrook for time, which is at once her enemy and her most valued resource, that she is freed, or compelled, to dispense with chronology altogether, to organize her book on other principles. As one condemned to an early death, she has no interest in, or obligation, to chronology; the passage of time is, among other things, an index of her declining vitality. Her style itself—a terse jumpy shorthand—suggests her sense of the compression of her lifetime. And much of her account is told in the present tense—for example, "my blood counts are in a slump" (105)—an obvious but effective formal device. At times too she writes her narrative in a nearly non-narrative mode. The chapters of this book are not so much units in a chronological sequence as varied responses to her progressive illness. Sometimes she proceeds by indirection, as when she interprets a teenaged daughter's resistance to getting her license as reflecting her attempt to keep her mother alive by continuing to depend on her; sometimes (more typically), her approach is bluntly direct, cutting through the gentility and sanitization of most illness narratives to enumerate the horrible side-effects of chemotherapy—including chronic retching and the loss of sex drive (far more of a deprivation than the loss of a breast). Sometimes she experiments, trying out the trope of illness as combat, self-consciously trying on the masculine role of the infantryman (Chapter 10).

Middlebrook's narrative also reflects the extremity of her situation—before her bone marrow transplant, she was given a 50 percent chance of surviving two years—in its deliberate departure from the decorum of the typical breast cancer narrative. For example, although narrators of illness sometimes criticize the conduct of physicians, friends, and acquaintances, they rarely find fault with that of relatives. Middlebrook, however, violates the taboo on criticism of family members to take issue with the responses of her sister—who remained distant—and her mother—who remained in denial. (Though hurt by the distance her sister keeps, Middlebrook candidly acknowledges that her cancer may create sibling envy, because it makes her the center of family attention [120].) More generally, Middlebrook takes advantage of the "privilege of the condemned" to indulge in behavior generally discouraged; she vents her anger, less at her predicament than at the failure of others to acknowledge its seriousness (Chapter 13). She violates the convention of being a "good patient" (not complaining) and illness narrator. (What she craves—rather than sympathy, much less admiration—is sheer interest, curiosity; she longs to be asked simply, "What's it like?" [135].)

But perhaps the greatest departure from convention in Middlebrook is her frank acknowledgment that her cancer will eventually kill her, sooner rather than later. (One referent of her subtitle, though not its primary one, is the near-death caused by intensive chemotherapy; during that crisis she underwent a radical dissociation from her body, "a poisoned wreck" [62], such that later she did not recognize pictures of herself in the isolation ward. Having had to rely on the witnessing of others to recall her to herself and thus to affirm the integrity of her existence, she narrates that episode partly in the third person.) Diarists, such as Elizabeth Gee, sometimes express or hint at resignation—and the death of a woman with cancer has been narrated in collaborative forms—such as *Cancer in Two Voices* and *Exploding into Life*—but no other retrospective autobiographical account with which I am familiar takes for granted *from the beginning* the eventual death of the narrator. This is not merely a violation of a narrative taboo, of course; in her daily life, in communication with friends and relatives, Middlebrook is frustrated, even enraged, by the refusal of others to acknowledge that she is doomed, as she believes and declares herself to be. (Her mother insists that in not hoping for a cure, her daughter is "not thinking right" [114], and Middlebrook suspects that after she dies some will hold her attitude responsible for the inevitable recurrence of her cancer.) While acknowledging the impossibility of narrating the event of her death, Middlebrook justifies her subtitle by self-consciously narrating the process of her dying. Her final gesture in the book, then, is to identify herself, eschewing euphemism and denial, as a "dier." In unwillingly but deliberately assuming that role eventually forced on all mortals, she pioneers as an autobiographer.

Despite its postcolonial impulse, much illness narrative is in many ways antimodernist in form (in its emphasis on plot and closure). Middlebrook's advanced account of her illness illustrates how such narrative conventions may fail to serve the needs of the ailing person—how illness experience may exceed or defy generic conventions and cry out for innovation. Indeed, in its evasion or subversion of chronology her book illustrates one drawback of the term *illness narrative*, which implies a work consisting of a single mode of writing organized as a story—if not strictly chronological in organization, at least based on and referring to a clear and coherent sequence of events. And it challenges the tyranny of the comic plot, the convention of an affirmative ending.

Terry Tempest Williams's *Refuge* (1991) is equally, but differently, advanced. One criticism leveled at personal narratives of illness and disability is that by nature—because they are *narrative* and because they focus on *individuals*—they tend to sentimentalize conditions that might better be looked at dispassionately—in other words, from a more political perspective. I hope it is by now apparent that breast cancer narratives to some extent resist this tendency, at least insofar as they are the product of feminist concern for a woman's disease. (In addition to asking "why me?," the more politically concerned narratives ask "why us?")

In discussing Feldman's narrative I remarked on the extraordinary extent to which, as a woman with breast cancer, she defined herself relationally. Terry Tempest Williams's anomalous *Refuge: An Unnatural History of Family and Place* (1991) goes even further in the direction of deindividualizing and desentimentalizing cancer narrative. Williams's book reads at first like a naturalist's dispassionate but observant chronicle of the gradual rise and fall of the Great Salt Lake—and an implicit critique of presumptuous human attempts to prevent or reverse the lake's flooding. Only gradually does Williams shift her focus to the cancer that kills her mother at fifty-four. And only in an epilogue, which flashes back to above-ground nuclear testing in the area, does Williams reveal her concern with the implication of environmental pollution in the various cancers in the last several generations of women in her family. The concern shifts from Williams's mother and grandmothers to her extended family and to an entire clan of one-breasted women, all of whom may have been delayed victims of the tests and/or of other environmental pollution.

In the end, then, *Refuge* is about breast cancer as an environmental crisis rather than as a personal calamity—a disease induced by arrogant human manipulation of nature. The book thus raises broader questions about the relation of men and women to the land and of citizens to their democratic government. Such a book resists easy categorization as an illness narrative—indeed, Anne Hunsaker Hawkins has dubbed it an "ecopathography"—because it reflects a different paradigm for telling the story of illness. Like Middlebrook's book, it advances our understanding of illness and expands the repertoire of ways to represent it.

The End of the Genre

Narratives of breast cancer constitute a distinctive, significant, and quite coherent new subgenre of American autobiography. As we shall see when we turn to narratives of AIDS, the prevalence of autobiographical accounts of breast cancer is noteworthy; women with breast cancer are taking their lives into their own hands, producing enduring accounts of their survival. Already the genre has its own history—from the diary of Alice James, which became a breast cancer narrative only incidentally, through the pathos of Isaac's *A Breast for Life*, to the politically aware, well-crafted, and innovative narratives of recent years. The nomination of Juliet Wittman's *Breast Cancer Journal* for a National Book

Award is a sign that the subgenre is coming of age and gaining recognition.

It is to be hoped that one day, having served its purpose, the form will be obsolete, like the slave narrative, and that the narratives will be of interest largely to historians trying to reconstruct women's experience in late twentieth-century America. But cancer is as much a natural as a social evil; although political mobilization and fund-raising may hasten progress toward a cure or preventative measures, and although some contemporary developments in treatment seem promising, cancer, unlike slavery, cannot be abolished by moral suasion, political mobilization, legislation, or war. Meanwhile, the continued incidence of breast cancer and changes in treatment strategies create a constant demand for new narratives, as informational appendixes or clinical details become dated. And, as we have seen, the form develops in part according to its own intertextual momentum; as in any genre later books may revise, correct, or build on earlier ones. As conventions become better established, so too does formal innovation become more possible and more desirable.

It is a critical commonplace today that culture authorizes autobiography—that is, that cultural forces determine what sorts of stories get written and published, who gets a life. But although culture may authorize autobiography, individuals write it. And regardless of whether their narratives are "failures" or "successes," we should not overlook the political significance of the act of autobiographical narration in the case of breast cancer. Whatever the choices these women make regarding treatment, prosthesis, or breast reconstruction, all have chosen to own their illnesses rather than to pass as healthy or physically intact. All enact narrative alternatives or complements to prosthesis and breast reconstruction—candid exposure of scars, literal or metaphorical, and the reconstruction of identity in all its fullness. In telling their illnesses they also tell their lives and those of others to whom they are related.

In her 1993 study of "invalid women" Diane Price Herndl argued that

the figure of the invalid woman at once unites the romantic ideology of woman as "body" (as opposed to man as "mind"), the Victorian stereotype of woman as weak and delicate, and the bourgeois ideal of woman as "conspicuous consumer" (who passively consumes since as invalid she must be served at all times). . . . She also stands in a specific relation to sexist definitions of women; she embodies the negative discourses about women. (10)

Although, as we have seen, narratives of breast cancer are not universally or uniformly counterdiscursive, they take a significant step toward refiguring women and illness. Indeed, in taking a "woman's" illness as an opportunity to write their lives, they tend to invalidate the discourse of women's invalidity.

Notes

1. This may be a function of the earlier detection of cancers, the result of better screening; the controversy over how to interpret such statistics is itself a sign of the politicization of breast cancer today. The good news is that in the 1990s death rates are falling for women younger than sixty-five, and especially for women younger than fifty (Love 271).

2. It is not, of course, a disease found only in women. Although its occurrence in men is rare (1 percent of the time), its rarity makes it particularly dangerous, for few men are concerned with detecting it. Of course, because of its cultural construction breast cancer has a different significance for men.

3. Even among these women, however, several narratives describe what appear to be medical bungles. For example, a physician dismissed Betty Rollin's initial lump as insignificant until a year after she discovered it; physicians changed Wadler's diagnosis and recommended further therapy when doctors at a second hospital examined her slides.

4. Toward its end *The Diary of Alice James* (1894) became a breast cancer narrative with the advent of an illness (diagnosed in 1891) that both validated and terminated James's long career of invalidity. Some remarkable writing marks that section of her diary, but although James is a significant precursor for contemporary women writing of their illnesses, she is not likely to serve as an exemplar because of the way in which she embraced her cancer as a vindication.

5. On the problematic term *memoir*, see note 3 in chapter 1.

6. These narratives, then, like most autopathography, have the odd implication that their author's lives as healthy people are unsuitable—or less suitable—subjects for autobiography. As slave narrators typically ended their narratives when they achieved freedom (and thus produced "slave narratives" rather than full-life narratives), cancer survivors end theirs at some moment of resolution. Once the threat of illness recedes, the narrative concludes. So although recovery from illness, like escape from slavery, precipitates into writing lives that would otherwise go unwritten, the conventions of the subgenre also reflect the cultural limitations on who may write a full-life narrative.

7. Issues of visibility arise in this literature in a number of ways. As here, one has to do with the invisibility of the tumor and the idea that it can be mastered if seen. Another has to do with the visible scars of surgery and their disguise. And that is related to the larger issue of women as objects of the male gaze. Responses to the problems of visibility take the form of confronting the tumor, observing others' surgeries, seeking out photos (rather than drawings) of surgical scars and reconstructions, and choosing not to wear a prosthesis, thus identi-

fying oneself publicly as a cancer survivor. All these strategies resist the traditional passivity and invisibility of women with breast cancer.

8. The most common element, nearly universal, is opening with the scene of discovery or diagnosis, after which the narrative circles back to provide a summary of the narrator's life up to that point.

9. Juliet Wittman, for example, explicitly denounces Lawrence LeShan's theory of the "cancer personality" (Wittman 58) and rejects the battle metaphor (107). On the other hand, some of these authors still succumb to the tropical disease.

Interestingly, the word *cancer* does not figure as prominently in the narratives' titles as one might expect. It is more often mentioned in subtitles than in titles proper, and often it is present in neither, as though the authors (or their publishers) were subconsciously affected by the taboo against naming the disease.

10. In many ways—its claustrophobia, the reader's sense that the narrator is repressing conflicts about her domesticity, her hallucinations (after she comes home from the hospital drug dependent, she hallucinates that her house is exploding), her spiraling mental breakdown—the narrative reads like an updated nonfiction version of "The Yellow Wall-Paper" (1892), Charlotte Perkins Gilman's classic story of a woman's mental breakdown. It thus illustrates the Gothic potential of the illness narrative.

11. In addition to Isaac, a notable exception here is Betty Rollin, whose *First, You Cry* (1976) was a best-seller that was made into a TV movie. Rollin acknowledges her vanity and that she felt less attractive and sexy following her mastectomy. On camera as a journalist she wanted to, and did, pass as a two-breasted woman. But even she, who seems to have so fully internalized socially defined ideal body images, was willing to expose herself in print. Her book has recently been republished with a new introduction in which the author, who had a second mastectomy in 1984, asserts from her present perspective that she made too much earlier of the loss of a "mere" breast.

12. Though Lorde is evidently not worried by this, some danger exists that her writing will valorize one politically correct response to the loss of a breast, imposing an additional burden of guilt on women who for whatever reasons feel the need for prostheses or reconstructive surgery.

13. Anne Hunsaker Hawkins suggests that with the advent of materialistic culture, illness narrative has succeeded spiritual autobiography (31), but it might be more accurate to say that the later genre has perpetuated or revived the former.

14. A partial exception is Nancy Brinker's *The Race Is Run* (1990), which includes photo sequences of various patients. However, these patients are anonymous; their torsos are usually cut off at the neck. The sequences seem designed mainly to display the results achievable with reconstructive surgery. The artist Matuschka has become well known for her photos of herself with her mastectomy scar exposed; the *New York Times Magazine* published one such photo on its cover (August 15, 1993). Deena Metzger also produced a poster and postcards

using a photo of herself naked from the waist up, displaying a tattooed mastectomy scar. Unlike the images in *The Race Is Run*, Lynch's are not anonymous; unlike Matuschka's and Metzger's, they are in no way glamorized. The most transgressive autoportraits of a woman with breast cancer, however, appear in *Putting Myself in the Picture* (1988), by the British photographer Jo Spence. For a discussion of Spence see Smith, pp. 146–53.

15. Although there is some question as to whether her tumor was malignant, Fanny Burney (1752–1840) did have a mastectomy without anaesthesia and wrote a compelling account of it; see Epstein.

4

HIV/AIDS and Its Stories

> We seem to require of our bodies and our illnesses that they tell revelatory stories, and HIV infection in what have been dubbed "risk populations" has been read as an elective contaminant. This election comes as a result of a prior choice to reside in the realm of the abnormal. To become ill with AIDS is to have been sick all along.
>
> —Julia Epstein, *Altered Conditions*, 1995, p. 19.

Writing Of(f) People with AIDS

According to Susan Sontag, "Societies need to have one illness which becomes identified with evil, and attaches blame to its 'victims,' but it is hard to be obsessed with more than one" (16). Some time in the 1980s AIDS seems to have succeeded cancer as the most feared and stigmatic disease in the United States. Like cancer, AIDS is an illness whose symbolic dimensions are especially prominent and significant; it offers an obvious and extreme instance of the "cultural construction" of illness. Even within medical discourse AIDS is a rather indeterminate phenomenon because it is not in the usual sense a disease at all but a syndrome whose symptoms are diseases. Outside medical discourse, as we shall see, this inherently unstable term is invested with meaning by various metaphors and cultural narratives—all of which are hostile to those most at risk or already infected. This has obvious implications for personal narratives, which can resist, but not entirely ignore or escape, presumptions about HIV/AIDS; at best, such accounts are in the position of revising what are in effect prescripted narratives. This sense that their story is already scripted for them may inhibit people with HIV from attempting to inscribe their narratives.

Clinically, whether one "has AIDS" is a matter not only of seropositivity (being infected with HIV, the human immunodeficiency virus) but of having an immune system so weakened that one is subject to a number of "opportunistic infections," such as pneumocystic pneumo-

81

nia (PCP). Because the infections that exploit immunodeficiency are different in men, women, and children and in various parts of the globe, the clinical definition of AIDS varies with gender, age, and geography; in response to growing understanding of the diverse manifestations of late-stage HIV infection, the official classification of AIDS in the United States has changed substantially over time. Exactly what constitutes a clinical case of AIDS, then, is a matter of shifting definitions. Without any change in one's condition and indeed without any physical examination or tests, one's diagnostic status could change overnight because of a change in the official definition of the illness; one's condition could be *reclassified*, rather than *diagnosed*, as AIDS. This has significant implications for personal narrative, because the moment of diagnosis is typically presented as a crisis or watershed. (Mark Doty has noted "the telling grammatical distinction, the difference between *being* [HIV-positive] and *having* [AIDS], between a condition and a possession. AIDS is a possession one is possessed *by*" [139].) Because lowered immune response—as measured by blood tests that count T-cells (or CD4 cells)—is now a constitutive condition of AIDS, some cases present an element of election; that is, patients may be told they "qualify" for a diagnosis (Doty 207). This further complicates the event. On the one hand, a diagnosis of AIDS may entitle patients to some kinds of health care, services, and benefits; on the other, it may effectively, if not legally, disqualify them from finding employment or insurance. More important, a diagnosis of AIDS—considered, until the mid-1990s at least, to be tantamount to a death sentence—is an unwelcome and irreversible change of status.[1]

The question of the "progression" of HIV infection through stages is also problematic. On the one hand, many clinicians characterize HIV as having five stages—acute HIV syndrome (coincident with initial infection), a silent or latent (asymptomatic) stage, progressive generalized lymphadenopathy ([PGL] when lymph glands swell up), AIDS-related complex (ARC) or "symptomatic HIV infection" (distinguished by symptoms like diarrhea and weight loss), and AIDS itself (Schoub 31–34). On the other hand, the Centers for Disease Control and Prevention used a four-part classification in 1986 (omitting ARC), and in 1993 it issued a different, more complex classification scheme. Dennis Osmond, a San Francisco epidemiologist, emphasizes that the disease categories created by these official classifications are not necessarily sequential stages; HIV infection is perhaps best seen as a continuum, of which AIDS is the end stage (Osmond 1.1-7–1.1-13). Estimates of the percentage of those infected with HIV who will eventually develop AIDS have risen steadily during the course of the epidemic to approach 100 percent; increasingly, it appeared likely, though it was never known with certainty, that all those infected with HIV would progress to AIDS. And, until the mid-1990s, AIDS has been generally been considered to be invariably fatal. In late 1996, however, came what may be a breakthrough in AIDS treatment—not the long-awaited "magic bullet" (a certain cure) or a vaccine but combinations of drugs, including new protease inhibitors, that seem to suppress the virus effectively and indefinitely in many people with AIDS. Thus, as the end of the millenium approaches, there is some reason to believe that the end of the epidemic may be in sight.[2]

Even before this promising development there were those who argued that the assumption that AIDS was invariably deadly, though not susceptible of disproof, was unduly fatalistic and thus pernicious. For one thing, it assumed no progress in treatment and cure; it projected the past into an indefinite future, ignoring progress in the treatment of AIDS and significant increase in survival times. According to Cindy Patton,

The consistent confusion of a positive antibody test with an AIDS diagnosis and the failure to distinguish anti-viral treatments from treatments for opportunistic infections create an unnecessarily pessimistic interpretation of the idea that there is no "cure for AIDS." Coupled with images of PLWAs [people living with AIDS] in extreme pain or as romantically sick figures, the media obscure the reality that many PLWAs continue to lead full, "normal" lives. (1990, 27)

The idea that AIDS—or even HIV infection—is an automatic death sentence is the ultimate marginalization of infected individuals, a way of metaphorically writing off people with HIV/AIDS (not only because it implies their guilt). The consequences of the too-easy equation of HIV infection with death from AIDS are real; particularly in the earlier years of the epidemic healthy people sometimes preemptively committed suicide after diagnosis or even after a positive antibody test. The idea of HIV as a death sentence may foster an unwarranted sense of hopelessness not only in infected people but in those who treat them. Emmanuel Dreuilhe has given eloquent expression to the corrosive force of the idea of the death sentence: "The enemy is not so much the HIV virus itself—supposing that it is the only cause of AIDS—as it is the unshakable conviction of the media, public opinion, my father, all my friends and allies—when they're being honest with themselves—a conviction that a part of me shares: that AIDS, as the press keeps repeating, 'is an illness that is always rapidly fatal and for which there is no cure'" (1988, 8). Considering the long period during which HIV may be latent, the possibility that HIV may require cofactors to produce AIDS symptoms, the possibility that some strains of the virus are more deadly than others, and recent success in suppressing HIV with combinations of drugs, it may make sense to consider HIV, if not AIDS, a "chronic and manageable disorder." *Life* is a death sentence—we will all die eventually; for people with HIV "eventually" may be a long time—long enough to witness a cure or, at least, treatment that may ensure indefinite survival. A diagnosis of AIDS is no longer necessarily a condemnation to death in the near future. As Patton observes, "The cultural/ symbolic difference between a disease conceived as 'inevitably fatal' and a disease course which may run twenty years from infection to death, is significant" (1990, 65). Considering HIV positivity as a life crisis rather than a death sentence may make a real difference in the longevity and quality of life of those with the virus.

To put it different terms, the idea of the invariable fatality of AIDS encapsulates perhaps the most widely shared cultural narrative of AIDS; diagnosis with AIDS, or even testing positive, is thought to determine and considerably shorten the plot of one's life. Such a demoralizing scenario greatly problematizes individual narration of experiences with HIV/AIDS. HIV-positive individuals may see themselves prematurely as doomed.[3]

There is more to the cultural construction of AIDS, of course, than its clinical ambiguity and the presumption of its invariable fatality. Beyond the matters of what AIDS is, who has it, and what will become of them is the loaded issue of who gets it and how. As Christopher Taylor has pointed out,

While certain sicknesses do not engender illness metaphors because of their innocuousness, sicknesses that are contagious, life-threatening, characterized by bizarre or debilitating symptoms, or associated with abnormal behavior are likely to give rise to imagery embodying positive or negative sociomoral judgments. Moreover, these judgments are further reinforced when the sickness manifests a propensity to afflict members of society who are already marginalized for reasons of ethnicity, life-style, or socioeconomic status. (1990, 56–57)

This dimension of AIDS was evident from the beginning of its appearance in North America: the syndrome was first known in the United States as gay-related immune deficiency (GRID) because it was first diagnosed in gay men. Even after being renamed acquired immune deficiency syndrome, AIDS has continued to be peculiarly subject to metaphorical construction. Its association with male homosexuality and intravenous drug use continues to define AIDS; that is, its public perception in North America is much colored by its association with the marginalized groups who first "acquired" their immunodeficiency and the ways in which they acquired it.

One ramification of the hegemonic metaphors of AIDS has to do with the pertinence of the sick role. In the case of HIV/AIDS the sick role—a kind of cultural contract with the ill person—becomes highly problematic:

Beyond the circle of intimacy, the popular perception is that the infected person, no matter what symptoms are or are not evident, "has AIDS." The social interactional meaning of this ascription is that the future of the infected person is death from this terrible disease, and that the person is dangerous to others. Most people assume that the infected person should be under a doctor's care ... even though the disease is also perceived to be incurable. And certainly there is a widespread and recurrent demand that infected persons be relieved of obligations, or perhaps deprived of opportunities, for normal social interactions and role performance. Many people insist that asymptomatic HIV-infected persons be considered sick, because they are incapable of performing "normal" role expectations through "normal" social interaction without putting others in what is perceived as danger. To this end, many people continue to insist that the identity of those who are infected should be discovered and revealed. (Quam 1990, 31–32)

The stigma of HIV, then, may force one prematurely into a sick role; others may marginalize and isolate those infected.

However, in another sense the sick role may be denied those infected with HIV: "If the illness is perceived to be the result of some serious deviation from social rules and norms, then the ill person may be . . . treated as a criminal. . . . AIDS as a disease which is sexually transmitted is clearly included in this category of illnesses that are considered illegitimate. Indeed, debates about disease control often take on a rhetorical tone more appropriate to crime control" (Quam 33). Thus the public perception of AIDS tends to result in what Erving Goffman has called "spoiled identity":

In a now classic work, *Stigma: Notes on the Management of Spoiled Identity*, sociologist Erving Goffman defined what he considered to be three types of stigma. The first is an abomination of the body; clearly AIDS could be so categorized.[4] The second is a blemish of individual character; again victims of AIDS and other sexually transmitted diseases have traditionally been seen as lacking control, as immoral and promiscuous.[5] And third, Goffman identified the tribal stigmas of race, nation, or religion. This, too, has been a recurring theme in considerations of venereal disease—the notion that particular groups were especially prone to infection. Perhaps the sexually transmitted diseases carry a particularly weighty stigma because they cut through each of these categories; an undesired *difference*, of a sexual nature, that sets its victims apart. Victims of AIDS thus suffer the biological consequences of a terrifying, fatal disease as well as a deep social stigma. (Brandt 1988, 156)

Unlike the case with more common, less stigmatic illnesses, the first question in many people's minds after learning that an individual is

HIV positive or has AIDS is how he or she contracted the virus. Most people's response, conscious or not, is to determine the degree of responsibility (or culpability) of the person affected. The self-protective motive in such a response is to insulate oneself from the illness by attributing the other's infection to an unshared trait such as sexual orientation or promiscuity. But the effect is to treat seropositive individuals as somehow deserving their disease because of its roots in their behavior or their identity.

Like the presumption of fatality, the complexity of the sick role has implications for the production of illness narratives. Though HIV infection and AIDS may be seen as existing on a continuum, crossing from one condition to the other is generally construed as a radical, irreversible, and tragic transition. The cultural construction of HIV/AIDS inhibits illness narrative in different ways on both sides of that watershed. To be HIV positive is to exist in a liminal social space—between health and serious illness. Thus people who are HIV positive but asymptomatic may resist writing illness narratives because they are reluctant to identify themselves as infected, for fear of prematurely adopting—or being assigned to—the sick role. Once diagnosed with AIDS, however, the same individuals might be reluctant to write illness narratives for different reasons—a sense of hopelessness, symptoms that interfere with the sort of detachment conducive to autobiography, or simply desire to avoid or minimize the stigma of AIDS. As we shall see, then, the vast majority of AIDS narratives have taken the form of memoir rather than autobiography.[6]

AIDS is culturally constructed, or "written," as a series of narratives. One such narrative has to do with the origin and course of the worldwide epidemic. More widely held and more empirically based than the various paranoid theories about the origins of AIDS as part of a deliberate genocidal conspiracy is the narrative that locates the origins of HIV in African monkeys. Without wanting to dispute or suppress this account, one can see that the association of a deadly sexually transmissible disease with the "Dark Continent" may reinforce certain racist ideas. Thus a crucial gap in this narrative—how the virus was initially transmitted from animals to humans—has been filled in with "outlandish suggestions . . . of tribal rituals involving the splashing of monkey blood over human genital organs to enhance sexual performance or sexual intercourse with monkey as the possible route" (Schoub 15). A related metanarrative has to do with the progression of the disease in the "developed" world. Thus

reports of the epidemic in the West continue to speak about "leakage" from the initial identified "risk groups" of homosexuals, Haitians, heroin addicts, and later hemophiliacs into an amorphously defined but clearly white, middle-class, suburban, "decent," and, above all, heterosexual "general population," a population that is carefully delimited *against* the transgressive otherness of same-sex desire, racial difference, injection drug use, and illness. (Epstein 1995, 159)

In the context of contemporary American society another primary AIDS narrative concerns members of the group first and perhaps hardest hit by the epidemic, gay men. As Paula Treichler has said, "Whatever else it may be, AIDS is a story, or multiple stories, read to a surprising extent from a text that does not exist: the body of the male homosexual. It is a text people so want—need—to read that they have gone so far as to write it themselves. . . . The connections between death, sex, and homosexuality made the AIDS story inevitably . . . able to be read as 'the story of a metaphor'" (42). Like a number of other diseases (like cancer) that have a strong metaphoric dimension, AIDS tends to generate lurid narratives. The most influential narrative associates AIDS with male homosexuality and attributes acquisition and spread not only to gay sex but to promiscuity, and particularly to anal intercourse. Thus a diagnosis with AIDS, especially in a young unmarried male, is often assumed—in the absence of evidence to the contrary—to be a result of homosexual contact; revealing the diagnosis is tantamount to outing. As Sontag pointed out in her 1989 book, "To get AIDS is precisely to be revealed, in the majority of cases so far, as a member of a certain 'risk group,' a community of pariahs. The illness flushes out an identity that might have remained hidden from neighbors, jobmates, family, friends" (24–25). AIDS is seen not only as a disease of excess but of perversity (26). A history of homosexuality may be attributed to all males infected with HIV.

Just as HIV status and AIDS diagnosis ascribe a likely past to those infected, so too do status and diagnosis tend to prescribe the future—to prescript suffering from various disfiguring and incapacitating infections, loss of mental lucidity, and death. Thus HIV positivity, and especially diagnosis of AIDS, are often read in terms of a narrative sequence leading from promiscuous gay sex to illness and certain death. One dominant narrative of AIDS, then, reduces the individual to his sexual identity and condemns him to an early death from a harrowing illness. The story of AIDS may at once sensationalize one's past, "spoil" one's identity, and foreshorten or deny one's future. Thus may AIDS discourse add psychic insult to the injury of physical infection. Only from the perspective of a homophobic mainstream culture, of course, does the revelation of homosexuality "spoil" one's identity. From the perspective of the gay community AIDS has been a powerful closet door opener, on both an individual and a collective scale. The gay challenge to heterosexist assumptions has taken many forms, including life writing and AIDS narrative.

More than any other contemporary illness, AIDS tends to subject people to punishment and marginalization by means of what I have just described as hegemonic scripts or metaphors. One obvious consideration, then, in reading AIDS narratives is their relation to the prescripting of AIDS, the extent to which they confirm or challenge the dominant narratives. Various forms of representation of HIV or AIDS offer positive counterdiscursive potential. But not all media are equivalent; different media have different biases or capabilities built in to them. Though surprisingly little, to my knowledge, has been written on AIDS and autobiography,[7] the question of the representation of AIDS in particular genres—as opposed to general discourse—has attracted some attention. For example, Douglas Crimp has commented instructively on photography as a medium. In practice he often finds photographic treatments inimical to the interests of people with AIDS. In his 1992 essay he finds a CBS *Sixty Minutes* portrait gallery of people with AIDS guilty at once of violating the privacy of the ill—by exploiting their cooperation and physical weakness to expose their emotions and thoughts to an audience of strangers—and of reinforcing their isolation—by utterly ignoring the public and collective dimensions of the crisis (120). Despite the presumably sympathetic intentions of the producers, their treatment of people with AIDS further marginalizes them, according to Crimp. *They* are ill, *we* (the viewers) are not; *they* are passively exposed to *our* gaze. *We* live; *they* die (voice-overs specify when individuals died, so that in many cases the exposure is posthumous). The effect is to make "them" seem hopeless and pitiable.

Other aspects of photographic images of people with AIDS also disturb Crimp—the tendency to show them alone, in hospital beds (rather than in the company of their families or partners); the emphasis on the visible signs of disease (in particular, the disfiguring lesions of Kaposi's sarcoma). The effect is to reify their illness and underscore their isolation. The convention of representing a number of individuals in a "gallery" of portraits, rather than attending to them as individuals, reduces them to their condition as "cases," *victims* of AIDS. Crimp acknowledges that the photographic rendering of people with AIDS has some truth and wonders whether he is right to criticize the bleak picture photography offers of AIDS: "Do we really wish to claim that [such] photographs . . . are untrue? Do we want to find ourselves in the position of denying the horrible suffering of people with AIDS, the fact that very many PWAs become disfigured and helpless, and that they die?" Ultimately, however, he stands by his critique:

Certainly we can say that these representations do not help us, and that they probably hinder us, in our struggle, because the best they can do is elicit pity, and pity is not solidarity. We must continue to demand and create our own counter-images, images of PWA self-empowerment, of the organized PWA movement and of the larger AIDS activist movement, as the ACT UP [AIDS Coalition to Unleash Power] demonstrators insisted at MOMA [New York's Museum of Modern Art]. But we must also recognize that every image of a PWA is a *representation*, and formulate our activist demands not in relation to the "truth" of the image, but in relation to the conditions of its construction and to its social effect. (126)

Crimp concludes that "photography is a very impoverished medium for representing anything so complex as AIDS, as *living* with AIDS" (132).[8]

In comparison to the medium of photography, life writing has many advantages as a medium. For one thing, because it usually focuses on one individual at a time, it tends to resist stereotyping. For another, in written narratives photographic representation is optional and supplemental, and it is thus rarely present. This means that the reader's relation to the subject is not colored or determined by responses to visual signs of illness, such as lesions. But despite the advantages of life writing over photography as AIDS discourse—or counterdiscourse—thus far memoirs have far outnumbered autobiographical narratives. This is perhaps not surprising; as Stephen Greco has tersely put it, " Writers with AIDS just don't live long enough to make a book out of their experiences, or are too exhausted or preoccupied to work efficiently on one" (1989, 115). Furthermore, as Marilyn Chandler has pointed out, gay men with AIDS

are in a position of extraordinary vulnerability, far greater than that of the ordinary autobiographer who risks exposing private life to public view. For most, admitting publicly that they are carriers of the AIDS virus will significantly change the nature of their relationships with colleagues and friends. For many it involves disclosure not only of humiliating details of bodily illness, but also of sexual practices and lifestyles that have been subject to chronic misunderstanding and the butt of slurs and jokes for generations. (1991, 55)

But the alternative to autopathography is to have others write one's illness, and the risks of that are considerable: one's identity and fate are out of one's hands. The obituary—which is, after all, a news story—is a seemingly reliable form of life writing. Yet even that supposedly objective genre reveals the volatility of AIDS as a signifier. Until the late 1980s obituaries in mainstream media generally did not list AIDS as a cause of death (and thus, to the outrage of gay activists, underreported the magnitude of the epidemic). In some cases, this happened because the families of gay men sought to veil or deny the cause of death in order to conceal the homosexuality of the deceased. Without defending the practice of concealment Emmanuel Dreuilhe tersely stated one rationale for it: "From the moment someone is stricken with AIDS, all his previous accomplishments are retroactively annulled. Cut down in their youth or middle age, these people become entirely defined by their deaths" (1988, 99). Peter M. Nardi has noted the irony of attempts to conceal AIDS as a cause of death in young men: "the language used to explain early deaths among young men reconstructs the causes in an attempt to distance the deceased person from the disease and the risk group, thereby perpetuating those very stigma. However, as more and more people learn to decode the language, the obituaries ironically have the opposite effect of actually signaling AIDS as the real cause" (161).

Even when families or surviving partners have wished AIDS and homosexuality to be recorded, mainstream media have often suppressed the cause of death and refused to list surviving gay partners, thus significantly misrepresenting the lives of the obituaries' subjects (Alwood 270–72). In gay media, in contrast, obituaries and death notices have been open about the cause of death; indeed, because death notices are paid for and composed by survivors, they are a particularly democratic form of life writing. During the AIDS epidemic the gay death notice has developed into a distinctive genre. It is thus a significant form of counterdiscourse, but for the most part it reaches only a small, sympathetic audience.[9] (Ironically, the poor, who live and die in anonymity and who tend to succumb to AIDS more quickly as a result of inferior health care, are less vulnerable to posthumous exposure and dissection of their lives; their deaths do not warrant obituaries, and sometimes their families cannot afford death notices.)

Though far more limited in number, life narratives intended for a general audience would seem more conducive to counterdiscourse. Narrative by definition involves the passage of time; thus the medium offers an opportunity to display the process of anticipating, living with, responding to, and managing illness—as opposed to static deathbed images (or "before and after" images) of "victims" who are often selected, consciously or not, on the basis of certain physical features—emaciation, disfiguration—to ensure that they will be recognizably representative of AIDS. In the case of autobiography subjects control their representation; in the case of memoir subjects are represented by those who know and care for them. The likelihood of negative stereotyping would seem to be minimal. Nonfiction narrative is not the only genre for the presentation of AIDS, of course; much has been done in fiction, drama, and the essay—indeed, at least until recently, the best writing about AIDS has probably been found in these more "literary" media. But personal narrative has the potential advantage of recording real lives, true stories. For all that autobiography is understood to be fictive, as poststructuralist theory would have it, it is hard not to regard autobiographies or memoirs as more powerful testimony than more literary forms of representation. (Indeed, at times their liabilities as literature—naïveté, a sense of mission—may buttress their authenticity as testimony.) When a mother or sister or partner takes up the pen to memorialize a son or brother or lover and, even more dramatically, when people with AIDS undertake to narrate their own lives, the personal stake and commitment have some effect, no matter how sophisticated we are as readers.

At the same time, like any chronic illness AIDS presents serious obstacles to potential autopathographers. As noted earlier, the most obvious is the lack of energy to undertake, and of time to complete, a narrative. Another related problem is the issue of narrative closure. With acute illness the convention is to use cure or recovery as an occasion for closure, though comic resolution usually involves more than "mere" recovery from illness. With chronic illness this opportunity or occasion is not available; how then, does one conclude a narrative of HIV or AIDS satisfactorily? (As we have seen, the end of a course of treatment and the hopeful signs of remission are often used in the case of cancer. To an extent AIDS offers parallels, but recovery from one opportunistic illness, though it may resolve a crisis, is not the equivalent of open-ended remission.) As a not merely chronic, but (as-yet) incurable and deadly illness, AIDS presents a more serious and fundamental narrative challenge. As we have seen, the master plot of autobiography (and of autopathography) is a comic plot: according to some evident standard, the protagonist is better off at the end than at the beginning. But a disjunction exists, or would seem to exist, between the required or desired plot of personal narrative and the inherent or intrinsic "plot" or "story line" of AIDS—that is, decline and dissolution. This disjunction, I think, has been a powerful inhibitor of autobiographical accounts of AIDS.[10]

But the most powerful constraints on personal narrative may lie in the cultural narratives discussed earlier. Because by definition the point of view of personal narratives is that of individuals directly or indirectly affected by HIV, such narratives have the potential of countering hegemonic scripts. Writing one's story or that of a partner or relative offers an opportunity to rewrite the culturally dominant narrative; one may alter the inscription of AIDS by taking the pen into one's own hands. This counterdiscursive potential, however, is not always realized. For one thing, different "risk groups" have not been proportionally represented in personal narratives of AIDS. The general cultural constraints on whose experience is worthy of life writing would exclude many of these individuals even if they were healthy. Thus there are few narratives by or about individuals who contracted HIV infection through intravenous drug use. There are also few narratives by individuals who were infected through transfusion. (Indeed, one striking aspect of the accounts of those thus infected—for example, those of Arthur Ashe and Fran Peavey, discussed later in this chapter—is the extent to which they are exercises in self-destigmatization.)

As we shall see, most book-length personal narratives of AIDS concern men infected through homosexual contact. But few such narratives are autobiographical. And the difference between being directly and indirectly affected by HIV—in other words, between autobiography and memoir—turns out to be crucial. As a rule, memoirs written by relatives of gay men with AIDS tend unwittingly to reinforce the narrative of leakage and/or to reinforce negative stereotyping. However well intentioned, they sometimes reify the marginalization of homosexuals.

Literary narratives are prone to other dangers; thus Judith Williamson has suggested that HIV stories are inclined to fall back on the conventions of the Gothic and the sentimental—horror and melodrama: "Where the stress is on the *activity* of the viral monster, one might say that AIDS discourse is closest to Gothic horror, and when it is on the 'passive' (non-complaining) suffering of the 'victims' it moves over into Sentimentalism" (1989, 75). Although these might seem natural and unavoidable ways of representing AIDS, they are not. "Terror . . . and pity . . . are *not* the only emotions available to us (where is ANGER, for example?) but they *are* the ones produced through the centuries-old generic structures that dominate our popular culture, and within it, AIDS speech" (80).

The challenges and pitfalls facing AIDS narrators are many. As we shall see, not all have been up to the demands of the subject. But even failures can be instructive.

HIV/AIDS and Celebrity: Rock Hudson and Sara Davidson, *Rock Hudson: His Story* (1986); Arthur Ashe and Arnold Rampersad, *Days of Grace* (1993); Mary Fisher, *My Name Is Mary: A Memoir* (1996)

The response of most celebrities with AIDS is to deny it as long as possible, even unto death—evidence, if we needed it, of the stigmatic nature of the disease, regardless of the method of infection. Both Rock Hudson and Arthur Ashe typified this reaction in choosing to conceal their illnesses as long as possible. Once the word was out, however, both chose to produce narratives that acknowledged their condition, narratives in which the conventions of celebrity auto/biography come into conflict with the marginalizing effects of AIDS.

Neither *Rock Hudson: His Story* nor Ashe's *Days of Grace* is a simple AIDS narrative in that neither limits itself to following the course of the illness. Both books, however, were evoked in part by the public knowledge of their subjects' conditions, and both narratives represent, among other things, attempts to regain control of public images. Thus AIDS does not merely figure as the final episode in these two "lives"; in large part it accounts for their existence.[11] For better or worse these narratives acquire importance by virtue of their subjects' celebrity. In a culture seemingly obsessed with the lives of the rich and famous, the accounts of AIDS with the widest readership are likely to be those of the few celebrities who have acknowledged their illnesses.

Despite appearing in opening "credits" as coauthor with Sara Davidson, Hudson seems to have played a minimal role in the composition of *Rock Hudson: His Story*. In contrast, despite his enlistment of Arnold Rampersad, a prominent African Americanist, as a collaborator, Ashe seems to have written his book. Already the author or coauthor of several other books, and proud of his education and intellect, Ashe seems to have controlled the composition of his narrative; at least its voice and vision resemble those of the Arthur Ashe known to the public through various media over the years. (As if to quash any doubts, the book contains photos of Ashe at work.)

Although both books were in some sense collaborative in authorship, the two books belong to different genres. Focusing on his career and his ideas more than his private life or personal development, Ashe's book is more memoir than autobiography. Even considering Hollywood's liberal notions of authorship (and leaving aside the issue of the stage name of "Rock Hudson"), Hudson's book is a bit of a generic anomaly. Although he is credited with coauthorship, the book is cast as biography. Hudson's role seems to have consisted of giving some short initial interviews, then authorizing his friends to cooperate with Davidson, who functioned in effect as his authorized biographer. (Though Hudson proposed further sessions after the initial interviews, he soon realized he lacked the talent, discipline, and attention span that even such minimal involvement would require; he also was not well enough to have written the book.)

If Ashe's book authenticates itself with photos of its subject writing it, Hudson's book reproduces—following the title page—the note that gave Davidson exclusive access to sources close to Hudson: "I've always been a private person. I've never wanted to write a book, I've never let my house be photographed and I've never let the public know what I really think. Now that's changed—there's a lot I want to say and not too much time left. I want the truth to be told, because it sure as hell hasn't been told before. So I've asked those who know me best—my real friends—to work with Sara Davidson in telling my story" (3). The crucial sentence is the last, which reveals another important sense in which the book is authorized: those who were in Hudson's inner circle at the time of his final illness and death evidently controlled its content and point of view. That circle emphatically excluded—indeed, expelled—one former partner, Mark Christian, from whom Hudson was estranged. (Christian soon gained notoriety by suing Hudson and his advisers for conspiracy to harm him by not telling him Hudson had AIDS.)

Hudson's is very much a Hollywood story—mainly concerned with his movies and his mating. What makes it extraordinary as an authorized Hollywood biography is that his love life was largely homosexual; in this sense it becomes a genuine anomaly—a kind of surrogate coming out narrative. For even if his homosexuality was well known in the gay community and something of an open secret in Hollywood, Hudson had been closeted as far as the general public went. The book is *his* story not, as we have seen, in the sense that he tells it—his words are pretty much limited to short excerpts leading off each chapter—but in the sense that it is *his* version of his life rather than that of the studio's publicity department.[12] It is, then, an inside story—the story of life inside the castle that Hudson used to protect his privacy.

As much as Hudson hated the invasions of privacy that characterize celebrity life, and as much as he feared exposure of his homosexuality and illness when he still had a career to protect, once his illness outed him he seems to have wanted to compensate for having lived a lie. One irony of his assiduous, almost paranoid, protection of his privacy is that when the shroud finally fell, revealing his homosexuality, the public reaction was overwhelmingly positive. This is not to say that the shroud was not necessary but that it enabled him to acquire a popularity that would weather the retrospective—nearly posthumous—revelation of his homosexuality. The received image of his cinematic romantic life—emphatically and exclusively heterosexual—seems to have canceled out what he revealed about his actual sexual history, which was largely homosexual and far from monogamous—indeed, precisely the sort of sexual career that religious conservatives cite to demonize homosexuals. Even as the biography exposes the private life that he had protected so fiercely, it records the outpouring of support he received after the announcement of his diagnosis. Thus his friends report, "You're a hero around the world," "Ten times more popular than you ever were as a movie star"; "You've made the disease real—the world is tuned in to AIDS because of you" (291, 292).

Hudson's first acknowledgement that he had AIDS came in July 1985 (approximately a year after his diagnosis), after officials at the American Hospital in Paris, where Hudson had been taken after collapsing in a hotel lobby, announced to his entourage that "if they did not explain the actor's condition, the hospital would" (Shilts 577). Thus, like Ashe's announcement, Hudson's was designed to preempt and to some extent control the inevitable media frenzy. A brief statement, released through a Parisian publicist, acknowledged his illness but at the same time declared that he had no idea how he contracted it and that he was totally cured (Shilts 578). Despite the equivocal nature of this statement, the revelation of Hudson's illness was a watershed in AIDS history; indeed, Randy Shilts made this event the climax of *And the Band Played On*, his narrative history of the first six years of the epidemic. Virtually ignored by the mainstream media for more than half a decade, the epidemic suddenly became a major news story. (Even President Ronald Reagan, an old friend of Hudson's, could no longer ignore it.) Almost equally important, Hudson's announcement helped make AIDS a fashionable cause, at least in Hollywood, which has a large influence on public opinion; fund-raising took off. Hudson became a kind of AIDS poster-boy; his celebrity (and no doubt his image as a wholesome leading man) made AIDS safe for the mainstream media.

Though provoked by Hudson's sense that he might do some good by finally revealing his sexual orientation, the book is disappointing both as AIDS education and as gay biography. Considered as AIDS education, the narrative offers only a negative example: Hudson appears almost completely oblivious or indifferent to any risk in his behavior—to himself or others. Told by a doctor that, if he has sex, he should wear a condom, Hudson worries to a friend, "I've never worn a condom in my life. Won't I give the show away if I suddenly have to put one on?" (254) One should perhaps not expect the authorized biography of a figure whose politics were as conservative—and low profile—as Hudson's to assume a militantly gay-affirmative stance. But the narrative is notable for its singleminded focus on Hudson; it nowhere mentions colleagues, acquaintances, friends, or lovers with AIDS. It is as though he lived, contracted his illness, and died in a kind of sociopolitical vacuum—known by the gay community to be gay but deeply alienated from that community. Like many stars', his life was managed and arranged for him. In withdrawing behind his fame and money to live a self-indulgent life, he alienated himself from other possibilities. As he belatedly realized, he sometimes sacrificed promising or meaningful relationships for petty or careerist reasons. Although he managed to live a life at odds with his public image, he remained trapped by the discrepancy between the public and the private "Rock Hudson." Only in its authorization of an apparently candid and entirely unapologetic account of his sexual career could the book be construed as gay-affirmative biography. Davidson's third-person narrative fails to place Hudson's life and death in the larger perspective of gay history. The tendency of the star biography to isolate its subject from ordinary mortals here functions to disconnect Hudson's illness from the epidemic that was ravaging the gay community.

By his own account Ashe's early heart disease forced him to face his mortality. Thus the condition that led to the transfusion that infected him with HIV also prepared him to cope with a terminal illness. He was diagnosed with AIDS when doctors traced his difficulty manipulating one hand to toxoplasmosis, an opportunistic brain infection characteristic of AIDS. Because Ashe was not aware of his seropositivity until the eve of the operation that revealed the brain infection, he, like Hudson, did not have the usual warning period, and the staged narrative of "progression" was simply bypassed (or rather, undergone unaware). Exquisitely attuned to his image, his role in society, and the political implications of AIDS, Ashe was sensitive to the responsibility and the opportunity that his illness afforded him. Thus, as a responsible public figure, he lived out his life with AIDS quite openly—but only after stubbornly resisting his "outing" by the media. And in that resistance we can see his conflicted attitude about AIDS. Curiously, but revealingly, Ashe's book is far more tormented by his illness than Hudson's.

Ashe's narrative deals with AIDS at three separate points. First, in a kind of prologue he gives an inside account of what he calls his outing by the media and his strategic decision to preempt published reports of his medical condition by making his own announcement at a news conference. Then, within the chronological narrative that ensues he deals with AIDS at the moment of diagnosis and again at the moment of his public announcement of his condition. Although Ashe's handling of AIDS at each successive point is intended to minimize his illness, the very multiplication of these moments of reckoning with AIDS is finally counterproductive; AIDS pervades the narrative, threatening to crowd out or overshadow other issues more integral to Ashe's identity and values.

Ashe's account of his life after his retirement from competition is an exemplary narrative in a number of ways. One is in its explicit advocacy of the mainstream middle-class values that Ashe thinks Americans, especially African Americans, have lost sight of today—values such as monogamy, family togetherness, self-discipline, education, traditional morality, faith in God, and public service. So devoted is Ashe to these values that his autobiography reads at times like an autobiography in the tradition of Benjamin Franklin (but with more emphasis on family values). Clearly, one impulse behind the book—in view of Ashe's likely early death, of heart disease if not of AIDS—is the transmission of these values in his absence to the generation represented by his daughter, Camera. (This is most evident in the poignant epilogue addressed to her by name, but it is implicit throughout the book.) Infinitely thankful that he has not transmitted HIV to either wife or daughter and that he has the time to compose a testament, Ashe is intent on passing these values along without interference. The crux of his predicament as an exemplary autobiographer is that his having AIDS threatens to taint his moral character or at least his public image. Thus he feels compelled to establish that he contracted the virus through no violation of those values. His repeated insistence on his innocence compromises the book's message and mission.

Having an illness may not entail any obligation to avow solidarity—political or otherwise—with others who have the same illness. But Ashe's social conscience leads him to speak not only as a moralist but as an AIDS educator, and it is unfortunate that he repeatedly distances himself from other infected individuals. His low-grade homophobia works against his good intentions. His insistence on his exemplary life tends not only to isolate him from him many other people with AIDS but to subtly reinforce their stigmatization.

Ashe's reference to his being forced to reveal his illness as an outing—a term he obviously picks up from the media—is a case in point. It is more than a little ironic that he employs a term used of people whose homosexuality is exposed against their will, because *his* point is that, although he has AIDS, he is not gay. He wishes to extend the term's usage to the exposure of any private fact an individual wishes to keep secret. But his claim that his interest in avoiding publicity over AIDS had to do only with protecting his and his family's privacy is not completely convincing because of the precedent of his heart disease. Granted, media interest in his heart condition was far less intense than in his AIDS, but he had not insisted on his right to privacy with that life-threatening condition. In the case of AIDS both the media frenzy and his resentment of it had to do not so much with his physical health as with his image—which is to say with the possibility that his identity would be "spoiled" by AIDS. Once he made his announcement, however, most people seemed to accept his account. Unfortunately, the thrust of his announcement was to deny that the stigma of AIDS applied to him—to put distance between himself and others with AIDS, at least homosexuals—rather than to question the basis of the stigma.

Similarly, much of the energy of the narrative as a whole goes into establishing an image of Ashe that is incompatible with stereotypes of people with AIDS. The autobiographical implications of AIDS are different for someone who contracted the virus through transfusion than for someone who contracted it sexually. Sexually contracted HIV infection is bound to raise painful questions about one's intimate relations, even one's identity. Thus for a man infected through homosexual contact AIDS may activate latent conflicts about his way of living and loving. In contrast, for someone infected by transfusion the illness has nothing to do with "who" he is or his sexual history; the meaning of AIDS is in theory neutral. But the cultural construction of AIDS is such that it is difficult to treat the subject as open to idiosyncratic interpretation; like race, it comes with a preexisting script that the author must erase before he can write another.[13]

Although Ashe's illness need not provoke any soul searching about his past, he evidently feels the need to establish the lack of connection between his illness and his identity. Without flaunting his heterosexuality through sexual boasting he makes a point of his freedom from any taint. Thus, when the narrative reaches the moment of diagnosis, he answers once again the question of how he became infected with HIV— although his narrative has described no risky behavior. Like a defense lawyer, he takes up all the possible scenarios and dismisses all but one—his choice of a blood transfusion to hasten his recovery from an operation. (The subtext throughout is Ashe's association of AIDS with gay sex and apparent insecurity about his sexual orientation. These undercurrents help to explain his rather naive and homophobic account of the relation between tennis and homosexuality, male and female, and his reference to the suspicion among some family members, before his marriage, that he might be gay.) He seems concerned mainly to keep distance between himself and the stigma of AIDS and its association with homosexuality (229). So AIDS precipitates from him not a confession but an apologia, a declaration of his innocence.

For the most part, following Sontag on illness and metaphor, he strives to be matter-of-fact about AIDS, but late in the narrative he departs significantly from this approach: "AIDS is not a metaphor for me, but a fact; and yet I find it hard to avoid its metaphoric energy, which is almost irresistible. I reject the notion that it is God's retribution for the sins of homosexuals and drug abusers, as some people argue, but on occasion I find its elements and properties peculiarly appropriate to our age" (220). He goes on to speculate about a connection between AIDS and disturbing contemporary social trends, such as rising crime rates, the weakening of the nuclear family, and so on. His tone and implications are apocalyptic: "AIDS then takes on a specially ominous cast, as if in its savagery and mystery it mirrors our fate." He then draws back, however: "Surely we need to resist surrendering to such a fatalistic analogy. . . . I know that I must govern that part of my imagination that endows AIDS with properties it does not intrinsically possess" (221). But the damage has been done; Ashe has suggested a linkage between

AIDS and cultural decline. Of course, his case, as he construes it, belies his metaphor—except insofar as he is an innocent victim in a process of cultural decay and decadence. This passage in which he advances and then retracts an apocalyptic reading of AIDS suggests its undeniable power as a "tropical" disease; it reflects the way in which AIDS can distort thinking—a kind of cultural, rather than clinical, AIDS dementia.

Mary Fisher differs from Hudson and Ashe in that she was not a celebrity before she was infected with HIV; rather, she became a celebrity as a result of her infection. Nevertheless, like theirs, her example suggests that privilege and celebrity can substantially moderate the stigma of HIV/AIDS. Like the narratives of Hudson and Ashe, *My Name Is Mary* is a full-life narrative rather than a narrative focused on illness. Indeed, it is multidimensional in content and form—part confessional narrative of recovery with roots in her treatment for alcohol abuse at the Betty Ford Center; part memoir of her careers as an advanceperson for President Ford and later as AIDS spokesperson. (Ironically, she acquired her infection in the course of her postaddiction quest for normality in sobriety, marriage, and children; she attributes her infection to intercourse with her husband, Brian Campbell, with whom she conceived two children.) Tellingly, she synopsizes her life as a series of crises, the last and most serious of which is her seropositivity: "If your father abandons you, your mother might get you another one; you adjust, you cope, you rebound. If people discriminate against you [because you are Jewish], you may fight back. If you're an alcoholic, you might try to recover. If you're lonely, you could reach out to others. If you're childless, you could adopt. If you have AIDS, you die" (183). Like Hudson and Ashe, Fisher responded to the identity crisis of seropositivity by exposing her status and thereby increasing the visibility of the epidemic; like Ashe (and not Hudson), Fisher made a mission of representing people with HIV. Ultimately, then, the fact of her seropositivity provokes, justifies, and dominates the book.

One theme of her autobiography is her search for identity, self-respect, and purpose in successive arenas—work, marriage and children, art. Ironically, having a career was at first complicated by her privileged background; Fisher found she was being rebuffed because she "didn't need to work." In her infection, however, she acquired a distinction that finally removed her from the shadow of her wealthy and influential father. Although it threatened at first to spoil her identity, her HIV positivity focused her life after her second marriage had dissolved. In the prospect of invalidity, then, she found validation.

Given her contacts, she was uniquely positioned to become what she describes as "the Republican AIDS poster girl" (253). Her opportunity to speak of her seropositivity at the Republican National Convention in 1992 gave her national exposure and instant fame. The gist of her message, and its distinctive appeal, is that anyone can get AIDS and that it doesn't matter how; she is thus at pains to emphasize her ordinariness:

What had made my speech in Houston effective, what had (finally) disturbed the souls of a few Americans, wasn't that I was a hero but that I was common. And that's it exactly. I was "one of us" instead of "one of them," and I have AIDS.[14] What made me shocking wasn't my distinctiveness, but my ordinariness. I didn't look like America's caricature of AIDS. I am a regular person, a mom; I could be your sister. And that's the point. (257–58)

(Hence her title, which echoes the formula introducing the confessions of Alcoholics Anonymous.)

It took courage for Fisher to acknowledge her HIV status, even more to undertake to be an AIDS spokesperson within the Republican Party, where AIDS was a notoriously unpopular issue. At the same time, however, she finds herself caught in a contradictory position. To her credit she does less to distance herself from, and more to challenge, the stigma of AIDS than Arthur Ashe. But like him she was lionized for reasons that are inconsistent with her message. It is precisely because she does not fit the profile of the typical seropositive person that she is so easy to embrace. One senses in the anger of many of her powerful supporters a hostility not to the virus but to those who have spread it through American society: if it can reach people like Fisher, whom they like and respect, it has got to be stopped. Anger at her fate in no way guarantees concern for other more typical people with AIDS.

Although she wants to guard against garnering sympathy generated by her "innocence" and her privileged background, she inevitably has to exploit such sympathy. Thus she makes speeches with titles like "Make Me No Hero" and accepts awards for heroism that she acknowledges she does not deserve. What her career as an AIDS spokesperson, of which her autobiography is an extension, demonstrates is not that she is a hypocrite but that her role involves cultural contradictions she is powerless to overcome.

Her treatment of her husband suggests what she is up against. Her attitude toward him is protective; remarkably, she expresses no anger toward him and is supportive of him despite the dissolution of their marriage. Her deflection of reporters' questions about how he was infected with HIV—on the ground that the means of infection is irrelevant—is not, however, enough to guard against her being represented as his innocent victim. Her acknowledgment in the book that he was probably infected through intravenous drug use and of rumors that he was bisexual threatens to reinscribe the distinctions she wishes to erase between the "innocent" and the "guilty." For many readers what she reveals about her husband will suggest the need for even greater vigilance against those who threaten to infect the "general population" with a deadly virus. Her assertion that it doesn't matter how you get AIDS is morally sound, but it doesn't follow from her other major point, that anyone can get AIDS. Thus her book does not directly challenge the sources of AIDS stigma.

Although Fisher remains healthy, Campbell weakens and dies. The course of his illness is a minor thread in the overall narrative, but the inclusion of photos of him among the many that illustrate the book tend to marginalize him; among her family and a large number of celebrities (including Gerald and Betty Ford, George and Barbara Bush, and Henry Kissinger), he alone wastes visibly away. Despite her generosity toward him, and in part because of her wish to protect his privacy, he becomes a kind of shadowy background character.

Even as it capitalizes on her anomalous celebrity, her book attempts to reclaim her life and its meaning. That she is not more successful at destigmatizing AIDS is not Fisher's fault; she cannot altogether escape benefiting from the prejudices that she seeks to erase. She makes the admirable gestures of acknowledging her seropositivity and affirming solidarity with other people with AIDS, but her book cannot entirely resolve the contradictions of her position as "the socialite with AIDS."

Celebrities with HIV/AIDS may try to be exemplary, like Ashe and Fisher, but they are clearly not typical. For one thing, their medical treatment is generally good—as a result of which they tend to live longer. More important, as we have seen, they often qualify for a sort of outpouring of public sympathy denied most people with AIDS. (The surprise is that Hudson benefited from this as well as Ashe and Fisher.) In contradistinction to the moral many like to draw from tabloid stories of celebrities' misfortune—that the rich and famous are no different from us (just better off and better known)—these stories of celebrities with AIDS suggest that celebrities do not in fact suffer the same disease as ordinary people; popularity can provide a kind of immunity against stigma, if not HIV itself. Thus, whereas Ashe expressed great gratitude for the lack of prejudice or revulsion he faced, the sympathy extended to Hudson, Ashe, and Fisher exposes the monstrous public hypocrisy on AIDS. All received more attention and acclaim with HIV and in part because of it than they would have without it. (Indeed, the nature of the public response to Ashe's illness reveals how unnecessary and unseemly it was for him to devote so much textual space to distancing himself from stigma.) The written lives of these celebrities reveal much about the conflicted and complex construction of AIDS in contemporary America.

Setting the Record Straight: Conversion Narratives

Narratives of illness and disability rarely focus exclusively on bodily ailment or dysfunction; rather, they are usually also about other things in addition to, or in place of, those ailments. Illness and disability offer, but do not dictate, subjects for personal narrative; rather, they function as occasions for what may be wide-ranging discourse, a platform for treating other topics. The more tropical the illness, however, the more that prescribed agendas may intrude. This is perhaps nowhere as clear as in the case of AIDS, which, though it is by no means confined to gay men, remains associated in the minds of many with male homosexuality. Given one interpretation of AIDS—as God's judgment on male homosexuals—it should not be a surprise, perhaps, that AIDS has been the occasion for Christian conversion narratives, two of which I will discuss here: *Love Broke Through: A Husband, Father, and Minister Tells His Own Story* (1990), by Thomas B. Stribling with Verne Becker, and *How Will I Tell My Mother?* (1990), by Jerry Arterburn with his brother Steve Arterburn.

The similarities between these two stories are many. Both authors grew up in conservative Christian families in rural middle American settings; as young boys both experienced religious stirrings as well as homosexual urges; both did well in school and went on to college and/or graduate school; both felt the call of the pulpit; both dated women exclusively before turning to homosexual relationships for sexual gratification; both present themselves as never having been fully comfortable in the homosexual community; after, and in part because of, diagnosis with AIDS both contemplated or attempted suicide; both experienced conversion when illness and/or other crisis left them in despair; both were welcomed back into their families and their churches; both try to use their experience to benefit others by ministering, formally or informally, to others with AIDS. Underlying these multiple parallels is that both books are modeled on the biblical parable of the Prodigal Son (Stribling 34).[15]

In addition to similarities of content—incident and idea—are similarities in form. Both books are collaborative in authorship; both include supplemental texts that add testimony or endorsements by others. (One purpose served here is to authenticate the conversions narrated and to attest to the sinners' acceptance back into the fold.) Both rely for narrative structure on flashbacks; both begin with some crisis precipitated by illness in the near past and then alternate between the course of events that brought them to that nadir and the course of events leading from conversion. The moment of conversion occurs near the middle of the narrative, followed by the reaffiliation of the individual with the family and church and his flowering as a Christian and minister.

Because of their conservative Christian point of view it may be tempting to dismiss these narratives as homophobic propaganda in the culture wars. But it is only fair to note that both narratives explicitly reject the ultraconservative position that AIDS is God's judgment on homosexuals; by way of undermining that idea, both point out that the disease also kills "innocent" people—nonhomosexuals, including children and hemophiliacs. Indeed, both narratives argue that the hostility of the Christian right to homosexuals is counterproductive and, in effect, un-Christian. To the extent that the books have any credibility with conservative Christian readers they might actually have a moderating influence.

However, both narratives are quite saturated with negative stereotypes about homosexuals, and both explicitly condemn homosexual acts. Although they acknowledge that AIDS is far too clumsy and scattershot to be God's method of punishing homosexuals, they leave no doubt that AIDS among homosexuals is to be regarded as the symptom of a "sick" and depraved lifestyle. For example, an appendix to Arterburn's narrative, addressed "To the Person with AIDS," contains this passage, whose content suggests that its *actual* intended audience is (Christian) gay males, with or without AIDS: "God has set up such a perfect, natural world into existence that once any portion of that natural world is violated, whether by adultery or abortion or homosexuality or any other sin, there is going to be a price paid. . . . The wages of *sin* is death. God hasn't caused this to happen to me or to you. Sin has caused it" (154). So although these books assume a position that is less bigoted than that of some fundamentalists, they are clearly not tolerant of homosexuality. Thus, although Stribling insists that homosexuality is no worse in God's eyes than any other form of sexual sin—that is, any sexual acts outside the context of a loving marriage—he cannot imagine legalizing, let alone sanctifying, gay marriage as a way of eliminating the sin. Apparently, homosexuality has an intrinsic element of perversion that somehow makes it more repellent in God's eyes than heterosexual sexual transgression. The real illness that these books are concerned with, then, is not AIDS but homosexuality; AIDS may be incurable, but homosexuality, according to these books, can be conquered through God's grace.

Narrators of conversion are often wary of dwelling on their sins for fear of titillating readers and thus gratifying, rather than disciplining, their salacious impulses; Stribling and Arterburn are extreme instances of this tendency. Their discomfort with their homosexual pasts is such that they refrain from *any* explicit description of gay sex. For the most part they do not acknowledge finding any legitimate gratification in gay relationships. Almost inadvertently, however, in a chapter called "The Lie of the Double Life," Arterburn, trying to explain the appeal of

the "homosexual world," conveys his sense of welcome and acceptance, of a refreshing lack of aloofness or gamesmanship, in the gay
world (101). This is the only moment in either narrative that hints at
any nostalgia for the forbidden world. For the most part both portray
their gay "lifestyles" as urban, upscale, self-indulgent, and decadent—
lustful rather than loving, promiscuous rather than monogamous.

They generalize, moralize, and "depoliticize" male homosexuality—
seeing it as a matter not of "rights" but of "wrongs." Curiously, neither
man acknowledges having any clear sense of AIDS as a threat or danger
before being infected with HIV or diagnosed with AIDS; not surprisingly, neither displays any interest in AIDS as a crisis for the gay community. Both are emphatically "spiritual" autobiographies; they pay little attention to clinical details of illness or treatment methods. Religious
crises tend to displace opportunistic infections as threats to equilibrium.

Terminal illness has the power to provoke self-examination in anyone
and thus conversion in some; it may be as powerful a disincentive to
atheism as combat. But with Stribling and Arterburn it is clearly not the
terminality of their illness but its stigmatic nature—its being rooted in
what their religious training taught them was sinful behavior—that is
crucial. Had Stribling and Arterburn had some other terminal illness,
they would have been far less likely, in my estimation, to have undergone conversion, much less to have written conversion narratives. For
whereas premonition of impending death might raise concern about the
state of their souls, other illnesses would not have raised the issue of the
conformity of their lives to "scriptural mandates." Because of their upbringing, however, their diagnoses evidently brought to a crisis the conflict between flesh and spirit; the resolution was that, however alluring,
gay sex was obviously not worth its price. Although both men seem to
have been, somewhat awkwardly, out to their families already, their illnesses, by outing them more fully, shamed them into conversion *from*
homosexuality. That is to say, their physical illnesses paradoxically
"cured" them of their *real* (spiritual) illness. Redemption—in the eyes
of God and their families—required not only renunciation but denun-
ciation of their sinful sexual habits.

Both claim that conversion eases or erases homosexual desire, because
it substitutes the real thing—spiritual, selfless, and lasting love of an
immortal male (God)—for its perverse imitation—lustful, selfish, and
transient passion for a mortal male. As Prodigal Sons both measure their
spiritual status by their acceptance by their nuclear families. Thus both
emphasize the role of their families in encouraging their conversion
and offering support afterward. But neither claims to have been converted *to* heterosexuality. Instead, they pass from physical to spiritual
intercourse with other men. Although Stribling never explicitly re-

nounces his three close gay friends (none of them a sexual partner), those friendships gradually give way to new friendships with "masculine" (in other words, heterosexual) Christians. (Stribling dedicated his book to "the men of the New York Fellowship who, through Christ, gave me back my masculinity" [5].) Similarly, Arterburn, at least posthumously through his narrative, establishes fraternal relationships with others like himself. The evidence of this is the appendix, "A Word from Jerry's Brother Steve," which cites letters in which other gay men, conflicted over their homosexuality, responded to the 1988 edition. One letter, for example, denies the distinction between author and reader: "There are so many similarities between your life and mine. While reading the book, I often wondered if perhaps I had not written what I was reading; or I wondered how anyone could know the things that I have felt and thought for so long" (196).

The conflation of homosexuality with sin and spiritual death is quite clear and consistent; conversion offers the narrators redemption from a state of sin to eternal life and, not incidentally, restoration to their supportive, though homophobic, families. Their plots are not merely comic, then, but triumphal. Illness and impending death fade away before the reality of salvation and the prospect of sanctification. Indeed, one narrative includes an element unique in my experience of life writing. A third-person postscript carries the narrative beyond the moment of death, reporting quite matter-of-factly that the author stands before God: "On September 6, 1989, with Peggy and his parents at his side, Tom took the last breath of Cedar Rapids air his diseased body could hold. A moment later, he stood in the presence of his heavenly Father, alive and whole" (Stribling 198). These narratives, then, stand at one end of a continuum of illness writing, the pole at which the physical is entirely subordinated to the spiritual.

Stribling's book is slightly more liberal on homosexuality, and he bravely calls for the church to minister to people with AIDS (whom he assumes are gay men)—rather than to condemn them or to seek only to convert them. Arterburn too calls for churches to be as welcoming as his was—not to alienate but to win back unhappy or conflicted homosexuals. Part 2 of Arterburn's book, following the narrative of his life, consists of appendixes addressing the "problem" of homosexuality. Although it urges parents to reject the behavior, not the person, its objective is to describe what parents can do to discourage or prevent their boys from growing up gay—such as discouraging effeminacy and providing male role models. (The emphasis on effeminacy reveals the stereotypes underlying their theorizing about homosexuality, for neither author characterizes himself as effeminate; on the contrary, both were seemingly quite "all-American" and dated women as well as men.) Where many illness narratives contain resources for those afflicted with the condition on which they focus, it is significant that most of Arterburn's material has to do with homosexuality rather than AIDS. The rationale is that prevention of homosexuality will prevent AIDS, but the implication is that preventing homosexuality is desirable as an end in itself.

The most interesting aspect of these books as discourse about homosexuality is their twofold theory of homosexuality. On one level is the theological interpretation; homosexuality is clearly the work of the devil, if not a matter of demonic possession, and as both narrators somewhat self-aggrandizingly suggest, the devil works hardest to seduce those with the most potential as God's servants. (Such a spiritual economy enables sinful pasts to be "converted" into glorious futures.) On a more mundane level, however, homosexuality is a function of bad upbringing and the physical or sexual abuse of children (in this case, boys). Young men fall into the trap of homosexuality because their families, teachers, and churches have failed them. In particular, young men seek sex with other men to fill a void left by an absent, distant, or feared father. In Stribling's case his father is literally absent because his spiritual awakening causes him to go off to study for the ministry; this makes young Stribling easy prey for sexual aggressors who offer physical intimacy. In Arterburn's case one source of his yearning for male love is a family history of fathers' physical abuse of their sons. So these narratives are not uncritical of patriarchy. Both narrators suggest that all was not right in their families—that fathers should be more than sires, disciplinarians, and breadwinners; they should be available and emotionally supportive to their sons. Yet both families are forgiven, as well as forgiving, and it is particularly significant that Arterburn's narrative is not only narrated with the help of one brother but framed by his mother's foreword and his father's postscript.[16] The nuclear family is reconstituted in the narrative's form as well as its plot, the other members' testimony flanking that of their dying member. This editorial apparatus authenticates the reaffiliation of the son with his nuclear family, his recommitment to family values.

Stribling goes so far as to suggest that both his homosexual urges and a kind of childhood conversion experience were rooted in his desire for his father's affection: *"Maybe if I accept Christ and become a minister, I'll be more like my father and he'll pay more attention to me"* (39). Such a yoking of his yearning for sex and for Christ risks reducing his later conversion to a final bid for his father's affection; it plays into the hands of those who would see religion as a projection of unresolved or unrequited infantile desires. But in context it is part of the rebuttal to the idea that homosexual desire is inborn, "natural," and therefore not wrong. Homosexuality is the result not of innate proclivity but of preventable institutional and personal failings. The "contribution" of the church to their homosexuality is not the intolerance of its teachings but the failure of its members to live up to them; Arterburn, at least, cites his molestation by an older boy at church camp and later by a male choir member.

Like most conversion narratives these books have a strong exemplary and even hortatory impulse; that is, they aspire not merely to narrate individual conversions, nor even to affect the conduct and attitude of their readers toward homosexuals or those with AIDS, but also to inspire further conversions. (Stribling in fact narrates having done so [177].) This means not only bringing sinners to Christ but bringing homosexuals to Christ, which is to say, getting them to renounce their sinful bodily urges and commit their souls to God. (It means, for most, celibacy.) Wittingly or not, Arterburn's appendix on "The Hope of Forgiveness" gives a Christian twist to the idea of coming out: "There is no need to spend your life trying to compensate for a past that went awry. God wants you to come out of the past. He is counting on your coming out of the past to help others discover the reality of His forgiveness" (170). One must come out of the closet in order to come out of sin; confession of homosexuality is a necessary part of salvation from it.

The many close parallels between the two narratives and their mutual derivation from the parable of the Prodigal Son reveal their profound conservatism. Far from demystifying AIDS, they demonize it by ascribing it to a willfully sinful way of life. They are conservative not just in terms of their contemporary cultural politics but also in the sense that they treat AIDS as an ancient script that is divinely, rather than biologically, determined. The narrative of a late twentieth-century epidemic is simply a new version of an old story. Rather than calling for new forms of autobiographical narrative, then, this new illness requires only the grace to see its underlying truth; once AIDS and homosexuality are rightly seen, autopathography virtually writes itself, following an eternal and literally canonical paradigm. The fact that these are two of the very few autobiographical accounts of AIDS suggests the appeal of the conversion paradigm, which supplies a comic plot where none would seem to be available. The more daunting the disease scenario, perhaps, the more a potential autobiographer requires a secure refuge from which to narrate his or her illness. As we shall see, however, the conversion paradigm need not be based in traditional Christian theology.

New Age Spiritual Autobiography: George R. Melton with Wil Garcia, *Beyond AIDS: A Journey into Healing* (1988)

From a skeptical perspective Christian conversion narratives by gay men with AIDS represent a failure of nerve or, to put it somewhat more positively, a sort of Pascal's wager (the proposition that it is reasonable to bet on the existence of God, given the disparity between the great benefit of being right and the negligible cost of being wrong). Infected with HIV, afflicted by guilt and the stigma of homosexuality, these men surrender their (now spoiled) sexual identities, renouncing their pasts in exchange for psychic relief and eternal salvation. They resign themselves to the death of the body in return for the eternal life of the spirit. A less radical conversion informs what we might call the New Age spiritual autobiography of AIDS, an example of which is *Beyond AIDS: A Journey into Healing*, by George R. Melton with his partner, Wil Garcia. The title reflects the theme of the book, which is that the individual can move beyond illness into healing by adopting the right frame of mind toward his ailment—and, in the case of AIDS, toward his sexual orientation. In this Arminian conversion scheme there is no need for conviction of sin nor radical infusion of grace. As Melton puts it, rephrasing Edgar Cayce, "It was only . . . in my own mind, that forgiveness needed to occur. Salvation was as simple as forgiving oneself!" (30)

In addition to Cayce, the authors base their views on the teachings of Carl Simonton and especially Louise Hay, who is well known (or notorious) for urging people in seminars and books to "heal their lives" and thus to "allow" their bodies to recover from AIDS. In this view, once one accepts responsibility for one's illness—understands that one has somehow "chosen" it—one can relinquish it. Once the mind gets out of the body's way, the body can recover from even the direst infection (*Beyond AIDS* 33). In Melton's case this involves reconceptualizing

AIDS as a message from my body. It was trying to tell me that I was dying from the distorted ideas about myself I held in my mind. AIDS was my body's attempt to bring my understanding into a greater alignment with life.

I was not dying of AIDS! Instead, by my limited attitudes and understanding about life I had been unconsciously committing suicide all along. AIDS was only making me aware of what I was doing. . . . A seemingly impossible shift was becoming the greatest teacher about life I had ever encountered. (54)

Wisely, or perhaps shrewdly, the book stops short of claiming outright that AIDS can be cured or even survived; rather, the frontispiece asserts that it doesn't matter whether "this journey culminates in a physical healing of the body or a healing into death." (This will be news indeed to many people with AIDS.)

Like many illness narratives espousing an explicit philosophy of illness, this one comes complete with endorsements by "experts" or sages; one is spiritual, the other medical, but they agree that the mind is the key to healing. The preface by Louise Hay lauds Melton and Garcia as among those "who are indeed healing themselves from the dis-ease called AIDS" (i). The foreword, by Laurence Badgley, a Santa Monica physician and author of *Healing AIDS Naturally* and *Choose to Live*, declares that "the true cause of AIDS is not the relatively weak HIV virus but comprehensive immune system weakness occurring as the result of a modern lifestyle which included prescription and illicit drugs, poor nutrition, promiscuity, negative attitudes, and an impoverished spiritual nature. With a shift in attitude, proper nutrition, and focused spiritual concerns, a person's revitalized immune system can abolish the milieu which fosters opportunistic infections, including HIV" (ii). The foreword ends with an exhortation: "Aspiring survivors, go out and take charge of your life, and as you do so you will take charge of your immune system. . . . Generate a new reality. Avoid those who would disempower you in your search for healing. . . . Always remember that your Self is the only One who can make it happen" (iii). However inspirational it may be to some, such an approach to AIDS (and other illnesses) defines those who continue to suffer from disease as morally and spiritually deficient—deviant, irresponsible, lazy.

Even for a spiritual autobiography, this book operates on a high plane of abstraction; in form as well as content it consistently privileges mind over matter. The narrative is not concerned with physical symptoms, opportunistic infections, and blood counts; rather, it focuses on a spiritual quest for peace that will bring healing. The book is divided into two parts—the former largely narrative, the latter purely expository—but even the first part is mostly about ideas, the search for an understanding of AIDS that will salvage self-esteem *and* promote healing (which turn out to be the same thing). The narrative is highly intertextual in the sense that the central activity is reading; it's about the books and ideas that make a difference. The narrative, then, consists of far more summary than scene. Indeed, one of the few realized "scenes" is the attendance of the coauthors at a Louise Hay workshop on Fire Island that confirms much of what they have been reading (56–57). The effect is to distance the reader from the circumstances of their lives—their jobs, friends, relationships.

At one point Melton reports that writing down his early life was of great importance to him: "By acting on the intuitive hunch to write down my life story, I had set in motion a process much larger than I could imagine at the time. Writing had unleashed memories and images of my past deeply buried in my unconscious. One by one they now came into remembrance. These memories were laying the groundwork for my own healing" (24). At another he comes to accept his responsibility for the rift between him and his father and is reconciled with him: "In that moment of forgiveness an entire chapter of my past was completely rewritten. An experience I had believed to be true for over thirty years, in an instant was transformed. In its place came the realization that in truth it had never happened as I remembered. There was no one to forgive except myself" (61).

But neither the narrative of his early life nor the "chapter" about his father appears in the book; they are means to an end rather than ends in themselves. Although he tells us that his illness precipitated a complete rewriting of his past, as well as his present and future, we have to settle for Melton's allusion to it. This gives a secondhand quality to the book; the refusal to include these therapeutic narratives undermines the book's explicit advocacy of autobiography as therapy. It suggests how a narrowly instrumental view of autobiography-as-healing may at once stimulate and restrict illness narrative.

The book's kinship to conversion narrative is evident in the narrative's climax or turning point, which is Melton's dream-vision of his healing, which he describes as an ecstatic orgasmic experience (67). From it follows a conviction of his wholeness and worth, the redemption of his body as well as his soul: "I had touched that place deep within me where the reality of my wholeness had remained forever untouched. And from that place would wholeness now manifest into my physical body, its path unblocked by any remaining obstruction" (68). Thus body is sublimated into psyche, orgasm into organic wholeness. Renouncing his regimen of smuggled drugs, Melton finds himself healing spontaneously and miraculously: "In the months that followed, the healing that had occurred instantaneously on the level of spirit, began to be made manifest throughout my physical body. Slowly, my body became aware of what my heart already knew. My blood tests reversed direction and began an ascent towards the range of normal" (69). The narrative, whose chronology begins with Melton's diagnosis with AIDS and Garcia's with ARC (AIDS-related complex—that is, symptomatic HIV infection), ends with the remission of symptoms in both—a double comic resolution.

One issue in HIV/AIDS narratives is how, and how fully, gay lives are represented. In Christian conversion narratives, as noted earlier, the depiction of gay sex and life in the gay community is largely stereotypical; they find no joy or community, only depravity and compulsion, but they gloss over even those rather than describe them in graphic detail. Melton's narrative, although it does not involve such a complete revolution in behavior and attitude, depicts even less of the "before" picture, except in the most general terms. Here the crucial transition is not to revulsion at past behavior, which then becomes too distasteful to depict; rather, it is disengagement from the body itself. Thus Melton excludes homosexual acts from the narrative not because they are sinful but because they are merely physical. The pleasures of the body prove to be too transient and trivial to narrate. Once again, illness narrative, which might foreground bodily experience, in fact retreats from it.

Christian conversion narratives concede the fatality of AIDS—and on some level they confirm that death is the price of homosexuality—but they offer eternal life in return for renunciation of past sins. The New Age paradigm offers a better deal: salvation *and* healing without renunciation of homosexuality. It is worth noting, I think, that both Melton and Garcia had quite strict religious upbringings—Melton in the Church of the Nazarene, Garcia in the Roman Catholic Church. In a sense both were ripe for the more conservative conversion scenario that we saw in Stribling and Arterburn. But in their absorption of New Age ideas about the mind/body relationship, they succeed in deflecting their guilt from homosexuality as such to a particular decadent form of it, "life in the fast lane"—drug use and anonymous sex with many partners. Even before their illnesses, and in part because of the specter of AIDS, they had begun to withdraw from the fast lane. Insofar as their illness and their reading confirm the danger and error of their former lives, their narrative echoes those of Stribling and Arterburn. Their view of homosexuality is more nuanced and subtle, but as Badgley's foreword implies, AIDS is still attributed to mental errors, bad habits, or character flaws rather than viral infection. The narrative still blames individuals for their illness and holds them accountable for their recovery. Thus the premise that illness is a personal failing is the basis of the promise of self-healing.

Still, the New Age approach demands not so much renunciation of the body and one's past as affirmation of the spirit and one's future. And a decisive shift in treatment modalities. Thus the two protagonists move from the drug underground—smuggling black-market drugs back from Mexico—to the therapeutic frontier, where they try crystals and channeling, only to move on to even more spiritual techniques. One major trend in the narrative, then, is the shift from physical to spiritual constructions of illness.

Stories such as this one must be seductive to many. The New Age view of illness seems to appeal especially to affluent individuals who are used to controlling their lives; New Age philosophy tells them that even illness is ultimately in their control. Illness represents not bad luck or infection with microbes but rather overemphasis on the body or abuse of it. These narratives are in some fashion counterdiscursive; certainly, they challenge the "scientific medical blueprint" or script for AIDS, which is that it is invariably fatal—essentially a matter of viral infection, from which all else follows. Any ray of realistic hope in the face of this epidemic is more than welcome, but the New Age approach to AIDS seems not to earn its optimism; rather, it seems a function of denial, if not delusion. Though the book's dedication functions as a kind of disclaimer, it seems somewhat disingenuous in light of the implication of the narrative that follows, which is that these two men healed themselves physically as well as spiritually—indeed, that their spiritual growth allowed or even caused their physical recovery. Their book may be downright dangerous insofar as it discourages others from treating their symptoms—the opportunistic diseases that constitute AIDS. As Mark Doty has noted, the philosophy of self-control, though seductive, may in effect inhibit growth, insofar as "the spirit's education [is] effected by what is out of our hands"; "we trivialize pain if we regard it as a preventable condition the spirit need not suffer" (157, 159).

And their counterdiscursiveness is far more forthright with regard to medical discourse than with regard to religious discourse. For although Melton emphatically rejects the idea of AIDS as God's judgment on gays, he does attribute AIDS, in effect, to a sick, if not guilty, lifestyle: "We [gays] have been afraid to look within at the cause for fear AIDS is a judgment on our sexuality. It is not. It does speak to our loveless use of the body, however. AIDS is offering us an opportunity to change" (118). My point here is not that there is no fault to find with the lifestyle they describe but rather that, although the virus is easily spread in such a culture, it is not *caused* by that culture. To say so verges on blaming the victim; although this approach shifts the blame from sexual orientation to sexual activity, from homosexuality to hypersexuality, it reinforces harmful stereotypes and will encourage others to see gay men as having collectively "chosen," and thus deserved, their illness. (And of course, if AIDS is susceptible to self-healing, there is no need to fund research for drugs or other treatments.)

The problem, as Melton sees it, is excessive carnality. AIDS is a function and a signal of overinvestment in the body. This view is clearly more generous than that of the Christian right, which demonizes homosexuality, but Melton placed the entire responsibility for overcoming this stigma on the individual—as though cultural inscriptions of homosexuality could be left intact and merely ignored. The antidote to physical narcissism amounts to a kind of spiritual narcissism.

Melton's New Age approach to AIDS leads to some questionable and dangerous conclusions, such as that unsafe sex is that which is not spiritual: "When the creative energy of orgasm passes through our bodies, it is the loving connection in the heart that transforms it into a life-enhancing experience. This is the truest meaning of safe sex" (127). (The safest sex, of course, is Melton's ecstatic orgasmic experience of redemption and healing—sex with one's soul.) Such thinking has obvious problems. And the characterization of homosexuals as *hyper*sexual does

not fit well with the larger claims about a global crisis in which gays exemplify a suicidal lifestyle: "The simple fact is this planet can no longer
support the level of destructive unconscious behavior we have been responsible for in the past. It has begun an unstoppable process necessary
to bring about planetary healing. . . . No one will escape this tide of
change. It is the coming of Christ-consciousness" (144).

Beyond AIDS, then, like so many AIDS narratives, inscribes the epidemic within an apocalyptic global scenario. Conversion narratives,
whether orthodox Christian or alternative New Age, tend to perpetuate
the mystification and moralization of illness—precisely those attitudes
that Susan Sontag incisively criticized in *Illness as Metaphor* (1978) and
Aids and Its Metaphors (1989). Illness often precipitates a look inward, a
reassessment of one's life, but conversion narratives often involve a projection of personal illness onto the world at large; the significance of illness is constructed in terms of well-known (and well-worn) plots derived
from other hegemonic scripts. Such books may offer hope to others—
primarily, those who already subscribe to the myths or metanarratives
these works inscribe—but as illness discourse they tend to be retrograde.

Family Plots: Relational AIDS Memoirs

> Sisters and Brothers: Narratives of Reaffiliation—Susan Wilt-
> shire, *Seasons of Grief and Grace: A Sister's Story of AIDS* (1994);
> Barbara Lazear Ascher, *Landscape Without Gravity: A Memoir
> of Grief* (1992)

> I had to leave my family to be gay.
>   —John Preston, *Winter's Light*, 1995, p. xvii.

For reasons suggested in the introduction to this chapter AIDS is an illness particularly resistant to autobiographical treatment. The AIDS autobiographies discussed thus far take advantage of the means of infection (Ashe), celebrity (Ashe), or of the conversion paradigm (Arterburn,
Stribling, and Melton) to negate the stigma of AIDS. On the whole, however, AIDS autobiographies are quite rare; even narratives of living with
HIV are uncommon. Significantly, although the vast majority of the
several dozen book-length AIDS narratives in print concern gay or bisexual men, they generally take the form of memoir rather than autobiography. They are written, then, not by the person with AIDS but by
someone close to him—a sibling, spouse, adult child, parent, or partner.
(These are particularly good examples of "lives" precipitated into print
by AIDS. Had these men died of almost any other cause, it is unlikely
that they would have been memorialized in writing.) However, not all
the potential narrator positions have been realized in published narra-

tives, as far as I know. I am unaware, for example, of any full-length narrative by the brother, husband, or son of someone with AIDS; the lack of such narratives is itself suggestive.[17]

One relationship that is well represented is that between a gay male with AIDS and a concerned sister. Two such narratives in particular—Susan Wiltshire's *Seasons of Grief and Grace* and Barbara Lazear Ascher's *Landscape Without Gravity*—illustrate the rewards and risks of sororal narrative. Neither book pretends to be a full biography of the ailing brother, nor does either focus exclusively on his illness; the sisters live at such distance—geographical and otherwise—from their brothers that they cannot report firsthand on the course of the illness or give a comprehensive account of their brothers' lives. One consequence of this is that their narratives tend to present a somewhat sanitized account of the illness, offering a minimum of clinical detail. If narratives of HIV/AIDS can be divided into those that universalize and those that particularize, these narratives are among the former. They focus not on the particular circumstances of illness but rather on the cost of losing a family member to AIDS; they are about grieving rather than about living intimately with the illness on a day-to-day basis. (AIDS narratives by partners or caregivers are more likely to particularize, in two senses; they are likely to include gruesome details of AIDS and to refer AIDS to the context in which HIV infection was contracted—usually, the gay community.)

In the case of AIDS memoirs, as opposed to AIDS autobiographies, the death of the subject can provide closure. But although the early death of a family member provoked the books by Wiltshire and Ascher, in neither does the brother's death alone provide narrative closure. As their titles announce, each focuses on the author's grief as a survivor; the plots are determined not so much by the course of the illness, with its tragic denouement, as by the course of grief, which is far less definitive in its conclusion.[18] Wiltshire remarks on the odd relation between grief and death in the case of terminal illness: "Six months, they say, typically constitutes the initial period of mourning. I had passed six months of intense grief [after John's announcement of his diagnosis]—*and I still had John*" (109). Ascher has a maternal metaphor for this; for her, grief is like a baby: "Grief comes to live with us as though we'd given birth to it. And, like a baby, it changes shape, size and personality, but it's ours. It's here to stay. Eventually it will come around a little less often and make less of a mess" (55). One function of both narratives, then, is to explore the dynamics of grief in the case of AIDS—when it is partly anticipatory and may be compounded by feelings of blame and guilt.

Families that generate AIDS narratives can be located on a continuum. On one side they are flanked by those families so shamed or traumatized by the presence of AIDS in their midst that they seek to deny or suppress the truth. Indeed, they may reject or abandon the person with AIDS. On the other side may be families that do not consider the death of a member with AIDS sufficiently remarkable to be narratable—as most illnesses and deaths go unpublished. The few families that generate AIDS narratives do so as a way of coping with an unexpected illness and complicated grief associated with a family member who was loved but also marginalized. In the case of the two narratives under examination here, at least, the narratives come from families in which the homosexuality of a member was an issue; the narrative is in part the resolution of that issue. (Once again AIDS is conflated with gay sexuality.)

We have seen in the Christian conversion narratives of Stribling and Arterburn a drastic form of reaffiliation with the family, based on the parable of the Prodigal Son. On the manifest level these sororal narratives—and family memoirs in general—are the polar opposite of the narratives of self-reaffiliation by Stribling and Arterburn. Here the gay member does not have to "earn" his reaffiliation with his family by undergoing conversion and renouncing what he has been; rather, the family accommodates itself to, or comes to terms with, his homosexuality. Indeed, the family takes the initiative in reconciliation, reaching out through an intermediary. (This agent may even seek to atone for the family's treatment of its gay member.) But if, like John Preston, many gay men have to leave home to be gay, the question arises as to whether and on what terms they can go home again. As healthy heterosexuals sororal narrators write from a position of relative security with regard to the epidemic. As "family narratives" these books quite literally represent the family's "terms": they tend to encode or enact family values that are sometimes at odds with those of the member being reassimilated. Sometimes, then, these narratives of reaffiliation reveal residual blind spots in the way they appropriate and recount the lives of gay men with AIDS.

In practice, individuals, not whole families, generate such narratives. As a subcategory of family narratives sororal narratives are gendered in specific and interesting ways. At first glance, the undertaking of such projects by women seems wholly conventional, reflecting the conditioning of women in patriarchy as nurturers, expressers of emotion, negotiators of family conflict. But there is more to it. In both cases the narrator is an older sister who for one reason or another feels a special bond with a younger brother who turns out to be gay, and both sisters have their own motives in volunteering as memorialists. In both instances, then, the act of memorializing is not as self-effacing, nor as compatible with patriarchy, at it might seem.

The gendering is more explicit in Wiltshire's narrative. The heart of her book is her edited diary of the twelve seasons of her brother John

Ford's illness—from diagnosis to death. In turning to the diary form she characterizes it as a female, even maternal, form; indeed, she locates her journal within a female tradition in her family[19]: "When our daughter Carrie was born, my mother shared with me the five-year diary she had kept during the years surrounding my own birth thirty-four years earlier. . . . I started keeping a journal on the day of Carrie's birth in 1976, and I keep one still" (65–66). Like her mother's diary, Wiltshire's journal of her brother's illness monitors a crucial transition in the life of a family member. In this case, however, she mothers her brother, and she marks the last, not the first, phase of his life. Like her mother, moreover, she presents the diary to its subject—on what she expects to be, and what proves to be, his last Christmas.

Wiltshire devotes her journal, and her narrative as a whole, to reconstructing her brother's role in the family hierarchy. Ignored or belittled as the baby of the family, and scorned to some extent for his homosexuality, John had become a high achiever in public life and politics. John Ford had had important posts in the Agriculture Department in the Reagan and Bush administrations before resigning to become a lobbyist for family farms. His resignation was prompted in part by disgust with Reagan administration policies and pronouncements on gay issues; he underwent a kind of political conversion, from the Republican politics traditional in his family to the Democratic politics of his sister, thus tightening their bond. Now his sister, in the role of family chronicler, rewrites family history, placing the two youngest children—her brother and, not incidentally, herself—at the core of the narrative. *Her* story is thus at odds with the official but unwritten family *his*tory. In rebellion against the family's patriarchal and Republican politics she plots with her brother to place a gay Democrat at the "head of the family"; she also underscores her mother's leadership in the family crisis. In choosing to serve in what might be seen as the conventional female role of official family mourner, then, Wiltshire also becomes a self-appointed revisionist family historian.[20]

As such, Wiltshire is commendable for her candor and grace. On the one hand, she is open about disagreements within the family and the disapproval of some members for John's "lifestyle" (which extends beyond his homosexuality to his financial extravagance); on the other, she gives the more conservative family members credit for changing. Despite its altruistic dimension, her act of public mourning is, as Wiltshire recognizes, also a gesture of (healthy) self-aggrandizement.

If their distance from the site of infection saves Wiltshire and Ascher from lapsing into the Gothic (in Williamson's terms), both also avoid the sentimental, as well—if only because they see its danger so clearly. Rather than idealizing their brothers, Wiltshire and Ascher work through their grief by reexamining and reconstructing their relationships with them and indeed the dynamics of the whole family. The central gestures of both narratives, then, are reassessment, recuperation, and rapprochement. As open-minded as both sisters are about their brothers' lives, however, both write ultimately as family members, and the act of reaffiliation often rests on heterosexist biases. There is, then, a sense in which the narratives plot against the gay brother, or at least take liberties with his life. This is perhaps most evident in the way each narrative elides the brother's relationship with his partner and with the gay community in which he chose to live. It is not coincidental, I think, that these two books concern brothers who are involved in long-term relationships. Such relationships establish a basis of connection with their married sisters. Unfortunately, in the process of reinserting their brothers into the heterosexual nuclear family, both narratives tend to uncouple them from their long-time companions.

This tendency is perhaps more marked in Wiltshire's case. Although she seems to be on good terms with her brother's partner, Doug, he remains oddly peripheral in her vision; had John been a married heterosexual, it is doubtful that his wife would have been assigned such a minor role. That hypothetical sister-in-law would have had gender and heterosexuality in common with Wiltshire; Doug has neither. Even so, his role is smaller than it probably should be. (Were gay marriage legal, one wonders what effect the legitimation of their relationship might have had on his role in the narrative.) One measure of his marginalization is that he is never given a last name. (His appearance in photographs in the text suggests that his last name is not suppressed in order to protect his identity or his family's privacy.)

More disturbing is the treatment of his death from AIDS, which is nearly simultaneous with John's: unbeknownst to John, Doug lapses into a coma before John dies, and Doug dies only a few hours after John. Wiltshire remarks on the sudden acceleration of Doug's illness—as if to catch up with his hitherto more gravely ill partner. "They lay side by side at home, where they wanted to be. It was as if they had joined hands to cross the line together" (179). According to Wiltshire, John dies "surrounded by people who loved him"; this phrase presumably includes Doug, though he is not conscious at the end. One wonders whether, and in what sense, the same could be said of *Doug*; apparently, his family—that is, his blood relatives—are not in attendance. On the one hand, the narrative acknowledges his place at John's deathbedside, as one of the loving inner circle; on the other, its utter omission of any details of *his* death, burial, or memorial thrusts him into the background. The circle is centered narrowly on John. It does not seem to occur to Wiltshire that Doug's sudden unexpected steep decline may in any way be a function of a need to compete for John's attention with the hovering Ford family, especially his sister.

As her treatment of John's political conversion suggests, Wiltshire is eager to challenge homophobia. Indeed, she sees the scholarly book she is working on at the time of her brother's illness, on the Bill of Rights, as in part a refutation of "the claims of the religious right that the United States is constitutionally 'a Christian nation'" (116). But climactic moments like the treatment of Doug's death expose the incompatibility of the narrative of sororal grief with the narrative of AIDS in a long-term homosexual relationship. The bond between the gay partners—so complete that their doctor affirms that the virtual simultaneity of their deaths is a function of their inability or unwillingness to live without one another—is more than this sororal narrative is able fully to comprehend and express. Wilshire acknowledges and even honors the relationship up to a point, but in the end Doug's death is elided. The problematic status of in-laws, who are family but not blood relations, seems to be exacerbated with gay couples; they're virtual out-laws.

One subtext of the book is the way in which homosexuality isolates individuals from their families, especially when it's secret but even when it's not; the narrator unconsciously reclaims her brother from Doug and the gay world in which he chose to live. Although she is introduced to his friends and seems comfortable with them—even remarks upon their speaking of themselves as "sisters"—she leaves them and his gay life mostly out of her account. That Ford did not tell his sister he was gay until he was thirty-four, though he had known it when he was seven, suggests that much of his life was simply inaccessible and perhaps incomprehensible even to his self-proclaimed "littermate." Despite its obviously heartfelt love and homage to her brother, this sister's narrative tends to realign his life with a unit from which he was quite independent; in addition to the tragedy of his death, then, there is the tragedy of the unacknowledged incommensurability of his way of life and that in which he was raised.

One irony is that a member of the power elite is unable to tell his story himself. His clout in the Republican administrations depended on his veiling or denying his homosexuality. When he was out of government, his illness prevented him from writing an inside account of those administrations and provoked his sister's memorial book. The result is tantalizing in its hints at a life not entirely knowable by his sister, a story that AIDS suppressed.

The issue of the timing of death raises similar issues in Ascher's narrative. The death of her brother, Bobby Lazear, occurred earlier than she expected—on a Caribbean island where he and his partner, George, were attending the wedding of George's sister. Lazear's death came while Ascher was still in the process of trying to "reconnect" with him; to this end they had planned reunions in New York (her home) and New Orleans (his). She realizes that the planning of these reunions may have been a function of denial of his impending death on both sides, an aspect of anticipatory grief (10–11). But although she suggests that the gravely ill sometimes manage to forestall death until some milestone is passed, she does not quite acknowledge that Lazear may have done that. She is troubled by his not sharing his death with her: "Now, even as I resent that he denied me this last visit, I begin to understand that perhaps bearing his own pain took all his strength and spirit, leaving none to bear the added burden of my own. Or perhaps this was his great act of kindness, to spare me the sight of my baby brother dying. Or, perhaps it was more sinister than that. It is perfectly possible that in the end he could not put his trust in my love" (90).

Later, she comes to believe that in concealing from her the imminence of his death, "He was . . . protecting himself. He feared, George now tells me, that we would rush down to take control, and he wanted to control his own destiny. He was right. Once I knew that Bobby had AIDS, I tried to control even from a distance" (124). Her soul-searching is candid, but the one possibility that Ascher does not consider is that Lazear simply had other priorities, that there were others whose feelings mattered to him more, whose presence comforted him more. Perhaps Ascher had more to gain than her brother from her attendance at his deathbed. Perhaps he found sufficient support in the gay community—an affiliation of sexual orientation and culture rather than of blood.

Her sense of significant dates is entirely oriented to her family's history rather than that of Lazear's partner, but the timing of his death may have been a function of his identification with his partner and his family. George remarked, "If I had written the perfect scenario of how Bobby should have died, it would not have been as perfect as this. He died in my arms, he wasn't in a hospital, he had had a wonderful day" (20). In a sense he and Bobby did write the scenario together. It makes no sense within the Lazear family chronicles into which the narrative seeks to reinscribe Bobby, but it does in the context of George's family history, in which the wedding was a major event.

If anything, Ascher's narrative is at first a more desperate narrative of recovery than Wiltshire's. Ascher acknowledges that from childhood Bobby seemed temperamentally a strange, somehow foreign, presence in the family, someone she at once admired and feared for his emotional flamboyance and nonconformity (14). When she learned he was gay, it simply confirmed her sense of his being somehow alien; there ensued a subtle but undeniable silence within the family on the subject, the virtual erasure of him from the collective family self-portrait: "As years passed many of my friends did not know I had a brother" (16). When she inferred that he was taking no precautions to protect himself from AIDS, she wrote him out of the family history: "He had embraced recklessness as a lifestyle. . . . When it was clear that his profligacy did not abate I turned from him, as if to say, 'Okay, if you're going to kill yourself, I'll abandon you first'" (19). Her estrangement from her brother gives Ascher's memoir of grief a greater intensity than Wiltshire's; it is charged with the guilt of rejection. The narrative, then, is in part an atonement.

Initially, she had been appalled to learn at Bobby's funeral, from someone who offered to say Kaddish, that Bobby had used his last name to pass himself off as Jewish in New Orleans—more of his flamboyant self-dramatization. But groping to express her outrage at Bobby's death at thirty-one, she finds herself thinking in terms of Nazis and the Holocaust and wonders, "What was the holocaust-as-metaphor for Bobby? The holocaust which, according to his tale, had destroyed most of his family. What was his pain beyond words?" (105–106) At this point she begins to understand his death in the context of the life he chose and to understand the way in which her account of her grief brings another, alien perspective to bear. Thus, without fully acknowledging, much less vanquishing, her homophobia, she does come, in her grief, to the point where she can let go of Bobby, cease trying to rehabilitate and reclaim him:

There were others who knew and, yes, loved Bobby better. I was important in his life, but not central. In forgiving myself, I have to accept that. There is a form of aggrandizement in remorse as though things would have been completely different if the mourner had done what had been left undone. The fact is that I might be suffering fewer regrets now if I had performed the "if onlys" then but they might have made no difference in our relationship. (117)

So although other aspects of Ascher's recovery from her brother's death provide the narrative's comic plot—the consolation found in religion, the grief work undertaken in self-help groups—the most important may be the narrative's working through of her relationship to her brother, with its grudging but ultimately selfless relinquishment of her sororal claims on her brother's body and soul.

Both sisters grieve honestly and openly for their dead gay brothers. Facing the uncertain deadline of AIDS, both attempted to repair damaged relationships while their brothers were alive. But the sisters undertake the major work after their brothers die, through the reconstructive project of memoir writing. To different degrees they manage to accommodate their brothers' homosexuality in their narratives, but their difficulty in acknowledging their brothers' partners suggests the power of the heterosexual family as a literary convention as well as a hegemonic cultural paradigm. A telling detail here is Ascher's noting with some surprise the tenacity with which George held on to the urn containing Bobby Lazear's ashes before and during the funeral (88). His behavior is not so striking, given that the remains are destined for burial on Lazear family property at a great distance from New Orleans. The nuclear family quite literally reclaims and relocates the body of its errant member.

At best these universalizing narratives may reinforce the sense in which we are all living with AIDS, despite greater prevalence to date among the well-known "risk groups." For they document the intrusion of AIDS into their insulated, if not "immune," families. Ascher remarks: "We are not alone in our anger, grief, and disbelief. The horizon fills with parents burying their young. Fewer and fewer of us are allowed the smug certainty that AIDS had nothing to do with our lives. Soon, each of us will have a child, brother, friend, friend of a friend, a distant relative who is doomed" (2). This passage may represent in microcosm the challenges of AIDS narratives by family members. Ascher's manifest meaning is that no one is finally immune to being touched by AIDS. But her language posits only male (and presumably gay) casualties; she does not so much universalize as overgeneralize from her family's instance. More tellingly, the point of view implied by the pronouns actually keeps the infection at a distance: "we" will all be bereaved but not ourselves infected and "doomed." Family narratives of losses to AIDS supply an important perspective—and often, as here—powerful testimony about the epidemic, but their point of view has obvious limitations.

> Young Wives' Tales: Carol Lynn Pearson, *Good-bye, I Love You*
> (1986); Elizabeth Cox, *Thanksgiving: An AIDS Journal* (1990)

Perhaps surprisingly, one of the narrator positions represented more than once in AIDS family memoirs is that of the wife or ex-wife of a man who is infected through homosexual contact. Obviously, this position is more complicated than that of a sister, who is not threatened in the same ways by her brother's infection. Two narratives nicely illuminate the difficulties of writing about AIDS from this perspective: Carol Lynn Pearson's *Good-bye, I Love You* and Elizabeth Cox's *Thanksgiving: An AIDS Journal*. A crucial difference between the two cases has to do with the temporal relation between the narrator's awareness of her partner's homosexual behavior and her marriage to him. Pearson knew of her husband's homosexual urges before she married him, whereas Cox was surprised and devastated to learn that her husband's mysterious illness was a result of homosexual encounters. As a result, Cox's is by far the more volatile narrative.

Like Gerald Pearson, the man she married, Carol Lynn Pearson is a Mormon. Armed with faith, they both thought that Gerald could put his homosexual inclinations behind him when they agreed to marry. (He had repented, and that should have been enough.) When it became clear to both that Gerald could not so easily suppress his homosexuality, the marriage became tenuous. They moved from Utah to the more liberal environment of California in the hope of working out their differences. Finally, however, seeing her marriage as a fraud, and unable to accept Gerald's continued infidelities, Carol Lynn Pearson insisted on a divorce. Quite capable of supporting herself and their four children, she was generous in her support of Gerald as well (financial, as his career faltered; emotional and logistical, as his health failed). When he was well, she welcomed him and his successive partners into her home; when he became too ill to live alone, she took him in and nursed him. The plot of this narrative, then, quite literally inscribes reaffiliation; indeed, it is reaffiliation that gives it its comic resolution.

As the autobiography of a Mormon wife, the book is significantly counterdiscursive in its critique of Mormon patriarchy; at one point Pearson even associates Gerald's preference for male sexual partners with Mormon sexism. (Gerald used the former Mormon practice of polygamy to rationalize his extramarital relationships with men [55].) What she doesn't reckon with, however, is the extent to which Gerald's desire to marry may have been a function of the Mormon view of homosexuality, the extent to which he may have seen marriage as a refuge from, or cure for, his sinful urges. Citing Brigham Young's adage that "A single man over the age of twenty-one is a menace to the community," she acknowledges that "Gerald felt the pressure to marry even more than I did" (11), but she doesn't fully take into account the extent to which Mormon heterosexism may have warped Gerald's sense of his worth and role in life and thus deformed his life narrative as well as hers.

Pearson vividly expresses her shame and anger upon discovering Gerald's continued homosexuality. And though ultimately her ideas and emotions dominate the narrative, she does voice Gerald's position on homosexuality. Indeed, the middle of the book stages a kind of debate on homosexuality and its implications for their marriage. The practical resolution is their leaving Utah for California, where they could address their problems under less forbidding scrutiny. The philosophical and moral resolution is equally equivocal. She comes to see Gerald not as a sinner nor as willfully hurting her and abandoning the family; rather, she sees his homosexuality as a powerful force each of them has to deal with separately. So she does reject the orthodox Mormon position for a more liberal one, but she has great difficulty accepting that Gerald's goodness and generosity are compatible with homosexuality.

Although the narrator's Mormonism is remarkable for its feminism and unorthodox in its matriarchalism, her narrative—loving as it is toward Gerald as an individual—finally represents homosexuality as a sterile, self-indulgent, and finally self-destructive choice. The narrative does "matronize" Gerald somewhat; the point of view is very much that of a woman who functions as a single mother, not only to her children but also to her ex-husband. Even when he is liberated from his marriage, Gerald's homosexual relationships, like his creative and financial projects, tend to fail after initial enthusiasm and optimism. She sees him as immature and irresponsible—not having to work steadily at relationships or jobs because so little else depends on them. Carol Lynn Pearson provides little or no sense of a gay community, much less of its mobilization against AIDS; when she takes her husband in during his final illness, the implication is that he has no other resources—either individual or collective. In this account, then, the salient fault of homosexuals is not deviant sexuality but arrested development; they are not so much decadent as juvenile and delinquent. Gay males are not men but boys, not husbands but narcissistic lovers, not providers but idealistic projectors; they are profligate in various senses of that word. ("Gerald was a spender and I was saver, both financially and emotionally" [38].)

Although the narrative is not explicitly Christian in its perspective, the underlying plot is a variant of that of the Prodigal Son, in which Pearson sees Gerald's excursion into gay culture as a colossal and deadly mistake. Even without AIDS homosexual life proves unsatisfying. With AIDS it proves to be suicidal. Here, however, the narrator welcomes the Prodigal Son back into his family without his having to renounce his homosexuality; no conversion is required. In the end, indeed, the narrative stages a remarkable ecumenical gesture. The epilogue ends with Pearson envisioning a reunion with Gerald in heaven, where they will be "sealed as friends forever" and where "Whoever is in charge of us will walk with us and will help us to sort out the mysteries and help us to complete the healing" (227). The narrative, then, is an act of forgiving as well as memorializing; one can only wish that the forgiving were not necessary. Gerald's life as a homosexual remains at best a mystery, at worst a flaw, to his ex-wife. Overall, the view of homosexuality here is less affirmative than that in either of the sororal narratives. But considering her conditioning as a Mormon and her painful history as a wife, Pearson seems to have made a significant accommodation to her husband's sexual orientation. Despite some stigmatizing of homosexuals, her narrative enacts a revision, if not an utter rejection, of the orthodoxy that crippled her husband and caused great pain to both of them. Compared to static photographs of AIDS "victims," this book does individualize a person with AIDS; it endows him with a family, a career—a life.

As the narrative of the episode that ends the life of her husband and begins her life as a single mother, Elizabeth Cox's *Thanksgiving: An AIDS Journal* (1990) is generically ambiguous in a couple of senses. First is the issue of its immediacy. Its subtitle identifies it as a journal (unlike Pearson's account, which is written from a single retrospective point of view). Cox organizes most of it in dated entries that she groups by seasons, or around holidays, over the period of less than two years from Keith Avedon's diagnosis to his death. One function of its serial composition, perhaps, is that it has more harrowing details of AIDS symptoms than most of the other narratives discussed here. The virus attacks vulnerable organs—in her husband's case, his lungs and eyes particularly; he is spared worse "symptoms"—total blindness, for example— only because Avedon and Cox finally decide to end his life. Thus, the journal, like Avedon's illness, has sudden and violent ups and downs. The journal form minimizes, although it does not eliminate, hindsight: every spiking of fever is a crisis, minor only in retrospect. Despite these attributes of frequent serial composition, however, the text is clearly a revised journal, more literary in its language than most, and the undated entries in the long first section seem to have been written from a single retrospective viewpoint.

Another generic ambiguity has to do with its fluctuation between being a biographical account of Avedon's illness and an autobiographical account of a crisis in Cox's life. It would be accurate but insufficient to say that the book records his suffering, whereas it expresses hers, for the difference between the representation of her experience and that of his goes well beyond that between subjective and objective, first- and third-person, points of view: after AIDS intrudes on their life, the journal replaces her husband as her confidant. The revelation that her trusted mate has contracted HIV through sex with other men destroys beliefs—in his fidelity, his heterosexuality, the safety of their lovemaking—that have sustained her as a wife. The disease destroys the emotional security that her marriage had afforded her and consigns her to a devastating isolation from, and with, her dying mate. To protect their young son (and themselves) they decide to confide Avedon's diagnosis only to family and a few friends. The marriage, once idyllically cozy, begins to feel claustrophobic when they are alone with their secret. She is both nostalgic for and suspicious of the cocoon in which she had lived.

The journal is at once, then, a chronicle of the marriage and an escape from it. Just as there is much that he has not told her, there is much she cannot now express to him—her anger at his betrayal of her, her fears of living on her own. And in that sense her writing is a betrayal of him, of their intimacy and sharing: "And the worst part of these days is that I can see in Keith's eyes that his worst fear is that I will start to think and feel all the things I just wrote down" (162). So although Avedon's illness determines the narrative's scope—it begins with his first mysterious crisis, which lands him in intensive care, and ends with his death—the journal's matter and manner have to do mainly with Cox's struggle to adjust to the new life-script AIDS thrusts upon her—in which she feels like Avedon's life-support system: "My job was to be Keith's lifeline— to keep talking to him, keep touching him—to pull him back to me, pull him away from death" (18).

As a deadly illness AIDS replaces one's indefinite future with a fore-shortened and harrowing prospect. (In this case, the first correct diag-nosis—after much misdiagnosis—of Keith's condition is coupled with a prognosis that fortunately proves incorrect: that he will not survive more than a few days.) In Cox's case, because of her ignorance of her husband's extramarital sex life AIDS also robs her of much of her past. Even as AIDS takes Keith Avedon's life literally, then, it takes Elizabeth Cox's metaphorically. The relationship she had thought she and Avedon enjoyed proves to be a fiction; she is simultaneously denied the future she had anticipated with him and the past she remembers. Thus, she, perhaps more than he, is cast adrift by AIDS: "The home I longed for, the life I had lived, no longer existed—and never would again" (35). When in the immediate aftermath of his diagnosis she first learns of her hus-band's "homosexual past" from his sister, Cox's first impulse is to lash out at the "craziness" of his family—to project this unfamiliar and un-palatable aspect of her partner onto his family, his blood. Yet she strug-gles to convert her anger and rejection into sympathy: "I refused to feel anything for myself. Instead I tried to turn the part of the tragedy that was mine alone—my feeling of betrayal and pain—into a new source of compassion for Keith. . . . Why hadn't he told me? It was because he was ashamed. And that was what hurt. That was the tragedy. Keith who should be so proud had had to suffer with a sense of shame" (24). She quite rigorously devotes the journal she keeps to the overwhelming de-mands of the present; at the same time, it aspires to heal the rupture in her life narrative—to allow memory to adjust to the necessary revisions of the past and to enable hope to project the thread of her life narrative forward. Her writing is a determined attempt to recreate a coherent life narrative in the face of bereavement and disorientation.

If the resolution of the plot is in one sense the death of her husband, its climax is their joint decision to end his life before the ravages of the disease made him unrecognizable. The book gives surprisingly little at-tention to the legal and moral implications of her husband's decision to end his life. It comes up rather fast; we have little access to Avedon's thinking about it, and Cox seems to accede to his decision rather readily, without much deliberation. At this point her agreement cannot be attributed to wifely acquiescence, for Cox had learned to take more and more responsibility as her husband got sicker. One significant trajectory in the narrative is Cox's transformation from Avedon's intimate partner to the giver and manager of his home care. She becomes an administrator and mother figure to her husband. Thus her agreement is partly a function of burnout. Many readers will desire a more probing discussion of euthanasia, but the episode will feel right to many others—which is to say that Cox will have succeeded in suggesting the horror with which both of them contemplated the continuation of the downward trajectory of Avedon's condition. Fundamentally, however, the decision to end Avedon's life is a matter of reasserting control over their lives. Another benefit of this decision has to do with its mutuality; if only temporarily, their interests and intentions once again coincide. They can collaborate for the last time on something of vital importance to both. With the decision taken, they can ritualize death. The decision not to fight any more also means a restoration of their privacy: no more intrusive visits from caregivers.

A delayed effect of this decision is the publication of the journal. Having helped Avedon to end his life, Cox may feel authorized to publicize the agony that he wished emphatically to keep secret. The course of his illness was complicated, in a way, by his not seeing himself as homosexual. Because he did not identify himself as gay, he did not take full advantage of the gay support network, although he did use the services of the Gay Men's Health Crisis; unlike gay friends he never integrated AIDS into his self-image (176). And although she too is at pains to deny that he is gay, an idea that is inconsistent with her sense of him, herself, and their relationship, Cox is increasingly unhappy with Avedon's insistence on privacy. After his death his life reverts to Cox's control, in a sense.

Although in a coda she justifies writing the book in terms of her son's need for a faithful narrative of his father's life and death, which he was too young to understand, it is not necessary for her to write, let alone publish, this narrative. The act of revising and publishing the journal, then, seems not primarily a form of grieving, although it does enact her mourning, much less the creation of a permanent testament for their son; rather, it seems a resumption of control over her and her son's lives—from Avedon, who, six years older, was always the dominant partner; from the public, which insists on misunderstanding and stigmatizing people with AIDS; and from AIDS itself. Cox had found therapy limited because "everything that is said in that office is about AIDS.

As if we are defined by being victims of AIDS, not people who had a life before AIDS, who want to continue living as complete human beings, who need to fit AIDS into our lives, not our lives into AIDS" (85). Her book is part of her reaction against the way in which AIDS took over their lives.

Although, obviously, the book wouldn't exist without AIDS, which threatens to dominate it, the narrative attempts to contain illness within a larger shared life. Although dedicated to her husband's memory, her book is finally the testament of a survivor—a woman made an auto/biographer by biological accident. Its composition is a significant role reversal, for it had always been Avedon, the musician, who after his bout with polio was "obsessed with creating his life" (34) and who would allude casually to the time when he would "write the book" about his life (5). In the beginning her decision to link her life with Avedon's was not a decision to form her own life so much as to reject the one she thought had been chosen, or prescripted for her, by her affluent family background. In her decision to write his illness she not only memorializes him but creates herself; like many women before her she becomes a life writer in part by serving as her husband's biographer. She discovers her voice in the silence after marital dialogue ends.

The resulting book is less his story than hers, then. While Avedon was alive, the journal served as the repository of that part of herself that the marriage could no longer contain; publishing the diary is a posthumous fracturing of the cocoon of the marriage from which she emerges as a transformed being. (She asks at one point, "Have I no identity but wife to Keith, mother to Luke, caretaker to both?" [99]) As a survivor she can tell the story Avedon had wanted suppressed; in a way, she posthumously "outs" him as a person with AIDS—and, indeed, as a person with a homosexual past. At the same time, she acknowledges and rehearses the process of living on alone, registering and negotiating the divergence in their life narratives. More important, she reconstructs the family unit with a coherent meaningful past that will underlie her future and her son's.

The dynamics of uxorial narrative, then, are distinctly different from those of sororal narrative (and, as we shall see, from those of narratives by gay survivors); surviving spouses have a good deal more at stake in their partners' illness than sisters, at least when AIDS is associated with gay sex. For both Carol Lynn Pearson and Elizabeth Cox their partners' illness represents in some way a violation of the marriage contract. And thus the illness infects their lives as well as their partners'. AIDS paradoxically both binds them to and alienates them from their straying partners. The resulting illness narratives are also auto/biographies of relationships. As is typically the case with AIDS narratives, AIDS is not represented merely as a physical illness; another topic, usually homosexuality, threatens to dominate the narrative. Indeed, the response of the narrator to her partner's homosexuality is generally the prime force in shaping the narrative—overtly or covertly.[21]

The Sins of a Father: Susan Bergman, *Anonymity: The Secret Life of an American Family* (1994)

As a memoir Susan Bergman's *Anonymity* is a conspicuously fractured, rather than linear, narrative; she tells little in chronological sequence and provides the reader with little orientation as scenes shift. Rather, the book juxtaposes shards of a family's life shattered by the discovery of the secret homosexual life, and resulting illness and death, of the head of the family, the author's father. The narrative ricochets among three time frames: the author's childhood and adolescence, her parents' courtship and early marriage, and the tragic aftermath of her father's death. *Anonymity* is thus not a narrative of illness in the usual sense; after all, Bergman was hardly in a position to witness her father's illness, which he successfully disguised or concealed from his family. (Don Heche died in 1983, relatively early in the epidemic, and in addition to the fact that the family was wholly ignorant of his homosexual life, the symptoms of AIDS were not so well known then as to give him away.) Moreover, in the years immediately after his death the family preserved his secret as much as possible.

But it is precisely for these reasons that *Anonymity* (1994) is such a revealing AIDS memoir. In its painful disclosure of a catastrophic secret illness it points to many more stories of illnesses never revealed; like the tip of an iceberg, it signals the presence of an invisible mass: those closeted AIDS cases in which the person with AIDS and his family are in deep denial. Precisely because AIDS is off to the side, being suffered in secrecy—passed off as cancer, pneumonia, and the like—this narrative may serve to represent what often shuns representation. It may epitomize the veiled AIDS death, in which the illness of some respectable family man is either misread because of its obscurity or misrepresented because of its stigma.

Like most family memoirs of AIDS, then, the book is less a straightforward narrative of illness than a narrative provoked by illness; AIDS is the nagging inconsistency that threatens to destroy the life of the all-American family and thus demands to be reckoned with so that the survivors' lives can go forward. The way ahead, the book implies, lies through the past. Instead of a narrative of bodily dysfunction, then, the book tells a story of family dysfunction resulting from the secret life that gave rise to the illness—and of the aftereffects on the family of discovering that it had lived a kind of collective lie. Much of the book concerns events in the lives of the widow and her children in the decade following the death of Don Heche; the book broods on the cost of his secrecy to his family.

By the time Heche died, leaving a widow and four children, he was somewhat estranged from his family. Suffering from mysterious illnesses, he had drifted off into a netherworld of medical treatment, recuperation with "roommates," and mounting debt. The book begins by suggesting the shock with which Heche's death ruptured the family's self-image: "It was not until my father died that we found out about his other life. Then our other lives began" (vii). Still reeling from the impact, the author gives vent to extreme anger at times: "Your father dies: you wish you didn't think, Good riddance" (16). Indeed, Susan Bergman's shock and anger at the discovery of her father's secret life are sometimes expressed as naked homophobia: "GO TO HELL, DADDY. Go to hell every single fucking jack he ever fucked or was fucked by, the zillion Grand Central Station royalty men's room flight attendant Times Square suicides. I don't mean it. I mean it, but I could never say it to your face" (18). Bergman comes by her homophobia "honestly"; she learned it at the knee of a father who raised his children in the same strict religious context that drove him deep into the closet. Thus the beliefs he grew up with and instilled in his offspring served later to indict him not only for "perversion" but also for hypocrisy.

One of Bergman's undeniable motives in writing the family's life is to out her father posthumously—to take revenge against a man who took advantage of biblical patriarchalism to hide his betrayal and selfishness:

The homosexual father prays before dinner and compares his calamity to Job's. The homosexual father sits in group therapy with his confused children and unsuspecting wife and discusses phantom trouble. The homosexual father is so frightened of his daughter's ordinary development that he finds a way to torment her for menstruating. . . . The homosexual father disapproves as his daughters flirt with older men. The homosexual father lives as though his were the only life. (17)

The danger of such a narrative, of course, is that it will become a kind of *Daddy Dearest*, burdening a defenseless parent with responsibility for all the tragedy and dysfunction that befalls his family after his death (including the bulimia of one daughter and the death of his teenaged son in a late-night single-car accident). Worse, the book may condemn not only her father but the entire gay community to which he seemed to have defected. But two things finally move the account beyond the blaming of family dysfunction entirely on the hypocrisy and homosexuality of the father. The first is that the author is eventually impelled to investigate—however tentatively and incompletely—her dead father's secret life; her motive here is no longer to condemn but to understand and share the life he so carefully hid from her. She interviews and gives voice in her narrative to various gays and lesbians who shared his secret. (His life was "double" but not symmetrical; he seems not to have had to conceal his straight life from his gay friends as carefully as he did his gay life from his family; presumably, this was part of the appeal of the gay world.) From this perspective his secret life looks less sordid and desperate, more companionable and affectionate; the daughter is able to sense part of its allure as a relief from the fundamentalist straight-jacket of his upbringing. (She is never, however, able to understand the appeal of sex for its own sake, and she portrays homosexuality as hedonistic and extravagant.)

At some point she is able to understand that the alternative to his secrecy might have been worse, that his secrecy protected the family—and especially his wife—from a revelation that might have been more damaging than the lie, one too destructive to contemplate; thus she appreciates belatedly that her father's secrecy may have served to protect his cherished family and not just him. Indeed, she comes to see that although his secrecy was a betrayal, it was not a desertion; secrecy was the price her father was willing to pay to remain connected to the family he obviously loved and needed. The lie was not only self-serving, though it was that; it was also a backhanded, but profound, compliment. It gave the entire family something all the members wanted and needed—at great cost to him.

Part of the price he paid was the support of his family in his final illness; by denying the nature and the gravity of his sickness, he deprived himself of the care he might have had, punishing himself in a kind of preemption of the judgment he felt they would be justified in exacting on him—or that he may have expected after death. Bergman comes to understand this by getting to know the woman who did take him in out of sheer compassion: "Her humble kindness toward him both consoles and convicts me. The savage deterioration of body and mind—couldn't I have seen that and put aside whatever grudge I nursed? . . . This is what I could have offered him—in her face, in the generosity of her touch, my father had been able to observe the most innocent and natural sorrow, that of bereavement" (162).

The second aspect of the narrative that moves it past revenge and talk-show accusation is the narrator's gradual turning from the sins of her father—and the depiction of the family suffering, as if from a hereditary curse—to the patterns of simulation and dissimulation in her own life, from childhood lies and exaggerations and her secret affair with one of her high school teachers to her unconfessed marital infidelity. She sees finally that she is repeating her father's dishonesty and hypocrisy—without even the excuse of homophobia to justify her secrecy—and sees that she must confide in and confess to her husband if she is to free herself finally from her father's shadow. It is not so much that, by doing so, she can regain the high ground from which to judge her father unhypocritically as that she realizes that she can never overcome her anger so long as she is guilty of the same faults—that her anger is partly a matter of displacement and projection.

She sees that her father's betrayal is extreme but not unique, that "transparency" is not easy for anyone to attain. She understands too that she is implicated in his subterfuge—that the entire family colluded in living a lie and that the time for that has passed. So the narrative turns dramatically from the rhetoric of indictment to the rhetoric of confession. In phrases that echo its beginning, with its image of lives broken in two, the narrative ends with her on the verge of confessing her infidelity to her husband: "This was the last day of my life as I knew it. . . . He could tell in the stillness of the pause between his question and my looking back up at him that his life was changing too" (198). She decides to do so despite her fear that he will leave her and take the children; evidently, he did not. (The book is dedicated to him.) The book ends, then, as it began, at a watershed—at the brink of a truly new life that this written life has brought into being. In writing the life of her family, and especially of her problematic father, she has been inspired to right her life—to move it and herself in the direction of transparency or consistency that she professes as ideal. Soul-searching results in her doing what she realizes her father must have wanted to do, unburdening himself to those betrayed. The narrative, which leads up to the narrator's confession to her husband and plea for forgiveness, finally offers clemency if not absolution, amnesty if not amnesia. In her confession to her husband she confesses *for* her father and thus forgives him.

That she does so does not mean that she condones his homosexuality; nothing in the narrative suggests that the author has changed her mind about that. But at least she has seen the hypocrisy—and un-Christian nature—of her recriminations against her father. So this book has an odd relation to AIDS discourse and illness narrative. Because of her father's passing off of his illness as other nonstigmatic ones, *Anonymity* is an AIDS narrative only obliquely, incidentally, and retrospectively. But it is a record of a life lost in some sense because of homophobia and recovered by his daughter, an example of a life precipitated into print by the intrusion of AIDS. Don Heche was outed, finally, by his disease. His daughter finalizes and formalizes the outing—but not ultimately in a vindictive manner. This family history—focusing on betrayals and dysfunction—is devoted finally to an expression of candor and transparency. Susan Bergman's concealments and deceptions teach her the insidious power of secrets: "What happens when the secret begins to keep you? You are no longer the one who fondles it, but when you sit it grasps you by the neck, when you rise it gnaws your heart raw with the dread of discovery" (190). Confession is the antidote to the poison of possession by a secret. To her surprise, one point of contact between her and her father is their secret adultery; to her credit, the point of communion between them is her confession and forgiveness.

> Parental Narratives, Maternal and Paternal: Barbara Peabody,
> *The Screaming Room: A Mother's Journal of Her Son's Struggle*
> *with AIDS* (1986); H. Wayne Schow, *Remembering Brad:*
> *On the Loss of a Son to AIDS* (1995)

In the growing literature of personal accounts of AIDS the position of a parent of a person with AIDS has been represented a number of times. Some of these, like Elizabeth Glaser's *In Search of Angels* (1991), have to do with children infected with HIV at an early age, whereas others have to do with the illnesses of grown children. Two narratives in the latter category suggest how the position of a parent may be inflected by gender; at least in the two examples under consideration, the maternal approach differs significantly from the paternal one. The mother's account, Barbara Peabody's *The Screaming Room*, focuses narrowly and intensely on her son's last months of life, his suffering, and especially her emotions as his sole caregiver; the book is powerfully and in the end somewhat claustrophobically body oriented. The father's account, Wayne Schow's *Remembering Brad*, attempts to place his son's illness in the broader context of his family, church, and culture; it is more oriented to intellectual and moral values, and it is the more reformist in tenor. The mother's book represents and enacts emotional catharsis, articulating and exorcising physical and emotional pain; the father's enacts an anguished process of moral and spiritual questioning.

As one might infer from its title, *The Screaming Room* is a harrowing memoir of AIDS, probably the most agonized and agonizing illness narrative considered here. It consists of Barbara Peabody's edited journal of the last eleven months of the life of her son, Peter Vom Lehn, who died of AIDS at twenty-nine. The narrative acquires intensity from its short chronological span, its narrow focus on his illness, and its point of view—that of a mother who devoted herself to nursing her ill son. An artist and a divorced mother of four grown children, Peabody had the resources—the time, money, and space—to take her ailing son in, and she functioned without assistance until close to the end of his life (at which point she called on a local AIDS project). Cautioned by friends and her ex-husband that she might be doing too much by herself, she insisted that she was neither obsessed nor heroic but merely a mother, a woman whose being is inextricably bound up with her children: "In these last heartbreaking days, I have come to realize what it really means to be a mother, to fight for your child. Peter, all my children, are part of me—my body, my soul, my life. All else is nothing" (27). The ethos and the pathos of the narrative, then, are those of an embattled mother fiercely protective of her threatened son.

Like most illness narratives, this one represents a best-case scenario in that the family of the ill person has adequate money and insurance and is collectively supportive. *The Screaming Room* (1986) is nevertheless a distressing narrative for a number of reasons. For one thing, it is a pure illness narrative in the sense that it focuses quite exclusively on the course of the illness from the diagnosis of PCP (and thus AIDS) to Vom Lehn's death within a year. Although the first chapter provides some background on the family history, Peabody makes no attempt to provide a comprehensive pre-illness biography of Peter Vom Lehn. Moreover, during the period narrated no other plot emerges from, or is grafted onto, the illness story. Such a singular and unrelieved focus on illness is in fact rare in illness narratives. Indeed, it is a good, if rare, example of a published illness narrative that does not aspire to be a biography.

Another reason the book is upsetting is that it documents in graphic detail the many symptomatic illnesses that afflicted Peter Vom Lehn: wasting syndrome, rectal lesions, herpes sores, deterioration and eventual loss of sight in both eyes, terrifying seizures, dizziness, dementia (with attendant hallucinations and occasional paranoia), as well as relentless, humiliating, and debilitating diarrhea and incontinence. As sole caregiver Barbara Peabody did not distance herself from her son's bodily ailments and his pain; as author she does not spare the reader the gruesome details of his illness. Thus, of all the narratives discussed here, it is one of the most "bodily"—one of the most attentive to physical suffering. Whatever its other virtues as an account of illness, this frank narrative is a salutary reminder of how sanitized most illness narratives are, how they minimize suffering and pain, how they insulate readers from contact with bodily fluids. (On the issue of incontinence Mark Doty has noted how "shit . . . interrupts every other interaction. . . . Like death, excrement is the body's undeniable assertion: *you will deal with me before all else, you will have no other priorities before me*" [233]. Nevertheless, his, Peabody's, and Paul Monette's memoirs are among the few illness narratives that do forthrightly acknowledge this aspect of AIDS.)

The Screaming Room is also quite unsparing in its account of the emotional toll that AIDS takes. With the advantages of his race, class, and geographic location (southern California), Vom Lehn got outstanding medical care; indeed, his mother gratefully acknowledges doctors and nurses by name. Nevertheless, her narrative vividly conveys the tedium of chronic illness: the countless trips to the hospital, interminable waiting for tests and their (often inconclusive) results, frequent and inexcusable delays in the administration of new treatments, frustrations of coping with impersonal medical bureaucracy and confusing paperwork, the staggering number of medications. Beyond that the book also suggests the underlying terror of dealing with AIDS—the frequent, often life-threatening crises; the sense of scrambling to respond to an illness that is not well understood, treating its symptoms with drugs whose side-effects are unpredictable; and the prevailing sense of futility.

As noted earlier, journals and diaries are particularly well suited for representing the dailiness of chronic illness because of their serial composition, which makes for immediacy, and their relative lack of hindsight, which makes for uncertainty. The convention of grouping entries into chapters when editing a journal for publication, however, works against the journal's structure, for the creation of larger units inevitably imposes a retrospective sense of order on the narrative. Peabody follows this convention only in the most minimal way; her untitled chapters collect entries in arbitrary chronological units (by months). It is significant that the division into chapters is derived from a neutral source, the calendar, rather than from any sense of order in the illness. This helps to retain the journal's sense of a lack of pattern, the sense that living with AIDS is a matter of being ambushed repeatedly by new and puzzling symptoms. At the same time, I think it reflects the willful shunning of an all-too-obvious structure, that of stages of disintegration. Both Vom Lehn and his mother were haunted by their sense of passing one-way "signposts," markers of decreasing mobility and independence: the onset of blindness; the need for a cane, then a wheelchair; the insertion of a Hickman catheter to deliver nutrition; and, finally, the use of a respirator. They shared a sense that AIDS, for all its ups and downs, has its own demoralizing underlying script; the division of the book into untitled chapters can be read as a refusal to subscribe to this generic plot. In its resistance to that script lies the narrative's tension—though it hardly qualifies as suspense—and an element of counterdiscursivity.

As is understandably often the case with narratives by caregivers, *The Screaming Room* ultimately serves the needs of the mother more than those of her son. In this instance the caregiver was working alone and largely in isolation with occasional visits from other family members. Peabody had no one inside or outside the household with whom she could regularly share the burden of her role. The book's title refers to her notion of a zone in which she could therapeutically and privately release her emotions. She hopes to find such a place after Vom Lehn's death; in the meantime such a room exists only in her imagination: "I carry my screaming room inside me. It has no doors" (124–25). By providing a psychic space in which she could express her grief, frustration, and anger, her journal evidently saved her; it enabled her to take care of her son without adding her pain to his. With its publication she fully and finally externalizes the screaming room.

An unusual feature of the journal is the inclusion of passages addressed to her son, set off in italics. Most sound as if they were added later, as she edited the journal after his death. As distinct from the rest of the journal, they represent both the insights of hindsight and the urge to express to her son things that she failed to say while he was alive. Though infrequent, these passages are particularly intense and poignant. Coming across these passages, the reader listens in on something even more intimate than the mother's private journal. If, while her son was alive, the journal was a private room to which she retreated to seek relief by writing about him, it also provides, posthumously, a place in which to speak to him, if only in her imagination. Indeed, it becomes a place where she can revive him by addressing him. With its division into two type faces, then, the revised journal marks its author's two conflicting impulses—to put her son's illness behind her and to continue a dialogue with him; to retreat from his diseased body and to reach out to his spirit.

As is perhaps appropriate for a book so attentive to the condition of the body, the epilogue presents the autopsy results, but the revelation of the multiple specific causes of death predictably brings little comfort. More significantly, the epilogue reports that virtually all other members of the family got involved in AIDS work; thus the book ends with some sense of compensation, though little consolation, for Vom Lehn's death. (The agreement of mother and sister, as they view Peter's body, that he looks like Christ, comes as a complete surprise in what is otherwise a remarkably secular narrative; if Vom Lehn is to be seen as a martyr, the narrative gives little previous sign of that.) The plot is comic only in the minimal sense that his death ends his suffering and begins to ease his mother's. The narrative's resolution is not his death so much as the catharsis it affords his mother:

"Oh, Peter . . ." I finally wail, and the tears come, falling on his hair, his tortured face, dripping on the pillow, his chest, his arms, as my whole body wilts, crumbles, caves in, I don't have to be strong anymore, the strengths built up during months and months of tension, of angry energy, dissolve, and I am just another mother who has lost her child, who holds his empty, wasted body in her arms and mourns, grieves, cries for loss of part of her own body and soul. (248)

Significantly, at the moment at which individuation ceases for Vom Lehn, it ceases for his mother; with his death she becomes, momentarily at least, an archetypal grieving mother.

The book does contain moments of pleasure, connection, and even joy, and Peabody makes clear that she found a sad kind of maternal fulfillment in devoting herself to her son's care. But the reader has little sense that either she or her son had any life aside from the illness. There is always the danger in a narrative by a caregiver that the subject, the ill person, will finally be objectified by being seen largely as a patient (even though not hospitalized). To some extent that happens here. Essentially, Peter Vom Lehn plays the role of patient, the sick son, and Barbara Peabody that of the self-sacrificing nursing mother. With its narrow and vivid focus on physical symptoms the book succeeds more as illness narrative than as life writing. The constricted scope of the narrative—bracketed by the moments of diagnosis and death—limits it as an account of the life of either mother or son. The book thus stands at one end of a continuum, an example of the parental narrative in which devotion to nursing is so complete that the process crowds out other dimensions of the subjects' lives.

The narrative gives little sense of how Peter Vom Lehn thinks or feels about his illness. Although he never loses his humanity or his will to live (until close to the end), it's not clear what he had lived for and continued to wish for. The journal provides Barbara Peabody with a screaming room, but her son seems to lack one; his emotions seem entirely bottled up, not finding release even in his support groups. Emmanuel Dreuilhe has claimed that "AIDS is above all a mental illness, not so much because the virus may affect our brains as because it forces upon us such isolation and anguish that it drives us mad" (6). Regrettably, one inadvertent effect of Peabody's narrative choices is to isolate her son in his sickroom. Indeed, the narrative contains some hints that he feels smothered. One such clue lies in his defensiveness when he tells his mother that if his health permits, he intends to move into an apartment of his own; another is when he writes enigmatically on a Mother's Day card: "Now let *me* know what I think!"

One element conspicuous in its absence is any reckoning with Vom Lehn's homosexuality. Although his mother acknowledges that he is gay, she does not allow his homosexuality to figure in the narrative in any important way; once he moves in with his mother, he has little or no independent social life. The effect of his illness is not only to sever him from his gay friends back in New York but effectively to desexualize him. Part of this is perhaps merely a reflection of the way in which his illness tends to drive the mother and son back into a regressive relationship. In particular, his chronic diarrhea and his dementia infantilize him (in different ways). By doing little to counter this regression, the narrative tends to reinforce it. Limited as it is to the last stage of Peter's life, during which he was increasingly dependent on her, the narrative literally enacts the paradigm of reaffiliation—in which the homosexual son is welcomed back into the bosom of the family—only to die there. As usual with this pattern, reaffiliation effectively ends the son's homosexual life, but in this case reaffiliation is not contingent upon renunciation of homosexuality.

Still, this book is powerful and moving testimony. And its focus on suffering in the final stages of AIDS can be defended as counterdiscursive in its portrayal of the sheer horror of AIDS, a call for attention to the plight of the people with AIDS—an indictment, implicit as well as explicit, of those who stigmatize, or who abandon, the ill: "Most of you will abandon them, leave them to die alone, terrified and despised. First, you can't accept their homosexuality, and next, you can't face dying and death. I look at Peter, his face pale and lined. No one deserves this, no one" (113).

In contrast to *The Screaming Room, Remembering Brad*, by H. Wayne Schow (1995), is not in any strict sense an AIDS narrative. Although its central section consists of a sample of Brad Schow's journal entries, only the last several of these register his illness and even then minimally and reluctantly. (His final entries welcome his impending death without actually naming his illness.) It is not so much a narrative *of* illness, then, as it is a paternal memoir precipitated by a life-ending illness. Had Brad Schow not died of AIDS, his father would probably not have felt impelled to write his son's life. That he did so is a testament not only to his grief for his son but to his growing sense of his implication in Brad's struggle to resolve the powerful contradiction between his homosexual urges and his Mormon upbringing.

One manifestation of the father's posthumous revision of his sense of his son's life is that the book is multigeneric and dialogical. Partly because its various sections present different kinds of life writing, no single narrative paradigm is able to dominate the whole. A prologue is followed by a brief biography called "On Tragedy and the Death of a Son." The two succeeding sections present entries from Brad's journals and excerpts from Wayne's letters to Brad. Completing the volume are an essay on Brad's final illness and its immediate aftermath, an essay on parental grief, and a kind of antiauthoritarian allegorical satire, "The Great Western Cooperative," aimed at least in part at the Church of Jesus Christ of Latter-day Saints.

Schow's sense of the lack of a single appropriate generic model drives him to this eclecticism. His son's life is such that Wayne Schow obviously cannot write it as the life of a Mormon saint; straightforward hagiography is not possible here. But the grieving—and aggrieved—father resourcefully finds in his humanistic repertoire a recuperative paradigm.

Thus in his paternal biography the professor of literature reads his son's life as the narrative of a tragic hero. The result is a kind of unorthodox hagiography that endows his son's life with redeeming ethical significance, not despite but because of his homosexuality:

If in the last analysis, I persist in seeing him as tragic, in seeing his ordinary life as more than ordinary, it is for the reason that he could not—or would not—accept the either/or premises that life thrust on him, would not give up on the one hand his natural necessity (and right) to be gay, including the extremes of his exploration of that identity, or on the other hand his need for respect from the idealistic culture that was formative in his development. (20)

The selection of entries from Brad Schow's journals, dating from his adolescence to the time of his death, offers a different perspective on his life. As a form of life writing the diary would seem inherently well suited for a closeted individual. (In this case, the irony is that Brad started keeping a journal at the urging of his seminary instructor.) But even in this private form Brad apparently held back; at least his father infers that gaps in his journal reflect self-censorship in deference to internalized standards of what, or who, he was supposed (in two senses) to be. One passage suggests Brad's painful awareness of the impossibility of sharing his whole life with a straight friend: "It becomes like trying to tell a story and having to leave out key elements. Great gaping holes. And because I am afraid of his reaction to such a revelation, I stumble on[,] trying to avoid making the gaps apparent" (68–69). This attests to the unavailability of autobiography as a form for him, at least so long as he is in the closet. At the same time, the journal entries do give Brad a relatively unmediated voice in the narrative compilation. As we have seen, it is rare for the person with AIDS to have even this much voice in a family memoir.

The journal entries give way to yet another form of life writing—a selection of passages from letters from father to son dating from the time Brad left home (and came out to his parents) in 1979 to his return to Idaho in 1983. Wayne Schow introduces them somewhat apologetically, acknowledging that he sometimes sounds like Polonius and even drawing out subtexts that run counter to his explicit messages. (For example, in retrospect he sees that his initial response to Brad's coming out—the suggestion that his homosexuality might prove to be a phase, not a lifelong orientation—was more a wish, even a subtle directive, than a prediction.) In effect, then, Schow exposes and repudiates his earlier homophobia; he points out how, beneath his seeming open-mindedness and the pose of a friend rather than a father, he nevertheless subtly sought to steer Brad back into the path of righteousness, to curb impulses he found threatening. (One form of subtle textual coercion was his pro-

motion of corrective life stories, such as C. S. Lewis's *Surprised by Joy*
[1956] or Benjamin Franklin's *Autobiography* [1818].) Wayne Schow's
letters, though sincere, well written, and rhetorically sophisticated, are
sometimes painful to read because of their occasional fatuity and their
evident futility. But this section becomes dialogical by virtue of the father's retrospective deconstruction of his paternal advice.

On the verge of death in his Mormon-dominated hometown of
Pocatello, Idaho, Brad Schow had insisted that there be no funeral service or even public announcement of his death, a gesture his father interpreted as a kind of (uncharacteristic) denial of his illness and of his
homosexuality—perhaps to spare his family, which had shared the truth
with only a few close relatives. His parents complied, but they also sent
a letter to hundreds of relatives and friends in which they frankly acknowledged Brad's illness and his sexual orientation and even criticized
the church for its lack of tolerance. *Remembering Brad* is a belated extension of this parental gesture, much more public and much more out-
spoken. The lapse of time between Brad's death in 1986 and the book's
publication in 1995 is indicative of the difficulty and deliberation with
which Wayne Schow came to grips with his grief, guilt, and anger.

Guilt is not a term he uses, but it seems appropriate, for the book as a
whole is, among other things, a spiritual autobiography of the father—
whose Mormonism was challenged and ultimately changed by his son's
conflicted lifelong attempt to resolve the contradictions of his "tragic"
predicament as a gay Mormon. Wayne Schow clearly feels that he did
not always ease his son's predicament and may rather, in all good con
science, have helped to build the closet from which Brad never completely emerged. What is remarkable about the book as spiritual autobiography is the extent to which the father's guilt is a function of his
Mormonism; his spiritual growth consists in deviation from orthodoxy.

The closeted Brad desperately sought dialogue with anyone. Although he found (which is to say, he created) in his journal a silent non-
judgmental confidant, he did not find there or elsewhere the affirmation he craved: "Since I do not feel that I could openly discuss what I
feel with anyone I know, this journal must lend its open, unjudging ear.
To be very honest, though, I wish this journal could judge what I write
once in a while. I guess what I'm looking for is complete acceptance of
such a life style. . . . I wish my journal could do that for me" (50). Nor
did he find true dialogue in his correspondence with his father. In practice Wayne Schow sometimes supplied both sides of an ongoing discussion of the moral and religious implications of Brad's homosexuality, reproducing and countering his son's views. And, as he came to see,
this was didactic or rhetorical, not spontaneous and mutual dialogue.

Strictly speaking, then, the book is not collaborative, nor does any section enact a literal dialogue between father and son. Still, taken as a whole the book does become multivocal. Having recognized in retrospect the way in which their correspondence, for all its professed mutuality, reflected the "built-in power distribution in our father-son relationship" (79), Wayne Schow did all he could to make his book less patronizing and monological. And, indeed, we hear not just two voices—those of son and father—but various voices of both men, deepening with maturity: the father's letters, like the son's journal entries, chart growth over time. Thus the book is dialogical insofar as it represents the father's growing willingness to listen to his son. Here, posthumously, he stages the mutual exchange that eluded them when Brad was alive.

Although the father controls the entire narrative, inscribing his son's life in the first chapter and circumscribing his son's journals with his own longer contributions, in the final analysis the father defers to his son in a crucial way. For he comes around in the end from his initial orthodox Mormon position on homosexuality to his son's liberal views: that homosexuality is not inherently sinful; that homosexual relationships, like heterosexual ones, should be judged by the fruit they bear; that the "question is not *whether* one is homosexual but *how*" (10). The book reflects Wayne Schow's growing awareness, beginning with his son's unsettling announcement of his homosexuality, that despite the father's advantage in years, experience, and (presumably) wisdom, his son's experience was quite beyond his ken—that he, the father, was always in the position of responding to what his son had already lived through or thought through: "Not the least Polonian aspect of my stance was the sense that he was racing ahead of me in his development, that I was trying desperately to catch up and influence what had already occurred" (80). Only posthumously—indeed, nearly a decade after his son's death—was Wayne Schow able to compose, assemble, and publish a set of texts that he believes does justice to his son's short life.

The book is remarkable, then, for the extent to which, though undeniably paternal (and though it takes parental liberty with a private diary[22]), the book avoids paternalism; indeed, it seeks explicitly and quite successfully to undo the author's paternalism and heterosexism (and the Mormon patriarchalism that underwrote both). By publishing the journal, Wayne Schow became the sympathetic judge that Brad once sought in it. In the end the father is able to put Brad's "tragic" life in a larger perspective: "Paradoxically, the world that was for us not long ago so far out of joint begins now to show some evidence of better alignment as a result of what has happened. . . . There is some satisfaction in knowing that this shortened life contributed to this adjustment of cultural consciousness, this opportunity to reassess our attitudes and values" (131).

Wayne Schow observes that AIDS has "become the most powerful closet door opener in modern history" (130); his book certainly opens a window on his son's life and his own. And it is exceptional in the extent to which it resists the typical pattern in family memoirs of AIDS of posthumously and unilaterally reaffiliating gay men with AIDS. Although Brad did come home to die, and although the book does restore Brad to a place in his family, flanking his writing with that of his father, it also lets him speak in his own voice and defers to his views. If anything, Wayne Schow constructs a book that metaphorically liberates his son, creating the space he sought in life—to be himself in all his complexity.

Though these two parents, Peabody and Schow, cope quite differently with their sons' illnesses and represent their relationships in diametrically opposed ways, both narratives suggest how powerful an event for a parent is the death of a child—particularly when the illness and the method of infection reflect behaviors or values inconsistent with their upbringing. Here, as in the narratives by siblings, spouses, and children of men infected with HIV through homosexual contact, the memoirs, in addition to narrating illness, raise moral and cultural issues. Indeed, the general trend of AIDS narratives, as we have seen, is to obscure the physical malady beneath or behind a screen of other concerns. On the one hand, the existence of so many family narratives reflects conscious resistance to stigma; generally, they represent a family's defense of its lost member. And family memoirs do have normalizing implications in their portrayal of gay men with AIDS as, after all, somebody's brother or son, father or husband. On the other hand, few of these narratives truly and fully challenge the hegemonic discourses of AIDS and of homosexuality. Because the enactment of reaffiliation in family memoirs is always on heterosexuals' terms, such narratives often misrepresent the lives they purport to commemorate.

Ultimately, family is the site of such narratives in part because the "lifestyle" through which the infection was acquired so profoundly challenges the family's integrity. The subtext of all family narratives, in a way, is the incompatibility of homosexuality with the nuclear family. Some narratives reaffirm, some challenge, the hegemony of the heterosexual model family explicitly; even those that proclaim their openness to homosexuality—because it seems an innate characteristic of someone dear to them—do not always manage to succeed in accepting its implications. They take advantage, one might say, of the vulnerability of the family member weakened by illness to reclaim him, willy-nilly. The embrace of the family (through a self-appointed agent) may be restrictive as well as comforting, subtly cutting the gay member off from his conscious voluntary affiliations. Wayne Schow's striking deviation from this pattern serves to underscore the power of the hegemonic pattern of reaffiliation.

It is perhaps significant, then, that in most of the narratives of HIV and AIDS to be discussed in the rest of the chapter, the nuclear family plays a small or marginal role.

Experimental Nonfiction: First-Person Narratives of Drug Trials— Paul Sergios, *One Boy at War: My Life in the AIDS Underground* (1993); Paul Reed, *The Q Journal: A Treatment Diary* (1991)

> This plague has attracted the inevitable swarm of AIDS researchers, officials, businessmen, and journalists, and they are the ones who have monopolized the media. We people with AIDS, who devote each waking moment to our own survival, have been unable to prevent those loquacious experts from stealing our thunder and robbing us of the only thing we have left: our illness.
>
> Like children whose guardianship is in dispute, or natives whose fate depends on the mysterious workings of distant colonial authorities, we huddle, dazed and terrified, while arguments whistle overhead.
>
> —Emmanuel Dreuilhe, *Mortal Embrace*, 1988, p. 3.

The preceding section focused on testimony from those related by blood or marriage to men infected with HIV through homosexual contact. Though reflective of the proportions of published narratives, such an emphasis neglects the crucial perspective of those at the center of the epidemic. They have not allowed their stories to be written exclusively by others any more than they have allowed their illness to be ignored by government and health-care bureaucracies. Indeed, among contemporary illnesses, HIV/AIDS has been unique in the extent to which it has inspired activism in those infected with or threatened by the virus. A complex underground has flourished, disseminating information about alternative treatments, distributing unapproved drugs or those not officially available, and even designing and running unofficial drug trials. HIV/AIDS thus offers a dramatic instance of the impulse among laypeople to challenge the authority of biomedical or scientific discourse and government policies—to recover power over their bodies.

This activism clearly disrupted what Cindy Patton (1990) has described as the prevailing division of labor in the AIDS "service industry" between "victims" of AIDS (homosexual men or otherwise marginalized individuals), who suffer passively; "volunteers" (generally, homosexual men or heterosexual women), who offer care; and "experts" (usually heterosexual men), who make policy and conduct research (20–21). This division of labor reflects various cultural hierarchies of knowledge and power as they come to bear on the AIDS crisis. In addition to other forms of activism, a number of gay men have been willing to put their bodies on the line, volunteering as subjects for experiments and drug trials—whether above- or underground. (Here the gay community has capitalized on its marginalized position.) Although controversial, this activism—an expression of a sense of urgency among those infected—has radically changed the way in which drug trials are run and accelerated the rate at which the Federal Drug Administration approves new drugs.

One by-product of this aspect of the AIDS epidemic has been personal narratives of drug trials. Individually and collectively, these narratives attest to the desire to resist confinement to the categories or roles assigned, as delineated by Patton. Two such narratives—Paul Sergios's *One Boy at War* and Paul Reed's *The Q Journal*—differ strikingly in their scope and narrative technique. In the first an HIV-positive man becomes a self-taught expert and underground drug-trial administrator. In the second a potential "victim" writes his account of his experimental drug trial—even as his case is written up in discourse he cannot control. Both accounts are counterdiscursive but in different ways.

Sergios's narrative is the story of a gay man who was diagnosed at twenty-two with ARC in 1983. Instead of, or perhaps as a way of, obsessing about his vulnerable condition and problematic future, Sergios threw himself into the quest for a cure. What began as self-therapy—enrollment in drug trials—grew into a compulsion to find treatments for AIDS-related illnesses and HIV infection. (His ambition is at once altruistic and egocentric; he will save himself by saving everyone.) Trained as a film producer, he gradually transferred his energy and attention to AIDS until he was working full time in the AIDS underground. Research on the virus becomes his vocation as well as his avocation and duty; without medical credentials or training he becomes an autodidact in AIDS-related science. In making the illness that threatens to take his life the object of all his attention and his energy, he makes a career, in effect, out of his seropositivity. The generic novelty of his book lies in the extent to which it is a memoir of his career rather than an autobiography—a remarkably impersonal account of his research in a field in which he is not merely a nonprofessional but an interloper.

Beginning as a not wholly compliant participant in an early official trial of AZT, Sergios moves gradually toward the position of underground test administrator. As such, he acquires an investment in preserving the validity of protocols and even in monopolizing information; ironically, in the AIDS underground he becomes a kind of establishment figure and rule enforcer. Sergios's position represents a kind of extreme case, then, of the assertive patient; by the end of the book he is actually designing studies, writing grants, and overseeing clinical trials. Yet, as immersed as he can get in the sometimes numbing details of immune system dysfunction, he is always aware of his personal stake in the research he describes. Thus, although impersonal and objective on the surface, the narrative has an intensely subjective subtext: the narrator's life is on the line.

The author's life narrative provides the backbone of the book. A quick summary of his first twenty years prepares the ground for the detailed middle section, which Sergios devotes to the technicalities of trials; the last few pages revert to contemplation of the author's situation. Sadly, the long middle section consists of a series of episodes with the same plot: a promising new treatment is devised and tested, but the results are finally disappointing. This pattern complicates the closure of the narrative as a whole; we know ahead of time that the narrative will not end on the triumphal note of the discovery of a cure or treatment, and thus we doubt that the narrator can provide a comic denouement for his story as a person living with midstage HIV. Indeed, his admission to the hospital and his diagnosis with AIDS, the crossing of a discouraging watershed, precipitate the narrative's closure. Thus we retrospectively see the long middle section as a kind of holding action; the momentum shifts, finally, to the virus, and the narrative quickly concludes, foreclosing an autobiographical account of AIDS.

This book has echoes of Scheherezade on two levels; both as researcher and as chronicler of experiments Sergios puts his energy into delaying actions. Eventually, however, the narrator must give up his research and his narrative to attend to himself and his new symptoms. In that sense, and in the sense that none of the treatments pans out, the plot threatens to be tragic. Indeed, the low point of the narrative comes in 1990 when, overcome by a vision of the futility of biotechnology and by fatalism about his condition, he attempts suicide (263). But Sergios resists the tragic trend of his story by suggesting that his narrative will ultimately serve as a chapter in a kind of triumphal narrative of the conquest of the virus. Although he may die of AIDS, and the research he oversaw may not have yielded the sought-after cure, it may prove to have been necessary, to have contributed—if only by ruling out worthless treatments—to the eventual positive outcome, in which he professes his confidence: "In the end, I knew biotechnology and man would triumph over disease, and young people would no longer suffer. I turned away from the pond and started back to my car, pulling my overcoat tightly around me, ready to face the gathering dark" (313).

One Boy at War functions as counterdiscourse in a couple of senses. First, it reports—not uncritically—on underground research from the perspective of a potential "patient"—which is to say, a partisan, rather than an "objective" science reporter, much less a scientist. That is, the point of view is that of a member of an opposition, or alternative, group. But in view of the narratives discussed earlier the book may be also counterdiscursive precisely because of the extent to which it characterizes AIDS as a scientific challenge. Scientism, with its careful methodical procedures and detachment, has sometimes enraged AIDS activists, who have seen the political and medical establishments as indifferent to the suffering caused by the epidemic. As a gay HIV-positive activist Sergios conducts his work with altogether "unscientific" passion and urgency. But his focus on HIV as an intellectual and technical problem severs the illness from the circumstances and means by which it is contracted; his book thus sidesteps the moralistic and metaphoric narratives of AIDS that sometimes color even sympathetic accounts. Sergios does not deny or conceal his homosexuality; rather, he treats it as incidental to the problem. The effect of his technical discourse—as well as shielding him from the prospect of his diagnosis—is to demystify AIDS, treating it as just another deadly viral illness. Here biomedical discourse represents a healthy alternative to the judgmental metanarratives of AIDS discourse. (One drawback, however, is that the book sometimes uses dauntingly technical language.) Thus in some ways Sergios's book is a throwback to those uncomplicated accounts portraying clinical researchers as exemplary modern heroes—"Men Against Microbes." He finds a redemptive metanarrative in biomedicine: science will triumph over the virus and, incidentally, over irrational cultural constructions of AIDS.

A radically different perspective on drug trials is provided by *The Q Journal: A Treatment Diary* (1991), kept by a participant in a trial of Compound Q, a drug derived from cucumbers and developed in China. The narrator, Paul Reed, a gay writer who had just lost his partner to AIDS, is trying to refocus his energies on his work and life. Part of this, inherent in being a seropositive gay male, is the transfer of his hypervigilance about health from his now-absent partner's body to his own. Although he explicitly frames the narrative as an account of a series of "infusions" of the experimental drug—and reports faithfully on the bodily effects of the chemotherapy—the book also functions obliquely as a journal of mourning. Reed does not deny or repress his grief; rather, he excludes it as too private for exposure even here. Nevertheless, it occasionally finds its way to the surface of the narrative. Sometimes it intrudes in sharp shards of pain, as when Reed finally summons the courage to sort through his partner's closet full of clothes (99). His sense of loss pierces his self-concern, even as it prompts it. At other times, it infuses Reed's frequent reports on what is as much psychic as meteorological weather.

As suggested earlier, because of its serial composition the diary or journal is especially conducive to conveying the uncertainty of living with a chronic and incurable condition. In a truly unrevised journal the writer of each entry does not know what the next entry will hold. If we allow a degree of editorial license, the writer knows no more than the reader about the future; the reader senses the uncertainty along with the narrator. So the form gives a good sense of the dailiness of chronic infection, the minor ups and downs—as much emotional as physical— even before the onset of opportunistic infections. It enacts a day-to-day approach to seropositivity. This uncertainty is, if anything, heightened with an experimental drug trial, where even those administering the medication are not sure how much to deliver or what to expect in the nature of immediate, let alone long-term, effects.

Unlike Sergios's book, which hopes to provide a chapter of the yet-to-be-written master narrative of the conquest of AIDS, Reed's book functions on a modest scale; it maintains a narrow focus on the dailiness of the narrator's life. This is not just a matter of selection and focus, however; the open-endedness of the journal form reflects the unpredictable course of the writer's life. The brevity and frequency of the entries—almost daily for a period of eight months—give a sense of the indeterminateness of the author's life and the volatility of his moods.

Indeed, the journal is ultimately less about the drug trial, which proves inconclusive, than about living on alone, resuming a life—even deciding that one *has* a life of one's own. The book gives a strong sense of the way in which, and the extent to which, the diarist is in effect writing his life: extending it in short tentative installments, reestablishing confidence that he has a life to live, and rebuilding some vital momentum.

Indeed, the hope that his experimental treatment encourages creates troubling uncertainty. Reed notes warily that "illness has a seductive power, in that it bestows a life plan of sorts. An AIDS diagnosis would imply all manner of things—a specific treatment plan in response to the opportunistic infection, a time frame for completing unmet dreams and goals, an excuse to quit work on disability leave, eligibility for an array of services, and an all-encompassing view of life" (14). Despite the grim implications of an AIDS diagnosis, it would at least clarify certain things; there might be some comfort in the decisiveness of the diagnosis and the familiarity of the script, whereas Reed is in a kind of no-man's-land between the death of his partner and his own diagnosis, between feeling ill (from side-effects of treatment) and becoming ill (with an opportunistic infection, hence AIDS). Having seen AIDS up close, he is not eager for its reality, but he candidly acknowledges what is too often ignored or denied, the appeal of an all-too-familiar scenario: "I see that, for anyone, the emotional response to Compound Q will include a grieving process, backwards as that may seem. One will grieve for the life being left behind—the 'certainty' of impending illness, the 'security' of knowing (vaguely) what is coming next, the sense of 'belonging' to a 'community' of illness, the lost 'privileges' that come with illness" (69–70).

The journal, which Reed terminates at the end of the first series of infusions, achieves closure in two related ways. One, which Reed strives to downplay even as it figures importantly in his sense of his condition, is that he receives favorable results on a viremia test; the level of HIV infection in his blood is virtually unmeasurable. Reed is careful to point out that this result cannot definitively be attributed to Compound Q— hence, the trial is inconclusive—and that it does not mean that his body is free of HIV infection. He is wary of offering yet another misleading claim of having reversed the course of infection (171). Nevertheless, he is obviously and understandably heartened by this result.

The second source of comic closure is his sense of having regained a future, a therapeutic gain that he attributes to his treatment with "Q" (123). Regardless of the ultimate success or worth of the drug (and, according to Sergios, "Not only was Compound Q not the cure for AIDS, but it probably held little potential to improve the condition of most ARC patients significantly" [231]), it had served his psychic need to project his life, one uncertain day at a time, into the future. Similarly, the journal tentatively extends his life, not just by its daily accretions but by assuming the continuation of his existence after the book ends. Reed may not triumph over HIV and avoid AIDS, but he has certainly benefited from his experimental drug trial. Reed's journal is modestly counterdiscursive in its representation of man who is positive in more than one sense; he is unafraid of death but unwilling to write himself off prematurely.

The Case Study: AIDS and Homosexual Self-Hatred— James Melson, *The Golden Boy* (1992)

In view of the dearth of AIDS autobiographies each perhaps looms larger than it should. In James Melson's *The Golden Boy* we have another example of an autobiography that probably would never have been written were it not for AIDS. In a remarkably short period of time Melson's life trajectory carried him from his boyhood in a small midwestern town to life in the urban fast lane. An ungainly boy who disciplined his body in puberty and emerged from adolescence as a stunningly handsome, charming, and talented young man, Melson went on to work as a model and a Wall Street banker and to enjoy travel and posh vacations. His book is the picaresque narrative, amusing at times, of an unabashed social climber who passes (as much as possible) as straight and, equally important, as coming from a more distinguished background than was actually the case. (In conversation he sometimes dropped the s from his name in the hope of being taken for a Mellon.) Although he was fond of boasting to friends, public disclosure was not his style. Had he not become infected with HIV, he would not likely have undertaken an autobiography. His diagnosis with AIDS, however, prompted him to question his values and made him want to leave behind a "permanent mark on the world. My legacy" (200).

One of his responses to his diagnosis was to rediscover religion; indeed, after studying for conversion to Episcopalianism, a denomination he found receptive to gay members, he underwent what sounds like a crisis conversion. Thus, as for Stribling and Arterburn, AIDS offered Melson not only an autobiographical stimulus but a genre, the conversion narrative. But his turn toward religion finally seems consistent with, rather than a reversal of, his earlier approach to life, shallow and self-serving. (Significantly, he narrates his conversion experience less vividly than some of his sexual encounters.) His choice of Episcopalianism seems to reflect its lenient admission standards rather than any sense of deep affinity between the institution and his beliefs or temperament. His conversion does not give shape to the whole narrative or control the point of view.

In terms of genre, then, *The Golden Boy* presents an unstable mixture of conversion narrative and picaresque narrative. The conversion functions only as a localized incident, offering a finally unconvincing claim to moral seriousness. Its effect is to declare that the picaro—who is, by his own description, skilled in "manipulation, exploitation, and deceit" (80)—grew up, but the narrative as a whole does not sustain that assertion. At the same time, the claim of conversion rather puts a damper on what is otherwise an amusingly catty, even campy, narrative of a life of utter self-indulgence. Finally, however, what makes this narrative so sad is not that its author died of AIDS but the gap between what it says and what it shows.

In addition to provoking his conversion, AIDS also effectively outed Melson. At least it caused him to level with his family; at work he continued to insist that he had cancer. He came out publicly and completely only with his book. But his narrative suggests that he had lived so long in the closet, had made such a habit of deceptive role-playing, that he finally didn't know just who he was. As he made his way in the big city, in addition to impressing his companions with his savoir faire and glamour, Melson remained concerned with his image back in his hometown, which he sustained by periodic letters home romanticizing his exploits. The following passage, in which he describes letters he sent to three distinct audiences describing his first visit to New York, suggests the complexity of his rhetoric of self-presentation:

Three carefully edited versions would be composedX: the first for Chicago friends—a steamy account of the previous evening's sex; the second for class-mates, highlighting the evening's glamour and my numerous social triumphs; and the third to my parents, reporting on the progress of my independent study on loft space development as a housing alternative in cramped urban settings. This would leave the first group seething with jealousy over my sexual con-quests and the second over my membership in elite society, while my parents would be reassured that I had not fallen in with the wrong people. (114)

The overall effect of Melson's autobiography is to suggest that he had become so adept at tailoring his self-presentation to particular audiences that he could not tell a straight story when he wanted to. So devoted was he to physical narcissism that when his looks and his body began to fail him—as a result of AIDS—he literally could not continue his narrative. Thus, although the book is in some important sense an AIDS autobiog-raphy, it is not an AIDS narrative. Though he acknowledges having shingles and diarrhea and retrospectively attributes them to his HIV in-fection, and though he acknowledges his diagnosis with AIDS, he can-not bring himself to narrate the course of his illness and his treatment.

Indeed, his major gesture as a person with AIDS is to distance him-self from other people with AIDS, whom he finds disgusting as well as depressing. Thus he remembers seeing, while still apparently healthy himself, someone obviously suffering from AIDS: "an emaciated, bald-ing figure with so many purple KS tumors he looked like a human Dal-matian. I shuddered in fear, wondering if and when my rather liberal sexual past would catch up with me" (181). The shocking thing about this sentiment is not that he felt it before his diagnosis but that he passes it along without qualification after his diagnosis. Similarly, other mem-bers of his support group repel him: "I was in the middle of a circus freak show. Did I now belong with this trash?" (191).

One of the most interesting features of this narrative is the manner in which the publisher frames and presents it. Published by Harrington Press in a Haworth Gay and Lesbian Studies series, the book is in some sense a sanctioned narrative, but those who present it realize that it is hardly affirming of gay life—that, in fact, it reflects the narrative of someone deeply conflicted about homosexuality, a homophobic homo-sexual. (The most defining feature here is the loathing Melson expresses for what he sees as pathetic aging "faggots." In one startling incident he brusquely shoves an older man who becomes too familiar in a Province-town bar; far from expressing regret for this in his narrative, he boasts: "It is one of the most treasured moments of my life, for it was the first time I stood up for myself like a man. . . . I had intimidated other men. I delighted in this sudden revelation of my masculinity" [102].) Another form that his self-hatred takes is disdain for those less handsome or well endowed than he. Although—or perhaps because—he was the butt of jokes as an overweight youth, the handsome Melson has no compunction about rejecting the short, the "swarthy," the plain. Having found in his newly disciplined body a source of power over other men, he exercised it cruelly at times. Having suffered rejection, he took revenge by spurning others.

In their attempts to rehabilitate Melson, to give his narrative social and moral point as testimony in the midst of the AIDS epidemic, the foreword by Lawrence Mass, M.D. (author of the first reports on AIDS to circulate outside the medical press; both reports were for the *New York Native*, a gay newspaper [Alwood 212, 215]), and the afterword by gay activist Arnie Kantrowitz take slightly different tacks. Both, however, present the narrative as a case study of a homosexual whose pathological narcissism and self-hatred are functions of cultural homophobia. Thus, according to Kantrowitz, "Melson's narcissism and his prejudices . . . are little more than a thin mask for his feeling that being homosexual is an ugly, unnatural, immoral thing; and all his glittering experiences in the gay world . . . did little to enhance his feelings of self-worth" (215).

At the same time, both Mass and Kantrowitz give Melson some credit for growth and self-transformation. In this reading the narrative traces a conversion-in-progress, not from homosexuality to nonerotic homosociality, as in the instances of Stribling and Arterburn, but from self-hating to self-accepting homosexuality. But, as should be clear by now, the conversion is at least tainted by its circumstances; in this case, an opportunistic approach to life is extended to the afterlife. Before the conversion has a chance to deepen, to reorient his life, Melson terminates his narrative; whatever depth the conversion may have later acquired is not available to the reader. The effect of the premature termination of the narrative—indeed, perhaps its premature undertaking—is to suggest that the turn to faith is inauthentic. His book is not a narrative of how AIDS reflects or reshapes his life; rather, it is about how AIDS ended life as he knew it. (When the party is over, life is over, even though he has a nagging sense that there ought to be more to it.)

Published autobiographies of any sort are rarely as inconsistent in viewpoint as this book; as I have argued earlier, autopathography is rarely begun until and unless the remission of illness and/or the resolution of related life issues allows for a comic plot. With AIDS, however, both the virulence of the illness (which in the early years of the epidemic usually killed infected individuals within two years of diagnosis) and the early age at which many are infected militate against the writing of autobiographical illness narratives. Despite, or perhaps because of, its flaws Melson's book highlights an additional obstacle to the writing of AIDS narratives in some instances. Melson's impulse toward autobiography and his weaknesses as an autobiographer both reflect the corrosive effect of AIDS on his self-image and his life narrative.

The breaking off of his narrative at the point of diagnosis underlines the impact and import of that event. The radical instability of Melson's narrative point of view—the vacillation between nostalgia for a life of carefree self-indulgence and his apparently sincere desire for transcendence—suggests what a profound existential crisis AIDS may pose to gay men who are conflicted about their homosexuality because they have internalized negative stereotypes. Such individuals may not be inclined toward the sort of religious conversion that requires renunciation of homosexuality, but they may not be so comfortable with their sexual orientation as to treat AIDS as a mere viral illness, like Sergios. For them, AIDS presents a particularly difficult challenge, a threat not just to life but to identity, a crisis of self-understanding and self-acceptance that may not be resolvable in the short time available.

A San Francisco Chronicle: Fran Peavey, *A Shallow Pool of Time: An HIV+ Woman Grapples with the AIDS Epidemic* (1990)

Fran Peavey's *A Shallow Pool of Time* consists of a journal followed by several essays about the effect of HIV infection on her, her community (San Francisco), and the human race. The journal is particularly interesting in that it begins as a chronicle of an epidemic that was happening around her rather than to her, only to become her "confidant" (31) when she discovers her seropositivity. Like most HIV/AIDS narratives by women, then, this one began as an account by someone not infected but rather concerned with the effect of AIDS on others; in that way, it is akin to the narratives by daughters, sisters, mothers, or wives of someone infected with HIV. However, her discovery of her infection changes Peavey's relation to AIDS and makes her account an anomaly. Because what she began as chronicle became a personal narrative in midstream, the apparently unretouched journal vividly reflects the author's change in status and thus in attitude toward HIV/AIDS.

Indeed, the journal demonstrates how the stigma of HIV/AIDS may pervade and "spoil" identity even when the individual's infection does not identify her as a member of a scorned "risk group." (Peavey attributes her infection to a blood transfusion necessitated by endometritis.) The immediate emotional effects of Peavey's discovery of her seropositivity are fear, dread, and even guilt and shame. This is surprising in someone who contracts the virus "innocently" rather than through gay sex or intravenous drug use. Her awareness of her infection with HIV seems to activate some latent sense of shame about her body. In part because her feeling of contamination is not something she is entirely aware of, the narrative illustrates the powerfully corrosive effect of infection.

The narrative effect of discovering her infection is the sudden narrowing of the focus of her journal. We know from her introduction and intermittent comments that she carried on her various jobs and avocations—as comedian, activist, environmentalist, and more. But the journal gives little direct evidence of her past and of the other dimensions of her life. Because she continues to be largely asymptomatic, the journal is not primarily concerned with clinical details and treatments but rather with the psychological and emotional aftershocks of her knowledge of her seropositivity. One dramatic index of the effect of HIV, then, is that her narrative gives such a constricted sense of her living with the infection. Her HIV status virtually monopolizes her "life," if not her life. Indeed, the virus creates a sharp rupture between her still active public life and her private life as recorded in the intimate journal. This is an unfortunate effect, as friends who read it before publication pointed out to her. But she is unapologetic:

"Well," I mused, "imagine how it feels to be embedded in the situation day after day. Of course being HIV+ is not all I do, and it's not even a very important part of who I am. I have my work. . . . And I enjoy play with many good friends. But please remember that this journal is about my experience with the new virus. I am chronicling an epidemic. As I step out of the newspaper headlines into real personhood with this virus, I may be preoccupied. Sorry about that." (93)

Despite its serial composition, the narrative is given overall shape by a couple of plots. Unlike Melson's, Peavey's infection with HIV cured her of prejudice; she hopes that journals like hers may provide others with a kind of vicarious "exposure" that will be healing for them as well. A related narrative line traces her growing sense of membership in a community that is vital although, or perhaps because, a deadly epidemic threatens it. Accepting that she has become part of a community by "virtue" of her infection, she avows her solidarity with other people with AIDS: "I realize that I did not decide to cast my lot with people with AIDS—in the United States, now mostly drug addicts and gay men—but . . . now I proudly stand with them. The killing must stop" (52). Rather than trying to distance herself from the stigma of HIV, she identifies with others infected with the virus.

The primary plot, however, has to do with negotiating a change in identity. More than any other HIV or AIDS narrative, Peavey's dramatizes the difference between being ill and feeling ill. Peavey finally takes the HIV antibody test, not because of recent exposure, much less because of symptoms—she has none—but because of new concern about past transfusions and because she wants to know her status as she enters a new relationship. Her immediate and pressing concerns are not about her health but about her identity and her relations with others (and not merely sexual relations). When her test results reveal her "status," her self-image changes instantaneously and fundamentally, without any change in her physical condition. It is not her seropositivity but her knowledge of it that so profoundly changes her identity and her life.

The immediate issue is, then, not survival but how—indeed, whether—to act out her status: she can still "pass" if she wants to. Urged to inform her past lovers of her status, she hesitates out of reluctance to change their lives the way hers has been changed. She fears infecting them with doubt at the very least—and dreads ending their innocence should they test positive—but realizes that telling them is the right thing to do. At the center of the narrative her test result poses a crisis of self-identification and also of relationality and responsibility. The crisis is eventually resolved by the disclosure of her status to older as well as newer friends on the occasion of her annual "General Accounting" of her life. She claims too that knowing of her seropositivity has made her more responsible. (While ignorant of her status, she had donated blood while in Afghanistan, a gesture that later haunts her). Thus the change in status, although it does not automatically or immediately stimulate personal growth, makes it possible.

One kind of exposure is behind her, but she finds another kind quite threatening. Readers may be surprised to find a woman who contracted the virus through the most "innocent" of means—transfusion—so afflicted by self-doubt and disgust upon testing positive. Indeed, the narrator herself is surprised: "I am shocked at the shame I feel when I talk about this virus inside of me. . . . They tell us where the virus comes from, but this secondary infection—shame—where does that come from?" (32). She never answers this question explicitly, but it appears that her socialization as a woman has made her self-conscious about her body—in particular, about menstruation. That she sees her menstrual blood as lethal reflects more than the danger of viral transmission through bodily fluids (44); the by-product of a healthy process has acquired, in her mind, a taint that she finds difficult to cope with.

One way of encouraging herself is to construct a hypothetical narrative explaining her infection: "A civic-minded man, probably gay, gave blood at a time when the technology could not distinguish infected blood from noninfected blood. I was given that blood by a doctor who was trying to keep me from bleeding to death. And now I have been told that there are antibodies to the AIDS virus in my blood. My body has done a very smart thing by making those antibodies. It shows that it is fighting the disease and probably winning. Go, body!!!" (34). Obviously, and understandably, she is here trying to construe her predicament as benignly as possible—to exonerate both the individual who supplied her infeted blood and the doctor who transfused her. This is patently a self-reassuring narrative; the blood donor is "civic-minded," her doctor is benevolent, her body is "smart." Even while her journal—as a *journal*—reflects, like Reed's, the nagging uncertainties of HIV positivity, here it contains its antidote—a kind of self-written life that relates past, present, and future as confidently and optimistically as possible. One antidote to seropositivity, then, is "psychopositivity," which takes the form of a wishful illness narrative.

Even toward the end of her journal, however, she acknowledges that she continues to struggle to reconcile her knowledge of her seropositivity with her self-image. As with Reed's journal, what degree of closure hers achieves has to do with the reestablishment of a sense of psychic and emotional equilibrium rather than with any change in her physical condition, which continues to be mostly asymptomatic (120). The equilibrium is a function of Peavey's having shared her news with friends and thus helped to create a supportive network in anticipation of later needs. She has to prepare those around her, as much as herself, for what is likely to happen.

Ultimately, then, despite its serial composition, the book achieves a comic plot—on several levels. First, Peavey is able to regain her composure, to integrate HIV into her life. Though, like a number of such narratives, this one ends before the onset of AIDS, this HIV journal is proleptic in that it suggests that she has the resources in and around her to deal with AIDS as well as HIV. (In an essay that follows we learn that, having calculated the extent of her financial and social support, she has secured drugs with which she can end her life [127].)

Moreover, the publication of the journal enacts a comic resolution of the issue of "spoiled identity." The act of going public is important; it is irreversible, like learning of her seropositivity, and it is exemplary, a model for others. Such was the political climate in California in the late 1980s, when she discovered her infection, that she made a practice of registering for medical tests under a false name. (Initiatives had been proposed that would have required the registration of people with AIDS.) In one of the essays appended to her journal, "On Secrets," Peavey confesses that her use of a pseudonym in dealing with bureaucracies deeply unsettled her sense of her identity and even of her health (128). What begins as a self-protective strategy becomes a self-divisive and self-destructive one; it heightens the alienation from her body initiated by her knowledge of her seropositivity. This is compelling evidence of how stigma compounds illness. This postscript to her journal underlines the role of her journal writing in keeping her self intact. The writing of the journal began to repair the breach within her identity; the publication of it under her name carried the process one step further. So the publication of the journal reflects a major step in her construction and presentation of self. The decision to publish under her own name represents an act of faith in a larger community and a real victory over the sense of shame and disgust that sometimes plagued her.

The last essay, "On Waiting," is a kind of meditation in which she generalizes her uncertain future to that of the human species, which seems vulnerable to new illnesses and ailments, perhaps because of environmental factors. Although it warns of coming disaster, this essay looks forward to a vantage point from which the species can look back. It does not provide, so much as it anticipates, closure, a time when the narrative of AIDS can be concluded with its cure, and "people learn to live together within reasonable limits of resources" (151). Like Ashe and a number of others, Peavey cannot resist the tropical seduction of AIDS; she concludes her journal with a kind of cosmic metanarrative of the disease in which her case is only a small chapter. Such a gesture, I think, attests to the power of illness to challenge one's comfortable presumptions and also to stimulate the desire for a larger narrative in which one's individual life can be seen as meaningful.

AIDS and Gay Auto/biography: Paul Monette, *Borrowed Time: An AIDS Memoir* (1988) and *Becoming a Man: Half a Life Story* (1992); Fenton Johnson, *Geography of the Heart: A Memoir* (1996); Emmanuel Dreuilhe, *Mortal Embrace: Living with AIDS* (1988)

> The project of our enemies is to keep us from falling in love.
> —Paul Monette, *Becoming a Man*, 1992, p. 25.

Though AIDS is not a "gay" disease, the vast majority of published book-length narratives, as we have seen, are concerned with AIDS in gay or bisexual men; surprisingly few of these, however, are written by infected men, their partners, or others in the gay community. Even fewer can be described as in any way affirming of gay culture; most subscribe in some way, or to some degree, to hegemonic narratives of AIDS and/ or homosexuality. Some of these accounts, as we have seen, are explicitly and deliberately homophobic (Christian conversion narratives); others reveal the limits of the very open-mindedness they seek to demonstrate (family memoirs). Only quite recently have gay men begun to tell the story of AIDS (as opposed to HIV infection) among them; even now, autobiographical accounts of AIDS are quite unusual. The dearth of gay-affirmative autobiographical accounts of AIDS says a good deal about the power of hegemonic views of AIDS (as well as the physical obstacles to autopathography); at the same time, a series of memoirs by gay men has begun to offer testimony from the epicenter of the epidemic, putting an end to a deafening silence. As a memoir by the partner of a gay man who died of AIDS, Paul Monette's *Borrowed Time: An AIDS Memoir* (1988) is a pioneering book here; a recent narrative in the same subgenre is Fenton Johnson's *Geography of the Heart: A Memoir* (1996). (Both Monette and Johnson had published other books—mostly poetry or fiction—before their partners, who were not writers, died of AIDS.) The rather considerable lag from Monette's memoir to Johnson's is suggestive of the taboo that these books violate. For they openly and eloquently express the "love that dare not speak its name." Although they are in some sense undeniably "narratives of AIDS" (to varying degrees), they are also memoirs of partners and of relationships—which is to say that they are love stories, if not romances. Like all relational memoirs, these narratives are at once biography and autobiography. But because of the nature of the relationships inscribed the line between auto- and biography may be much less distinct than it is in the relational narratives discussed earlier in the chapter. Even when they are outwardly conventional in form their concern with gay couples is a noteworthy cultural innovation.

Considered in relation to its predecessors, *Borrowed Time*, an account of Roger Horwitz's final illness by his partner, is a refreshing anomaly in its treatment of homosexuality; it is unambivalently and unabashedly affirming of gay life. Residents of West Hollywood, both men are at peace with their homosexuality and at home in the gay community. Though their relationship is not entirely monogamous, it is an enduring one, a virtual marriage—some ten years old at the time of Horwitz's diagnosis. Each man has long been out to his parents, who have had time to get over any initial shock and dismay; confronted with Horwitz's diagnosis, both sets of parents are thoroughly supportive through the ordeal of illness. In this narrative, then, the homosexuality of the central figures is something the narrative simply takes for granted rather than addresses—or skirts—as an issue, much less an embarrassment. And that difference alone makes *Borrowed Time* a breakthrough among narratives of gay AIDS.

As Monette fully appreciates, his book depicts medical care that is state-of-the-art, compassionate, and enlightened. Horwitz's doctors did not seem threatened by Monette's "grapevine" research on AIDS treatment nor by his aggressive advocacy on Horwitz's behalf. Indeed, through personal connections Roger Horwitz became the first patient west of the Mississippi to receive AZT; as such, "he was the miracle man, period. He had to be, because thousands of our brothers were about to follow him on AZT" (307). Horwitz's privileged access to the drug helps to endow his story with another dimension. It links it to the "treatment" narratives: one of its leitmotifs—like that of Sergios's book—is that of the long-awaited, highly touted "magic bullet" that fails. Far from challenging "medical discourse" or portraying physicians as insensitive or hostile, the book is dedicated to one of Horwitz's physicians, Dr. Michael Gottlieb. (In 1980, Gottlieb, an immunologist at UCLA, was one of the first researchers in the country to begin to investigate what came to be called AIDS [Shilts 42].) Indeed, it is Gottlieb who, upon learning that Monette is a writer, first suggests that he write about AIDS, because "nobody else does" (80).

The book is counterdiscursive, rather, in its rebuke to an indifferent or homophobic public and to inert or negligent government bureaucracies. Monette does not exempt himself from blame for stigmatizing people with AIDS, pointing out early on that the impulse to think in terms of a susceptible "them" and a safe "us" was powerful in the gay community as a defense against AIDS hysteria. His purpose is in part to raise the genre of inside storytelling from rumor and gossip to tragic or heroic narrative: "The story I want to tell is about heroism and sacrifice and love, but I will not be avoiding the anger. I watched AIDS become gossip, glib and dismissive, smutty, infantile. I gossiped myself. It was sometimes the only way to talk about it, but all the same it's a yellow and disgusting way" (19).

Monette foregrounds the difficulty of narrating illness because of the way it threatens one's sense that life has coherence, continuity, and extension. Among the sources for his account were his journal and Horwitz's calendar, but Monette sometimes finds these barren because they had seemed so inadequate or irrelevant to what was happening at the time. For example, he finds a gap in his journal after it reports Horwitz's diagnosis: "For a while my journal stood frozen around the two-word entry for March 12: *the verdict*. No reason to keep a record of what was over now" (87). Life goes on and hope revives, however, and Monette resumes his journal. But when Horwitz's condition worsens, their daily records again become spotty or trail off:

I have virtually no record of the next three months. Except for a few doctors' appointments, Roger's calendar is completely blank for the rest of the year, and he wouldn't even bother with a calendar for '86. Between then and the end of January there is a single five-line entry in my journal, and my daily calendar is as empty as Roger's, because I ceased to write my appointments down. . . . It was as if the whole idea of calendars had become a horrible mockery. (192)

AIDS interferes with their plotting their lives, in two senses. By making the future uncertain, it confounds planning. It also defies or deters immediate recording, which is also, after all, future oriented: "when you live so utterly in the present, the yearning to record it goes away. To write in a diary you have to hope to read it later—or to last long enough to make the appointment two weeks down the road" (192). Illness may so occlude the future that it undermines one purpose of a daily record—to preserve the present for future reading and reexamination; also, living under threat of death can become an end in itself, an all-absorbing enterprise that allows little perspective and little surplus energy for inscription. Having survived, Monette finds he can fill in the journal's gaps, but he elects not to erase its eloquent silences. He thus illuminates the way in which journal keeping and retrospective narrative of illness complement one another; each can render aspects of illness that elude representation in the other.

Judging by the favorable reviews, Monette was largely successful in his aim of making literature of an AIDS story. It helped that he was already a writer with poetry and fiction—and novelizations of Hollywood thrillers—to his credit, for the book succeeds as sheer narrative partly as a result of Monette's control of tone, pace, and generic conventions. Perhaps the most interesting and original formal gesture is that Monette ends his book simply and abruptly with Horwitz's death, toward which the narrative has inexorably progressed. The manipulation of pace is crucial here. From its opening words—"I don't know if I will live to finish this" (1)—the narrative has an undeniable sense of urgency, of time running out, and Monette noticeably slows the pace as he approaches the end, as if to delay the inevitable, to prolong Horwitz's existence—on paper at least. The writing is particularly affecting here, and the lack of any epilogue or coda prevents the reader from retreating too quickly from the event to its meaning; no consolation is offered. The effect is to convey utter and unmitigated bereavement, to enact the void in Monette's life caused by the end of Horwitz's. The unconventional termination of the narrative, before any funeral rites or memorial service, makes the book Horwitz's most powerful memorial.[23] Moreover, it forestalls any reaffiliation of Horwitz with his family; the gay relationship remains in the foreground, at the core of the narrative. Thus it is as much by exclusion as by inclusion that the narrative affirms the partners' intimacy, maintained at such cost.

Though the book reads as a seamless chronological narrative, it mingles elements of two established genres, the war story and the love story.[24] The book's jacket illustration of Menelaus carrying Patroclus from the battlefield at Troy signals that Horwitz and Monette are to be seen as warriors rather than victims; when one soldier is wounded, his brother-in-arms loyally and lovingly tends him till he dies. This trope, invoked at intervals, serves to counter the stereotyping of homosexuals as effeminate, selfish, and irresponsible. At the same time, the narrative inscribes a shamelessly romantic love story; here the durability of the relationship—and their quite bourgeois lifestyle—helps to contest stereotypes of gay men as promiscuous and impulsive, bent only on immediate gratification. As a whole the book is more tender than martial or militant in its tone; indeed, it is by and large intimate, even cozy, in feeling, for all that it documents a kind of doomsday scenario. Monette's subtle mixture of love and war enables him to valorize both gay love and a stigmatic illness—reconstructing AIDS as a kind of fatal lovesickness.

Although Monette's verbal and narrative facility make this reconstruction look easy, this is no small achievement. The book's most romantic conceit is suggested in Horwitz's remark to Monette: "'But we're the same person. When did that happen?'" (314). This gesture, along with Monette's discovery of his seropositive status during Horwitz's illness, makes the book in some sense auto/biography—a narrative of two lives that are one and one death that is two, a kind of *liebestod* (lovedeath). In this somber narrative of his partner's final illness, then, the gifted Monette wrote a kind of crossover classic, one that transcended the limits of his previous work in various genres, high and low, gay and mainstream.

Ultimately, however, the book's value derives as much from its inside point of view as from its literary skill. As a gay man, as a caregiver to a partner with AIDS, and especially as a man who is seropositive, Monette writes from a vantage unattainable, and even perhaps unimaginable, by a parent, sibling, child, or ex-wife of a gay man with AIDS, no matter how open-minded. For unlike the narrator whose relation is defined by the heterosexual nuclear family, this narrator has an intimate connection with the larger homosexual community that is under threat. One manifestation of this is the pattern of overlapping narratives of others with AIDS, which helps the reader view AIDS from various perspectives. First and foremost, the narrative offers a close-up look at AIDS by a caregiver (like that in *The Screaming Room*). As narrator, Monette attends almost as closely to Horwitz's condition as he did as caregiver. (Indeed, at times the author seems to be compensating—or overcompensating—for having missed signs and symptoms during the illness.) The unsanitized narrative immerses the reader in the couple's life and in Horwitz's predicament, detailing the many hospital visits and the various infections battled.

At the same time, it offers a kind of cross-section of a larger community. Monette finds himself fielding, and trying to shield Horwitz from, reports of crises and downturns in the condition of various acquaintances and friends. The presence of overlapping stories helps to define the psychological burden of living with AIDS, which presents an insidious double threat. On the one hand, the indeterminate and shifting borders of stages such as HIV infection, "pre-AIDS," and "full-blown AIDS" undermine attempts to insulate oneself psychologically from AIDS. On the other, it is hard not to abstract patterns from other illness stories and apply them to the one at hand; the reports of the myriad other cases tend to reify a generic plot that is a hopeless downward spiral. From all sides AIDS seems to thrust its morbid master plot onto Monette, who is hard-pressed to maintain his sense of authority. But these fragments of other stories, along with references to gay organizations mobilized to deal with AIDS, help to make Horwitz's story a powerful synecdoche, a making public of "the story of a kind of bond that the growing oral history of AIDS records again and again" (1988, 65).

By generating a single exemplary account of a person with AIDS, Monette begins to fill the vacuum decried by Gottlieb. Significantly, Monette's account portrays Horwitz's illness in the context of a meaningful life with his partner—unlike the all-too-familiar pattern of reaffiliation; more, it represents the larger life of the gay community. The community is not just the backdrop for Horwitz's story; it is the site of a collective engagement with the epidemic. Monette is unsparing about the indifference, selfishness, and denial characteristic of some individuals in that community, but he is also careful to note the mobilization of others against AIDS, "a community of the stricken who would not lie down and die" (103). His is a gay-affirmative narrative not just in its matter-of-factness about homosexuality but also in its affirmation of the community's efforts at self-preservation.

Monette, who died of AIDS in 1995, never narrated his illness. Perhaps, having narrated Horwitz's illness from the point of view of an HIV-positive partner and having in the process denied the distinction between his partner and himself, Monette felt his illness narrative would be redundant. He did, however, turn to autobiography in his next book. Though not in the narrow sense an AIDS narrative, *Becoming a Man: Half a Life Story* (1992) is in an important sense an AIDS autobiography insofar as it was impelled both by Monette's sense of his limited lifespan and his increasing politicization by the AIDS epidemic.

The second book is a prequel to the first, an apt complement: having narrated his life with Roger Horwitz in *Borrowed Time*, in *Becoming a Man* Monette narrated his life before Horwitz. In explaining the genesis of the latter book, he acknowledges that it was to some degree a corrective work. He acknowledges that the sense of liberation and fulfillment he found in his relationship with Roger, his first real love, may have led him to idealize that relationship, and he regrets seeming to have endorsed couplehood as the sole model of gay life (174–75). Despite his disclaimers, however, *Becoming a Man* risks reinforcing these tendencies, for its subject is the painful, protracted, and halting process of his coming out, which was completed and confirmed only by his relationship with Roger Horwitz, which taught him that he could have sex and love with the same man. By Monette's account this revelation transformed him; it made him and his life whole. Thus, just as *Borrowed Time* stops abruptly with the death of Roger Horwitz, *Becoming a Man* ends suddenly with his advent in Monette's life.

The title's reference to "half a life" can be read in a number of ways. On the literal level it reflects the limited chronological span of the book—roughly, the first twenty five years of Monette's life. (At the same time, it is probably inflected by his sense of his entire lifespan's being foreshortened by HIV.) But its major import is to characterize his life before Roger, his life alone in the closet, as a less-than-full existence—at best, "half a life." Indeed, he implies that it was less than that, a fraction of a fraction, for despite the sex he engaged in—with female as well as male partners—he characterizes himself during most of this period of his life as "bodiless" (38), "dead below the belt" (172), in a "frozen state" (173).

The powerful counterdiscursivity of Monette's account is suggested by the other half of its title, for the book simply and daringly equates Monette's achievement of mature masculinity with his acceptance of his homosexuality. For the first half or more of his life his sense of manhood and of his life story did not conform to available cultural templates; Monette felt he was not a man, at best a man with "no story" (1). When it came time for him to share his autobiography with the other members of his senior society at Yale, he could tell all but the single fact that made sense of the rest (156). Only in coming out did he discover that he had a story after all, one shared with lots of his "brothers"—a story of oppression and repression, falsehood and inauthenticity, eavesdropping and ventriloquism, faking it and passing. Courting the safety of invisibility, Monette had became a voyeuristic eye and sympathetic ear. (His ability to evoke confession from others is no doubt one key to his talents as a narrator.) His narrative is at once rich in personal revelations (deep dish) and in some sense generic—the story of his tribe.

Having come out, then, he tells a story that is all too common, in the hope that it may cease needing to be lived or told. Though not entirely new, the nonfictional narrative of coming out takes on a new urgency in the context of AIDS: "every memoir now is a kind of manifesto, as we piece together the tale of the tribe. Our stories have died with us long enough. We mean to leave behind some map, some key, of the gay and lesbian people who follow—that they may not drown in the lies" (2). Thus *Becoming a Man* is not just a narrative of one man's emergence from the closet; it is at once in some sense a validation (by uncloseting) of the "nonstory" of the closet and a gesture in the direction of destroying the closet once and for all. It is a blow against the compulsory invisibility of homosexual lives.

Writing his story means rewriting the family narrative encapsulated in the photo album of "'40s Brownie snapshots with scalloped edges" (4): "the pictures were lies" (30). His revisionist narrative is attentive to the dynamics of his nuclear family, including issues raised by having a younger brother with spina bifida—"*I had to be the normal one*" (29)—but he is careful to deny that his family made him gay (12). Monette's ultimate loyalty is to his tribe of gay men; this is a narrative of painful but finally redemptive affiliation with a marginalized minority. One manifestation of this is that the book omits what one might expect would be an obligatory and perhaps climactic scene—coming out to one's parents. The real achievement is coming out to oneself rather than to the world.

As may be evident already, *Becoming a Man* is a kind of counterconversion narrative. Like a conventional conversion narrative, the coming-out narrative traces spiritual torment, arduous efforts at "reform" that result in false assurance (Monette's attempts to go straight), and finally an abrupt and radical transformation, after which the narrative quickly concludes. This book, however, is the antithesis of the Christian conservative narratives discussed earlier. Whereas those narratives claim absolution from the sin of homosexuality, Monette's celebrates his deliverance from the guilt induced by the equation of homosexuality with sin. The conversion narrative and the coming-out narrative both represent homosexual self-hatred, but they overcome it in opposite ways—one by denouncing homosexuality, the other by affirming it. Like the conversion narrative, the coming-out narrative portrays the earlier self as a different person, a "dead self" (172); in this instance the Old Paul, tormented by guilt from the very dawn of eros, gives way to the New Paul, fulfilled by his discovery of a body-and-soul mate. The overall movement is from the hell of the closet to the heaven of his open life with Roger Horwitz.

Although he alludes to AIDS only occasionally, it haunts and impels the whole, which ends with Monette's feeling, "I'm the last one left, in a world where only the ghosts still laugh. But at least they're the ghosts of full-grown men, proof that all of us got that far, free of the traps and the lies" (278). The fact that the book won a National Book Award for nonfiction (1992) reflects both Monette's accomplishment and the progressive uncloseting of homosexual lives. Homophobia and AIDS have, in different but related ways, taken a huge toll in gay lives; counterdiscourse like this offers to repair some of that loss.[25]

A notable successor to *Borrowed Time* is Fenton Johnson's *Geography of the Heart*(1996), a memoir of his three-year relationship with Larry Rose, who died of AIDS in 1990. One difference from Monette's memoir is already evident—the relatively short duration of this relationship. Johnson and Rose were not able to be long-time companions; their relationship was still new when Rose's death cut it short. Another difference from *Borrowed Time* is in the narratorial point of view: unlike Monette, Johnson was not infected with HIV. Thus his narrative lacks some of the urgency of Monette's; it is populated with ghosts—Rose's and those of many gay friends but not haunted by the prospect of the narrator's death.

The narrative does, however, reflect the strains of the relationship's asymmetry. Impelled in part by a sense of the limits of his lifespan, Rose pressed Johnson for commitment; Johnson resisted, partly because commitment would bring the burdens of caregiving and the pain of bereavement. As it happened, however, the two agreed to move in together about the time Rose was diagnosed with AIDS. And ultimately HIV cemented the relationship that it had at first obstructed. In a gesture similar to Monette's the narrative suggests that the two men thought of themselves as one; an index of the relationship's development is that Johnson's great early fear—that Rose would infect him and then abandon him by dying (92)—was eventually supplanted by his fear that Rose's death would deprive him of a large part of himself (109). One burden of the narrative is to explain why both men—knowing Rose would soon die—regarded themselves as lucky. One of its achievements is that most readers will come to agree with their assessment: the two men learned from each other that love can encompass, if not overcome, the illness and death of a intimate partner.

The major formal innovation of this book is that, in addition to telling the stories of the establishment of the relationship and the erosion of Larry's health after his diagnosis with AIDS (about two-thirds of the way through), Johnson attempts to narrate or at least synopsize both men's lives before they met. Thus the long middle section, "Emigrant Sons," begins by alternating between the story of the incipient relationship and vignettes of the two men's pasts. Johnson devotes roughly equal space to both their pasts; as a version of auto/biography, a memoir in which center stage is shared by two protagonists, then, this narrative is particularly egalitarian. (He may have found a precedent for these "parallel lives" in Gertrude Stein's *The Autobiography of Alice B. Toklas* [1933], which brings the separate stories of Toklas and Stein up to the point of their meeting before narrating their life together.) Compared to *Borrowed Time* (whose subtitle accurately identifies it as an *AIDS* memoir), *Geography of the Heart* is more a memoir of Johnson and Rose, both as individuals and as a couple.

Although Johnson is interested in discovering broad parallels between his life and Rose's, he is also respectful of their differences. One such difference involves the ways in which they are emigrant sons. Rose was the only child of European emigrants, German-Jewish survivors of the Holocaust who settled in southern California, whereas Johnson himself "emigrated" to California from rural Kentucky, where he was one of nine children of Catholic parents. Although Johnson remained emotionally close to his large family, he quickly came to recognize the special intensity of the bond between Rose and his parents, who perhaps overinvested in their only child.

Geography of the Heart is particularly interesting in relation to patterns of family affiliation we have seen in earlier narratives of gay AIDS. We have seen sisters who, as memoirists, seem to slight their dead brothers' partners (Ascher and Wiltshire), a father who attempts posthumously to release his son from a closet he helped to build (Schow), and a gay memoir (Monette) in which nuclear families, though supportive, are peripheral. Johnson is an interesting novelty in that he reckons explicitly and tactfully with the triangular relationship involving gay men and their partners' families. This no doubt reflects his sense of coming late into Rose's life when his parents' claims (with all the burdens of modern Jewish history) had long been established (71). But it also reflects the Roses' generosity and openness to Johnson and their eventual acceptance of him. Before he would agree to live with Rose, Johnson insisted that Rose inform his parents of his diagnosis. Their appreciation of Johnson's willingness to commit himself to a man whom he knew was mortally ill altered the dynamics of the triangle: "In his mother's eyes I was transformed from a rival for Larry's love into an ally. To his father I became, not just a friend to his son, but a genuine son-in-law. Because of AIDS his parents welcomed me into what had been a nearly closed circle, a family unit walled off from the harshness of history. Because of AIDS I became a member of the family" (152).

The timing of Rose's death—during an impractical sentimental journey to France—appears to reflect his preference, on some level of consciousness, for dying as well as living with Johnson—rather than where his aging parents lived. Johnson appreciates both the compliment of the affiliation and the rapidity of Rose's final decline, which spared them a long ordeal. Rose died of a heart attack in the American Hospital in Paris with Johnson nearby. Though not kin, much less "next of kin," Johnson negotiated the cremation and the return of Rose's ashes to the States. Rose's double status—as only son and gay partner—was enacted in dual memorial services—one held (at the urging of Johnson, who gave the eulogy) for family and family friends in Hollywood Park Cemetery, where Rose's ashes remained, and one held for gay friends in the San Francisco Bay area.

Insofar as the narrative is written by Johnson, not by a member of Rose's family, the memoir affiliates or associates Rose with the gay community on two levels, as a member of a gay couple and as a member of a larger community besieged by an epidemic in which he is a casualty. At the same time, and to a remarkable degree, it recognizes and honors the way in which Rose had been shaped by his past and his parents' past; indeed, in a gesture that is not paralleled, to my knowledge, in the composition of any of the other AIDS narratives discussed here, Johnson submitted an early draft of part of his book to Rose's parents. Moreover, Johnson remained close to his "in-laws" after Rose's death. His narrative reflects this voluntary affiliation in the amount of space devoted to the Roses; the narrative thus suggests generous alternatives to the pattern of the unilateral posthumous reaffiliation of gay sons with their families.

Emmanuel Dreuilhe's *Mortal Embrace* (1988) is an even greater anomaly in the personal literature of AIDS; one of only a few autobiographical accounts of living with AIDS, it is the only one I am aware of that is not a conversion narrative. It is not exactly an AIDS narrative, however; it is a series of essays reflecting on AIDS rather than a narrative focused on the author's "case." Aside from occasional references to childhood years in Southeast Asia, a former wife of ten years, and a dead companion, the book offers little in the way of autobiographical disclosure or clinical detail. (Indeed, Dreuilhe characterizes diagnosis as a kind of anticlimax, because the great "collapse" [of his immune system] had occurred without his knowledge [94–95].)

He characterizes his book as a series of still images in the "manner of David Hockney's photographic montages, a complete series of images of the same sickroom: that mental room which now forms the confined universe of people with AIDS, a room we will leave only to die. All those snapshots with overlapping perspectives offer views that vary according to the day and mood . . . because our perception of our own condition is uneven and discontinuous" (5). Its avoidance of narrative serves to neutralize the apparently inherent plot of AIDS; the adoption at times of a first-person-plural point of view helps the book to transcend the individualism of most illness narratives. The book is most idiosyncratic in the degree to which Dreuilhe writes as one member of a large army: a lowly, nearly anonymous foot soldier. The book's unifying trope of AIDS as a war also helps Dreuilhe to justify or explain his lack of a single retrospective viewpoint: "Diseases, like wars, are diffi-

cult in the telling; those actually immersed in the struggle cannot communicate what they feel, especially in the beginning, when they lack all
perspective on what is happening to them—and the others don't know
what they're talking about" (138).

Unlike Monette's and Johnson's memoirs, then, this book is more
concerned with war than with love; indeed, it might as well be entitled
Mortal Combat. As we have seen (Chapter 2), the metaphor of illness as
war has been identified as one potentially hostile to patients' autonomy. What redeems the military metaphor here is that it is adapted by
a person with AIDS who knows exactly what he is doing. In his hands
the metaphor is at once earnest, angry, passionate, and playful; his
book is a resourceful, extended, and even exhilarating riff on a conventional theme. Among other things, then, the book is a literary tour de
force; its intellectual power is such that it revitalizes a tired trope and
puts it to counterhegemonic purposes. (This revival of a dead metaphor
is a death-defying act in more than one sense.)

The adaptation of the figure has a number of effects. To begin with,
while allowing that people with AIDS may be dying, Dreuilhe characterizes them as heroic warriors—much in the fashion of Audre Lorde's
image of one-breasted Amazons in her *Cancer Journals* (1980). The "sickroom"—the liminal zone inhabited by people with AIDS—becomes a
battlefield, a scene of struggle, rather than a site of isolation and invalidity, passivity and despair. Moreover, the trope of people with AIDS
as warriors helps to neutralize the stereotype of homosexuals as effeminate (and unsuitable for the armed forces). Rather than hedonistic,
they are represented as chivalric, disciplined, ascetic, and chaste.

Even more cleverly, Dreuilhe reverses the cold war image of homosexuals as spies and traitors; his warriors are not merely heroes but patriots. Of French background (the book was written in French), Dreuilhe
saturates his book with references to French history and literature. Patriotism is defined first—eccentrically but apparently innocuously—as
loyalty to one's body: "We have grown up in our bodies, they are our
native lands, and although we know their shortcomings by heart, we
have a natural affection for them, warts and all" (9). (It is only natural
that we should fight aggressively to defend them when they are threatened.) Thus he initially compares himself, a guerrilla fighting an in-
vading virus, to a member of the French Resistance.

But his version of patriotism is finally counterhegemonic. Late in the
series of essays Dreuilhe shifts his ground; at this point he defines his
patriotism as specifically homosexual, loyalty to a threatened tribe of
bodies: "The bombed-out ruins of this war aren't just our skeletal bodies, gnawed by worms and parasites, those insatiable vultures, but are
also the domain of gay sexuality" (117). Rather than "straight" nation-

alism, his patriotism assumes an anticolonialist dimension: "More than ever we must refuse to disown our native land, adopted though it may be; we must refuse to betray our friends. If the Afghans can fight fiercely to defend the desert they call home, then we ought also to fight for our beleaguered land, our homosexuality" (125). People with AIDS are transformed from marginal deviants to "true freedom fighters . . . struggling for our homosexual homeland" (137). Thus his trope works to convert a marginal status into a culturally validated one. (Though his strategy is, on one level, deadly serious, it has a playful aspect; certainly, it is self-consciously self-dramatizing, even melodramatizing. At times, indeed, it verges on boot "camp," and he occasionally undercuts his own "bravura kitsch" [150].)

Like much AIDS counterdiscourse, then, Dreuilhe's book is not primarily critical of medical discourse. (If the enemy is HIV, physicians and researchers are on the right side; indeed, Dreuilhe treats them as officers.) Rather, it is critical of hegemonic discourse of AIDS as a stigmatic, invariably fatal, and perhaps deserved disease. The trope of people with AIDS as combatants helps to enhance self-esteem in those infected, who may have internalized prejudicial stereotypes (36). His strategy helps to neutralize the Trojan horse of self-doubt, the idea that homosexuals are their own worst enemy (37). Dreuilhe's use of the war metaphor is calculated, then, to raise morale, to enlist support on the home front. It is also an act of demystification: AIDS is "only" a war (not a divine judgment). Even if his strategy does not slow the virus, it may restore confidence and pride in his nation: "We must cure ourselves, not by turning away from the poisoned well of homosexuality, but by drawing from it new reserves of spiritual strength, merely filtering out the dangers inherent in careless sexual activity" (154–55).

Near the end of the book Dreuilhe acknowledges that his book also has a personal, even selfish, agenda; it is in some way an attempt to save his life. On one level it is a "magical exercise," an act of "verbal exorcism," an attempt to externalize HIV by writing about it and thus cure himself. On a more modest level his book aims to communicate his illness to his readers: "I dream of indoctrinating and enlisting all those who read my words, so that they might save me" (139). Dreuilhe cannot, of course, attest to the book's effect on its readers. But insofar as this non-narrative book has any plot, it may lie in its claim that the act of writing has been an act of self-purification and even beatification (behind Dreuilhe's nomination of himself and his comrades to the status of heroes and patriots lie the conventions of canonization):

Even if I do wind up dying of AIDS, like all the others, I'm no longer afraid of it, because these pages have purified me, given meaning—at least for me—

to these last three years of care, grief, and mourning, a meaning that is intensely personal. I shall have died for a cause, faithful to the last: the acceptance of my strengths and weaknesses, my respect for my own homosexuality and that of others, the celebration of my personality, of the choices I've made, of my love for myself and, through myself, for all humanity. (150)

Like Monette's *Becoming a Man*, although through entirely different means, *Mortal Embrace* equates masculinity with homosexuality, maturity with self-acceptance, even self-celebration.

Instead of trying to purge AIDS discourse of metaphors, to achieve a kind of metaphorical disarmament as Sontag did with breast cancer, Dreuilhe seeks to commandeer metaphor and enlist it on the side of embattled patients. For this reason his is the most deconstructive—at once the most literary and the most political—response (in the form of personal testimony) to the dominant discourse of AIDS and homosexuality.

The Invisible Epidemic

As we have seen, relatively few accounts of AIDS are autobiographical.[26] (The personal literature of AIDS is thus markedly different from those of breast cancer and paralysis, which consist almost entirely of autobiographical narratives.) Instead, most personal narratives take the form of memoirs—relational accounts written from different perspectives tangential to the person with AIDS. Underneath the superficial diversity of perspectives, however, is a good deal of uniformity. For one thing, almost all the narratives concern gay or bisexual men. One consequence of this is that to a large extent AIDS is conflated in these narratives with male homosexuality. What unifies the accounts of their condition, unfortunately, are more or less prejudicial scripts associated with homosexuality. One of these is scripted by the Bible: the story of the Prodigal Son. The narratives of Arterburn and Stribling are modeled quite explicitly on this biblical paradigm, which they fuse with the paradigm of St. Paul's crisis conversion. Still others, without any manifest biblical allusion, use the underlying plot of the return of a straying son or brother.

These I call "narratives of reaffiliation." At best they have the normalizing effect of depicting gay men with AIDS as members of ordinary families. But their construction of AIDS is often conflicted or inconsistent. On the one hand, they are liberal in outlook and usually tolerant of homosexuality; their testimony typically represents conscious resistance to stigmatization. On the other hand, insofar as they collectively depict AIDS as afflicting only homosexuals, they associate it with the Other. The reaffiliation plot often implies, like the conversion narrative paradigm, that the gay family member has strayed into a way of life that is somehow fundamentally deviant. Often, there's something slightly patronizing or presumptuous in their posthumous appropriation of the lives of their gay member; at worst there's something unseemly in the implication that the gay family member may be reaffiliated because he has paid such a terrible price for his difference. And insofar as they portray their gay members as sick and dying, they tend to reinforce a marginalizing view of homosexuality and of AIDS.

Insofar as AIDS narratives have mainly been written by heterosexuals about gay men, the story of AIDS has been told generally from a significant, "safe" distance. (The same is true for deafness—though for different reasons.) Partly because so much AIDS narrative is done at one remove, it is rarely "body" writing. Narratives of AIDS are generally written literally from outside infected bodies. Most of it is not testimony of the experience of being ill. It represents illness secondhand, which is to say that it often misrepresents it. But the generation of so much narrative from a safe remove—and conversion represents one kind of remove from the homosexual body—suggests the powerful obstacles to AIDS autopathography.

The secondhand nature of much AIDS testimony is thus significant, especially given the amount of media attention the AIDS epidemic has received, and given the extensive literary and artistic response to it. Though AIDS is not a gay disease, its effect has been particularly catastrophic in the gay community—so much so that the Holocaust is often invoked as an analogy. At the same time, that community's response has been notably constructive—vital and activist—on a number of levels, social, political, and intellectual. Never before has the discourse of illness been so thoroughly and rigorously subjected to critical analysis, scrutiny, and counterdiscourse. Not coincidentally, gay critics have provided or performed most of this analysis. AIDS coincided with and has greatly stimulated gay studies in the academy and the gay rights movement in the world at large. So at work here is a larger phenomenon in which, on the one hand, AIDS threatens to inscribe stereotypes and prejudice on the bodies of gay men with homophobic vengeance and, on the other, has offered an opportunity for writing—and fighting—back on the part of a threatened and mobilized community.

As Cindy Patton has pointed out, "Every gay person can tell you this: our bodies are written by science. From at least the mid-nineteenth century we were scrutinized for visible differences—first our genitals, then our desires, our hormones, our genes, our perceptual apparatus, our moral capacity" (129–30). And especially in the early years of scientific investigation, as Patton notes, research depended on the cooperation and testimony of the gay population:

In the first few years of the epidemic . . . people living with AIDS spoke often and well into the black hole created by the refusal of the mainstream press to report on the epidemic. Science needed the speech of people with AIDS and their friends in order to unlock the "mystery" of AIDS—a Nobel-prize winning task. Many men (and some women) willingly gave evidence of their illness and of their lives, describing symptoms and answering long epidemiological questionnaires about the intimate details of rich and complex sex lives. But once science had its information it could no longer tolerate the speech of people living with AIDS. People living with AIDS wanted some information back: When would a cure come? What would the treatment be? What would it cost? But once the disease had been wrested out of the discourses of people living with AIDS, once HIV was discovered and could be made to perform in the laboratory without homosexual bodies, science no longer wanted to hear that discourse. (130)

As Patton goes on to say, the gay community did speak back in various media against the mainstream media. But as late as the mid-1990s written personal narrative has not played a major role in this; perhaps it does not seem the most urgent and accessible of media. At this point in the epidemic a survey of available book-length narratives of HIV and AIDS suggests that personal narrative is a site of contestation. For one thing, just as AIDS memoirs outnumber AIDS autobiographies, heterosexual writers' accounts of gay AIDS outnumber gay ones. The division between the sexual orientation of the typical narrator and that of the typical person with AIDS turns out to be significant. Far fewer gay-affirmative personal narratives of HIV and AIDS exist than one might think. Even the story of gay AIDS, then, has only begun to be narrated from the autobiographical point of view.

Despite high and in some cases rising infection rates, the story of AIDS in other minority communities—the African American community, for instance—has not even begun to be witnessed in personal narrative at all.[27] As with other illnesses the cases that get narrated are almost inevitably and intrinsically *not* representative of the majority. For one thing, only a statistically tiny fraction of cases gets committed to writing, let alone published. For another, those who narrate their illnesses, or have them narrated by companions or relatives, are generally not representative of the general population. They are typically upper-middle class—professionals by occupation—and thereby endowed with various assets and advantages—not least, adequate health insurance and competent, if not solicitous, medical care. Thus they tend intrinsically to be *best*-case scenarios. Their narratives, then, tend to underplay, if not to ignore completely, issues of money, insurance, transportation, housing, and transacting the business of paying bills and filing forms. This dichotomy between the typical case and those represented in print is perhaps truer of AIDS narratives than those of many other diseases, for two of the most heavily afflicted groups—gay men and intravenous drug users—tend to have different demographic profiles. As we have seen, AIDS among gay men has often been represented—though rarely autobiographically; AIDS among intravenous drug users has not been represented, as far as I know, in a book-length narrative. The moderating effect of income on AIDS is a great advantage in terms of longevity and quality of life. So although autobiography may be a democratic medium, and illness may be a universal experience, autobiographies of illness do not necessarily tell typical tales.

Their lack of typicality is significant and instructive. Whatever their virtues as individual narrative, the books surveyed here collectively serve to confine AIDS to the homosexual community—and to describe its role there variously. What is left out is the emerging demography of AIDS—its spread among the urban poor and its spread in other segments of the population. Thus the lags at work here are important—the chronological lag between transmission of the virus and awareness of that spread, so that our knowledge of HIV demography is always out of date, and the cultural lag or slippage between the manifestation of the virus in individuals and the surfacing of their stories in print (or other media). As a result, the gallery of people with HIV/AIDS in this chapter is in some ways entirely misleading. (Even Abraham Verghese's fine *My Own Country* [1994] is concerned almost entirely with gay AIDS patients.) There is, of course, danger in associating AIDS with the urban poor, another marginalized group, like homosexuals, only less vocal and powerful:

The danger is that preoccupation with the epidemic will diminish because of general disdain for problems of the poor or because of an ill-founded belief that the wall between the urban poor and the rest of society is less permeable than the wall between those who are bisexual or gay and those who are not. As fear recedes, the pressure for public education is likely to diminish as well. AIDS may once again become less about the conduct of all of us and more about public policy toward an already submerged class, one that is largely minority and largely outside the sympathies of the wider society. (Price 1989, 3)

Some books have begun to suggest the scope of AIDS in a cross-section of the population: "compilation narratives" (for example, George Whitmore's *Someone Was Here: Profiles in the AIDS Epidemic* [1988] and Steven Petrow's *Dancing Against the Darkness: A Journey Through America in the Age of AIDS* [1990]). In addition, testimony issues from the standpoint of the unrelated caregiver. As a genre, however, such works are vulnerable to the criticisms leveled against photographic surveys.

They may tend to de-individualize because they offer only vignettes of a number of cases; indeed, they tend to portray their subjects *as* cases. They may focus on particularly dire instances—late-stage AIDS. (Certainly, the quotient of unpleasant physical symptoms is much higher in compilations than in other narratives.) Still, these books are a beginning. And other media will obviously have to supplement written personal narratives.[28] But the stories of gay men need to be supplemented with those of a population more representative of those now infected with HIV. The proliferation of individualizing narratives has the potential to demystify the illness.

As we saw at the start of the chapter, dominant cultural narratives tend to write off people with HIV/AIDS. If they are already members of marginal groups, their viral status merely confirms it; if they are not, it tends to confer marginal status. They are written off to the periphery where they will contaminate no one—considered doomed, consigned to a living hell. Life writing about AIDS has the potential to contest that process; it is well underway, but much needs to be done. If "Silence = Death," testifying equals life.

Notes

1. On a larger scale, the statistical charting of the incidence of AIDS is also greatly complicated by the construction of the illness. A single decision may re-define thousands of cases into existence. Since issuing its initial "surveillance definition" of AIDS in 1982, the CDC (Centers for Disease Control and Prevention) has refined or revised the definition in 1985, 1987, and 1993. The changing definition of AIDS—which has become more inclusive over the years to recognize the varied manifestations of HIV infection in women, children, and intravenous drug users, for example—may suddenly and drastically alter the tally of those infected. Thus issues that might seem to be cut-and-dried matters of "fact"—such as the rate of infection, mortality rate, and survival times—are not at all simple to determine. For instance, the addition of a low T-cell count to the CDC criteria for AIDS in 1993 had the effect of lengthening survival times, because the diagnosis of AIDS could then be made before an initial opportunistic infection (Osmond 1.1-2–1.1-3).

2. According to the CDC, "AIDS deaths [in the U.S.] in the first half of 1996 were down 13 percent from the first half of 1995." The decrease among whites was 21 percent, whereas it was only 10 percent among Hispanics and 2 percent among blacks; deaths among men declined 15 percent, whereas deaths among women rose by 3 percent. The decline in deaths means that more people than ever are living with AIDS in the United States (223,000adolescents and adults, an increase of 10 percent since mid-1995 and an increase of 65 percent from 1993) (Painter 1A).

3. "Magic" Johnson's resumption of his career as a professional basketball player in early 1996, after a four-year retirement, may constitute a watershed in HIV/AIDS awareness. His return to the strenuous life of a pro basketball player should powerfully illustrate that HIV-infected people are not necessarily ill.

4. AIDS is typically marked on the body by its wasting syndrome and sometimes, in addition, by the lesions of Kaposi's sarcoma.

5. As this chapter will demonstrate, even quite sympathetic narratives of people with AIDS often characterize them as impulsive and self-indulgent—profligate.

6. See note 3, chapter 1, on the distinction between *autobiography* and *memoir.*

7. A notable early exception is Chandler, "Voices from the Front." Steven F. Kruger's *AIDS Narratives* (1996) came to my attention too late to be considered.

8. The insistence on being called not *victims* or even *patients* but *people with AIDS*—or people *living* with AIDS—seems to many a matter of denial, self-delusion, or political correctness, but these terms are significantly different ways of representing—relating to—people with AIDS. Some terms stigmatize and marginalize, others individualize and humanize.

9. On gay death notices see Harris's 1992 essay, "On Reading the Obituaries in the *Bay Area Reporter.*"

10. According to the "Hot Type" section of the *Chronicle of Higher Education*, a Vanderbilt University pathologist, Dr. Mahlon Johnson, who was infected with HIV during an autopsy, will publish a book in which he claims that his seropositivity has been reversed. The working title is *Working on a Miracle*; the publisher is Bantam. Although Dr. Johnson was never diagnosed with AIDS, the seven-figure sum reportedly paid by a mass-market publisher suggests the marketability of a "restitution story" associated with HIV.

11. Much of Ashe's book reads like an exemplary autobiography of his post-athletic career that he might have written had he not contracted HIV; nevertheless, the book we have is very much determined—perhaps overdetermined—by his illness.

12. The book's illustrations, however, are mainly "official" photos—studio portraits, pictures with co-stars, and the like. They include almost no snapshots; only one of Hudson's lovers appears, and that is his publicist and personal manager, who was reconciled with Hudson when he was ill and who no doubt helped to control the book's image of him. Ironically, their professional relationship had made it possible for them to travel together without raising eyebrows.

13. Revealingly, Ashe distinguishes sharply between his illness and his race in this respect: "Race is a more onerous burden than AIDS. My disease is the result of biological factors over which we, thus far, have no control. Racism, however, is entirely made by people, and therefore it hurts and inconveniences infinitely more" (126–27).

14. In fact, Fisher did not have AIDS when she spoke in Houston or wrote her memoir. Most of the time, however, she is careful to observe the distinction be-

tween HIV positivity and AIDS; thus in her epilogue she speaks of being "on the road to AIDS" (277).

15. At times Arterburn's narrative approaches an allegorical style—rather like certain scenes in Frederick Douglass's 1845 *Narrative*, where the dialogue and characters' names seem to carry transparent thematic significance. Thus Arterburn's "fall" begins when he visits a gay disco with a female friend. Returning to retrieve his Mastercard, which he "absent-mindedly" left there, he runs into a friend (named Randy) who asks, "What the *hell* are you doing here in this place?" (emphasis added.) Arterburn adds: "I had no idea just how appropriate his question was. It was hell, disguised as the most exciting place on earth" (83).

16. Arterburn's parents do not in any way respond to his accusations. His mother's foreword stresses his redeemed status while confessing confusion over how he might have become gay. As if in denial, they characterize him as having "returned" to a healthy family.

17. Jerry Arterburn's *How Shall I Tell My Mother?* does involve a collaboration between an ill man and his brother, but the brother, Steve Arterburn, is not the narrator.

18. Conscious of this, Wiltshire chose the diary as her medium in part because of its intrinsic provisionality:

> Another motive compelled me to tell of our struggle with this disease on a daily basis. I imagined myself writing not for me alone or even for John, but for every brother and sister who has a sibling with AIDS. I realized that if I waited until after John's death and recalled the past retrospectively, I could not avoid casting over it a mantle of coherence and an aura of understanding that it did not have for me at the time. And my companion sojourner siblings would know it was not true. (66)

She adds, "The only significant change I have made from my journal entries is the ineffably sad one of turning the verbs from the present tense into the past" (67).

19. She also relates it to the traditionally female art of quilting, which she characterizes in terms pertinent to the AIDS Quilt itself: "Quilts are formed from many pieces cut from other fabrics, but they are not whole cloth. They are a purposeful rearrangement of the scraps at hand. They are also a form of art that offers warmth and comfort" (150).

20. John Ford had his own revisionist narrative in the works—a novel about the "extensive gay network inside the Reagan administration, its ties with the thousands of gays in staff offices on the Hill, and how the two groups worked together, often on a non-partisan basis. The more personal side of the story was what happened—and what did not happen and should have—when AIDS came" (122). Although Wiltshire introduced him to a literary agent, Ford apparently never finished the book.

21. *My Name Is Mary*, discussed earlier in this chapter, represents a significant departure from the narratives of Pearson and Cox, for Fisher writes as a woman not only married to but infected by a man with HIV. The effect of

Fisher's infection is to make her, not her husband, the protagonist of the narrative and her book a full-life autobiography rather than a memoir of her marriage. Janice A. Burns's *Sarah's Song* (1995), which came to my attention too late for consideration, tells the story of her life with her husband, William Burns. He contracted HIV in an earlier relationship, she contracted it from him; both died of AIDS.

22. Brad seems not to have authorized the publication of his journals; apparently, his father did not conceive of publishing a book about Brad while Brad was still alive. But Schow may have found some warrant in a journal passage in which Brad declares his wish that his parents would read it without his permission, because it might ease his coming out to them.

23. Mark Doty's *Heaven's Coast* (1996) makes an instructive comparison here. Doty's book is strong on compensation; it concludes with a chapter summarizing the year following the death of his partner, Wally Roberts, and an epilogue entitled "Consolations." Moreover, it opens with a long meditation ("Coastal Studies") on Roberts's absence from Doty's life. The unifying trope, derived from Provincetown environs (and reminiscent of Thoreau's characterization of Cape Cod as an eternal frontier), is that of earth as "heaven's coast"; although mortals are confined to the shore, Doty suggests, bereavement offers glimpses of another dimension. This introduction gives way to a chronological narrative of the intrusion of AIDS into Roberts and Doty's life together. Thus, although the book is particularly invested in spirituality and compensation, it does not blink the realities of AIDS; indeed, putting the meditation before the narrative suggests that only when Doty had some healing perspective on Roberts's death could he undertake the painful but ultimately therapeutic task of telling their story.

24. For another perspective on *Borrowed Time*, see Hawkins, pp. 72–73 and 148–49.

25. For a more sustained analysis of Monette's books, to which mine is indebted, see Newtown.

26. This is beginning to change. Two recent additions to the autobiographical literature of AIDS are *This Wild Darkness: The Story of My Death* (1996) by the writer Harold Brodkey, and *Life Is Not a Rehearsal: A Memoir* (1997), by the conservative Boston talk-show host David Brudnoy.

27. According to Hanna Rosin, for example, "Blacks, 12 percent of the population, account for one-third of all AIDS cases. Three out of five new AIDS victims now are black, up from one in five in 1986. Black women are now fifteen times more likely to have AIDS than white women, and their children, eighteen times more likely" (1995, 21). And, according to Ann Louise Bardach, "Currently, blacks and Latinas make up 77 percent of all AIDS cases among women; the number of Latina cases is seven times higher than that of Anglo women" (1995, 30). Finally, according to Monroe E. Price, "Nine out of ten children who died in 1987 of AIDS in New York were minority children" (1989, 65). According to Painter, of new cases in 1996, 41 percent were among blacks, 38 percent

among whites, and 19 percent among Hispanics. Clearly, the *full* story of AIDS has not yet begun to be told in personal narrative; given these demographics, it may never be.

28. For a discussion of film as an interactive medium for AIDS narrative, see Egan's 1994 discussion of the film *Silverlake Life*.

5

Crossing (Out) the Border
Autobiography and Physical Disability

> Others resent [us] for this reason. We are subverters of an American ideal. . . . The disabled serve as constant, visible reminders to the able-bodied that the society they live in is shot through with inequity and suffering, that they live in a counterfeit paradise, that they too are vulnerable. We represent a fearsome possibility.
>
> —Robert Murphy, *The Body Silent*, 1987, pp. 116–17.
>
> Unless we die suddenly, we are all disabled eventually.
>
> —Susan Wendell, "Toward a Feminist Theory," 1992, p. 66.

Disabling Discourse

As a physical and existential condition disability is both related to and distinct from illness. The two are often related causally—illness may cause disability and vice versa—yet the two conditions are different conceptual entities. The common sense of the difference is that illness is temporary and can be moderated by treatment, if not cured, whereas disability is permanent and can only be moderated by rehabilitation. A more important difference for my purposes is that whereas most illnesses are not stigmatic, disability is, almost by definition; to use Erving Goffman's term, "spoiled identity" is ascribed to people with disabilities—as it is to people with cancer and HIV/AIDS. Society commonly considers disabled people the embodiment of trauma, personal disaster, or failure; ignoring the profound ways in which we are all interdependent, Western culture's individualism stigmatizes or blames those who fail to be "self-sufficient" (Connors 97). Thus people may shun disability as though it were contagious. Behind such a construction of disability are powerful—because unconsciously held—attitudes toward the body: "Our culture idealizes the body and demands that we control it. Thus, although most people will be disabled at some time in their lives, the disabled are made 'the other,' who symbolize failure of control and the threat of pain, limitation, dependency, and death" (Wendell 63).

Despite the stigma attached to it, the boundaries of disability are indistinct because of disagreement over what counts as disability and because disability can take so many forms. Some impairments are matters of physical form or appearance, some of function; some are stable, some "progressive"; some are congenital, some "acquired" or adventitious; some are severe, some moderate; some are obvious, some hidden, and so on. Disability is not marked on the body in the same ways as sex or race; indeed, it may not be marked on the body at all. Moreover, unlike most marginalizations "disability is the one minority group that anyone can join at any time, as a result of a sudden automobile accident, a fall . . . , cancer, or disease. Fewer than 15% of disabled Americans were born with their disabilities. . . . And since disability catches up with most of us in old age, it is a minority that we all, if we live long enough, join" (Shapiro 7–8).[1] Part of what makes disability so threatening to the nondisabled, then, may be precisely the indistinctness and permeability of its boundaries; the border is patrolled vigilantly by "normals" more out of fear that they may stray over it than out of fear of transgression by those on the other side.

The role of modern medicine in the construction of disability is crucial and complex. Twentieth-century advances in medical technology have made it possible for people to survive accidents and illnesses with impairments that would have killed them in earlier eras; thus modern medicine has quite literally created new groups of disabled people. Thanks to antibiotics and catheters, for example, spinal cord injury is far less often fatal than it was early in the century. (There were virtually no paralyzed veterans of World War I, but large numbers of wounded soldiers survived World War II and subsequent wars as paraplegics and quadriplegics.[2]) The medicalization of modern life has also created new diagnostic categories that are tantamount to new disabilities—for example, conditions like attention deficit disorder. Moreover, developments in medical technology enhance the functioning of people with various impairments to a degree that was unimaginable even fifty years ago. Thus modern medicine has at once increased the numbers, life expectancy, and quality of life of *disabled* people.[3]

Such developments are a function of a paradigm that regards disability as residing in some physical abnormality of the individual body and the role of medicine as analyzing, correcting, or compensating for that dysfunction (Connors 100–102). Ironically, however, people with disabilities, many of them beneficiaries of the medical paradigm, have begun to point out its limitations. As Rosemarie Garland Thomson has noted, although

medicalization in certain contexts has a role in managing some disabilities, it easily slips into paternalism, echoes stereotypes of dependence, and/or reinforces the sick role for disabled people. By contrast . . . a more politicized discourse is now emerging which interprets disability according to a "minority model," locating the major disadvantage of disability in prejudicial social attitudes and exclusionary institutions rather than in bodies that have traditionally been cast as aberrant markers of inherent inferiority and personal misfortune. . . .

Academic theorists . . . are currently interrogating the prevailing interpretation of disability as corporeal inferiority, recasting it instead as another form of embodied difference which, like race and gender, has traditionally been interpreted as inadequacy. ("Redrawing" 584)

In this political paradigm disability is a dysfunction not of the individual body but of the body politic.

Perhaps because their conditions—though various—tend to be chronic and marginalizing, people with disabilities have become politically organized and active. Indeed, we are in the midst of a historic movement for disability rights. In the last few decades people with disabilities have been increasing in visibility, independence, assertiveness, and political power—as well as in numbers. The increasing politicization of disabled people has to do less with sheer numbers than with changing consciousness. Although each has had its particular impetuses, the disability rights movement ranks with other civil rights movements—including the women's movement and the gay liberation movement—as major mobilizations of marginalized groups in the late twentieth century.

According to Joseph P. Shapiro, "Like homosexuals in the early 1970s, many disabled people are rejecting the 'stigma' that there is something sad or to be ashamed of in their condition. They are taking pride in their identity as disabled people, parading it instead of closeting it. This simple but iconoclastic thinking—that a disability, of itself, is not tragic or pitiable—is at the core of the new disability rights movement" (Shapiro 1993, 20). The passage of federal legislation mandating the end of institutional discrimination has punctuated the movement for disability rights as a civil rights movement. But like other such social movements, it has depended not just on pragmatic mobilization but also on "theory"—the analysis and deconstruction of discriminatory or marginalizing cultural hierarchies. Insofar as one element of the oppressive culture is discursive—the ways in which the disabled are talked about, written about, portrayed in electronic media—one response to marginalization by disabled people (like other marginalized groups) has been to challenge the prevailing terminology.

Much fun has been made of euphemistic terms like *differently abled* or *physically challenged*,[4] but the basis of discursive reform involves two significant distinctions. The first is between bodily impairments and social and cultural environments; the second is between the "individual model" and the "social model" of disability. According to Michael Oliver, the individual model of disability

locates the "problem" of disability within the individual and . . . it sees the causes of this problem as stemming from the functional limitations or psychological losses which are assumed to arise from disability. These two points are underpinned by what might be called "the personal tragedy theory of disability" which suggests that disability is some terrible chance event which occurs at random to unfortunate individuals. . . .

The genesis, development and articulation of the social model of disability by disabled people themselves is a rejection of all of these fundamentals. It does not deny the problem of disability but locates it squarely within society. It is not individual limitations, of whatever kind, which are the cause of the problem but society's failure to provide appropriate services and adequately ensure the needs of disabled people are fully taken into account in its social organization.

Hence disability, according to the social model, is all the things that impose restrictions on disabled people; ranging from individual prejudice to institutional discrimination, from inaccessible buildings to unusable transport systems, from segregated education to excluding work arrangements, and so on. Further, the consequences of this failure do not simply and randomly fall on individuals but systematically upon disabled people as a group who experience this failure as discrimination institutionalised throughout society. (1996, 32–33)

At times, then, the "cultural construction" of disability can be quite literal—as when the physical environment is built in a way that restricts those who use wheelchairs. (Such individuals are not confined *to*, but confined *by*, wheelchairs—or rather by the lack of curb cuts, elevators, and ramps available to them.) The critical distinction, then, is between the impaired body and its cultural site, for it is the latter that creates *disability*. Individuals with disabilities are handicapped or disabled by a physical environment that disadvantages them and a culture that excludes or stigmatizes them. (The physical exclusion from public life is consistent with their discursive erasure.) Although these terms may seem counterintuitive—to my ear *disabled* still sounds unduly absolute—their crucial counterdiscursive effect is to displace the "problem" of disability from impaired bodies to an unresponsive culture.

Autobiography: Enabling Discourse

Western culture, whether high or low, has not generally been kind in its representation of disability; literature often epitomizes disability as physical deformity and associates it with corruption, perversion, and obsession. Canonical secular literature provides demonic cripples such as Richard III and Ahab. In the Old Testament being blind, deaf, crippled, sick, or diseased is a sign of having done something to incur God's disfavor; sin brings on disability. The New Testament characterizes people with disabilities as cursed or possessed by evil (Shapiro 30). (The persistence of these attitudes underlies faith healing even today.) As Paul Longmore has observed, the conflation of deformity with evil expresses in a kind of shorthand a whole complex of unconscious attitudes about disability:

Giving disabilities to villainous characters reflects and reinforces, albeit in exaggerated fashion, three common prejudices against handicapped people: disability is a punishment for evil; disabled people are embittered by their "fate"; disabled people resent the nondisabled and would, if they could, destroy them. In historical and contemporary social fact, it is, of course, nondisabled people who have at times endeavored to destroy people with disabilities. As with popular portrayals of other minorities, the unacknowledged hostile fantasies of the stigmatizers are transferred to the stigmatized. The nondisabled audience is allowed to disown its fears and biases by "blaming the victims," making them responsible for their own ostracism and destruction. (67–68)

Of course, not all literary media are equally likely to stereotype and stigmatize disabled people. As a medium historically accessible to minorities of various sorts autobiography has significant potential for challenging the hegemonic discourse of disability. The British photographer David Hevey implies this in his 1992 analysis of the way in which his medium has traditionally reinforced the marginalization of disabled people: "Disabled people, like black people/people of colour, women, and so on, are aware that their bodies are constructed as the site of oppression. . . . In my experience of being a disability photographer, disabled people need space to tell the story, the journey, of their body and in doing so, reclaim and be proud of themselves" (117–18). Hevey attempts to position and represent his subjects in a way that calls into question the conventional portrayal of people with disabilities as passive and pathetic. But as his remarks imply, autobiography—which by definition involves *self*-representation—is potentially, at least, a more promising medium than photography in which to challenge the discourse of disability.

According to Robert Murphy, "The major goal of the handicapped movement is not to foster dependency, but to move the disabled into the mainstream of society as autonomous individuals. . . . The handicapped individual first must fight all his own impulses to flee back inside himself, to wrap himself in the mantle of his own impairment. He must overcome a sense of inferiority, he must break out of isolation, he must reach out to a world that does not welcome him" (1987, 158–59). Among literary genres, autobiography is particularly well suited for this endeavor. Because print, unlike photography, effectively masks the body, autobiography serves to deflect the gaze from a body that might otherwise trigger stereotypical responses. It thus removes one impediment to interaction in everyday life—which may remain an obstacle in film, video, and photography.[5] As a verbal rather than visual form, writing may offer a kind of neutral space for self-presentation and the renegotiation of status. Moreover, insofar as autobiography is the literary expression of the self-determined life, the genre that may be said to embody personal autonomy, it seems the ideal mode for contesting the association of disability with dependence. Writing autobiography, preferably without assistance, may enable individuals with disabilities to cross back over the border into the mainstream or, better yet, to cross out—or at least blur—that border.

According to Rosemarie Garland Thomson, Toni Morrison's disabled characters "deny the norm of the dominant culture . . . and create their own perspective, a kind of alternative psychological and physical order of self-authorized empowerment and dignity . . . a revised social order, one in which the hierarchies of value, the rules that define norms, and the processes of stigmatization have been rewritten" ("Speaking" 245). There is much to be said for counterdiscursive portrayals of disabled characters in fiction by nondisabled novelists, but disabled individuals may have more to gain by self-representation in autobiography. Autobiography, however, has its generic constraints. One is that it is generally regarded, poststructuralism to the contrary notwithstanding, as a species of nonfiction, a referential art that, to use Paul John Eakin's evocative phrase, "touches the world." Characters and narrators in autobiography are ontologically different from those in fiction, and the conventions of the form reflect this. The autobiographer does not have the same latitude as the novelist—certainly not that of the mythical novelist like Morrison—in constructing a world. Norms of realism generally govern autobiography, which is to say that the laws of nature and culture dominate the world of autobiography.

Autobiography involves a much more fundamental problem of self-representation for individuals with disabilities: that their impairments may impede or even preclude the writing of a such a narrative—at least without assistance.[6] In cases of severe impairment living a life may be hard enough; writing a life may prove impossible. The physical process may be too arduous to seem worth it. And getting a life published presents other obstacles. Although autobiography may be in theory the most democratic of genres, it is in practice not open to all. Historically, access to autobiography has required preexisting distinction—success or celebrity—and those have been parceled out unequally. Serious disability, especially if incurred early in life, may obstruct or preclude "normal" life—work or career, marriage or partnership, bearing and raising children—let alone the sorts of distinction that autobiography has traditionally required. The situation of disabled individuals is that their most obvious "distinction" is one that may disqualify them as autobiographers—unless it can somehow be made the focus for the book, the hook for the reader. But if the disability becomes the whole subject of the story, there is some risk of reducing autobiography to case study—reifying disability and thus reinforcing marginalization.[7]

By comparison, illness—at least acute illness—is relatively conducive to autobiography. It is a more universal experience and thus easier for readers to identify with. And whereas some illness narratives have a built-in audience of those at risk—for example, narratives of breast cancer—most impairments are not perceived in quite the same way. If they are associated with "birth defects," they don't threaten those who don't already have them; if they are caused by accidents, like much paralysis, their seeming randomness insulates potential readers. Moreover, there is the problem of the generic convention of the comic master plot. As we have seen, autobiographical narratives of illness have comic plots almost by definition: those who tell stories of illness have lived to tell them, and although not always cured, they generally write from the perspective of some sort of recovery or healing. Many disabilities are chronic and do not admit of cure or complete recovery. So it may be more difficult in the case of disability to find a vantage point for narrative, a safe distance from an ongoing and sometimes consuming condition. A comic plot may seem entirely inconsistent with the lives of those whose master status is permanent disability. Indeed, if chronic physical impairment—for example, paralysis—is perceived as stasis, it may seem incompatible with plot of any type—and thus seem unnarratable.

Given the pervasive stereotyping in popular culture of disabled individuals as monsters, criminals, and sexual deviants, we have much to gain from simple matter-of-fact accounts of what Irving Zola has called "ordinary lives" of people with disabilities. But the preference, expectation, or demand for triumphal plots will effectively silence many potential autobiographers. We are left with the paradox that those individuals with disabilities who represent themselves in autobiography may not in fact be very representative—in other words, typical—of those with disabilities.[8] Nor will various impairments be represented in proportion to their numbers. For various reasons disability is most frequently represented in the form of manifest physical disability, especially paralysis. Paralysis bids to become the paradigmatic form of physical disability, I suppose, because of its obviousness, extremity, and apparent intractability. At the same time, because it may so dramatically threaten one's sense of integrity and may so radically rupture one's sense of autobiographical continuity, it seems to call for compensatory or therapeutic narration.

Consider the testimony of Arnold Beisser, whose illness-related paralysis confined him to an iron lung shortly after World War II:

Suddenly there were great changes inside my skin, and what had been so familiar now became alien. What I called myself, my "I," resided inside a body, a space-occupying mass that had been so familiar to me that it required no thought. Beyond my skin boundary was the outside world. Inside was me.

But my body, which I had called myself, had changed dramatically from autonomous to dependent, from strong to weak, from rapidly moving to completely immobile. I had to rely on others for even my most elemental functions and activities. My spatial existence seemed more like that of a sack of flour than a human being. (1989, 21)

Beisser's paralysis profoundly alienated him from his body and thus himself. It is only by reference to his ongoing interior autobiography that he assures himself of his self-identity: "In spite of all this, I paradoxically continued to think of myself as the same person I had been. . . . The personal experiences that had formed my identity and history still lived in my mind. So it seemed to me that *I must* be the same person" (20).

Paralysis may have become the paradigmatic condition of disability not just because of its severe threat to selfhood, but also for gender-related reasons. Given that disabled women outnumber disabled men, the prominence of published narratives of male paralysis says much about the gendering of disability. One common gender pattern is the paralysis of young men from injuries in high-risk activities—like war and violent sports. These sudden accidental disabilities incurred by virile young men—soldiers and athletes—get more than their share of media attention. (Although he is no longer young, the identification of actor Christopher Reeve with the role of Superman makes his case a particularly interesting example here.[9])

Certainly, the need to use a wheelchair literally lowers a person's stature (and implicitly status), and the apparent uselessness of the lower body implies a lack of potency, sexual and otherwise (whereas in fact male and female paraplegics are quite capable of having children). A patriarchal culture may consider these deficits more costly, more tragic, when incurred by men. Indeed, according to Michelle Fine and Adrienne Asch,

Having a disability [is] seen as synonymous with being dependent, childlike, and helpless—an image fundamentally challenging all that is embodied in the ideal male: virility, autonomy, and independence. Yet this image replicates, if in caricature, all that is embodied in the ideal female: emotionality, passivity, and dependence. Concerns with "emasculation" may promote efforts directed toward those at the locus of the *masculinity/dependence* contradiction, not toward those at the redundant intersection of *femininity* and *dependence*. Certainly the social imperative seems to have been to study and rehabilitate the "wounded male." (3)

The prominence of male accounts of paralysis, then, may have much to do with the association of paralysis with emasculation, even feminization. The story of the disabled male is privileged because of the semiotic clash between the modifier and the noun, whereas the story of the disabled woman is ignored because of its apparent redundancy.

Like the story of illness, however, the story of impairment is narratable only when it can assume a comic plot. When impairment deprives someone of the appearance of autonomy and potency, that person's story is unwritable and unreadable unless and until he or she can claim some compensatory power and freedom. In a patriarchy, of course, such compensations are more available to men than to women. This helps to explain some of the lack of diversity in those who have narrated their physical disability. Although those who work with their minds are generally more likely to write autobiography than those who work with their bodies, this may be especially so among people with disabilities, for the vocations—and thus the self-respect—of professionals are more likely to survive their disability. The authors of the narratives discussed in this chapter are not very diverse in race, gender, or class; they are mostly white male professionals. As such, they were well positioned to become or remain economically viable despite their impairment; their intellectual power was able to compensate for their loss of physical power and control of their lower bodies. One significant pattern in their accounts is the redemptive shifting of emphasis from the body to the mind. Self-rehabilitation involves in large part redefining the self as more a function of mind and spirit than of the flesh. (Which is to say that it reinforces the cultural identification of men with the mind, women with the body, and the privileging of mind over body.)

Disability generally does not impose the sort of narrative scripts or plots that illnesses often do. At the same time and for the same reason—because it seems to connote statis—disability may seem to defy narrative because it offers little hope of a comic resolution, little prospect for closure in the form of physical recovery. It should come as no surprise, then, that one generic convention that crops up in various forms of disability autobiography is that of the conversion narrative. Consistent with the necessary shift of male generativity from body to mind, the generic formula of conversion also provides a narrative of restitution where none would seem possible.[10]

Disability and Spiritual Autobiography: The Paradigm of Conversion

> The Trope of the Fall: Oliver Sacks, *A Leg to Stand On* (1984);
> Leonard Kriegel, *Falling into Life* (1991)

In many ways *A Leg to Stand On* is an extraordinary narrative, gripping in its account of a solo hiking accident, vivid in its description of the strange (and estranging) deadness of the author's injured leg as a result of his fall. The book reflects thoughtfully on the complex relation between the mind and the body as Oliver Sacks explores the gulf between the outward appearance of his body and his subjective sense of being a single amputee. Nowhere have I read a more compelling description of what it feels like to be paralyzed—or, perhaps I should say, what it *doesn't* feel like, for part of Sacks's achievement is to communicate the paradoxical feeling of paralysis—the sense of senselessness, the alienating effect of the lack of feedback from his numb leg.

> I had imagined my injury (a severe but uncomplicated wound to the muscles and nerves of one leg) to be straightforward and routine, and I was astonished at the profundity of the effects it had: a sort of paralysis and alienation of the leg, reducing it to an "object" which seemed unrelated to me; an abyss of bizarre, and even terrifying, effects. I had no idea what to make of these effects and entertained fears that I might never recover. I found the abyss a horror, and recovery a wonder; and I have since had a deeper sense of the horror and wonder which lurk behind life and which are concealed, as it were, behind the usual surface of health. (13–14)

Sacks powerfully conveys how devastating any loss of control over one's body can be; coinciding with and ironically reinforcing his experience of paralysis is the experience of being assured by a specialist that nothing is wrong with his leg. Such overruling of his subjectivity "took away a foothold, the human foothold, I so desperately needed. Now, doubly, I had no leg to stand on; unsupported, doubly, I entered nothingness and Limbo" (108). In casually denying Sacks's reality, this physician reified Sacks's passivity as a patient, his dependence on the validation of his experience by medical authority.

Despite its explicit critique of such medical arrogance and of the neurology that underlies it, despite its vivid glimpse into the condition of paralysis, in the final analysis Sacks's book fails to reckon with, much less to counter, the stigmatization that accompanies disability. One contributing factor in his failure is the outcome of his case; because Sacks's paralysis proved only temporary, he speaks about disability from a position of restored function and status—all the more grateful for them as a result of their temporary loss. Unlike most of the books to be discussed later, then, his is a single-experience narrative written from the safe side of the border between disability and "normality." Whatever his intentions in this book, his brush with disability seems to have led him unconsciously to distance himself from a condition he found thoroughly alien and threatening.

One literary manifestation of this is his characterization of disablement using terms like *abyss, horror,* and *lurk* in the passage quoted earlier. Here and throughout his book Sacks relies on the lexicon and the rhetoric of the Gothic and the grotesque. Fantastic Gothic images appear, for example, in Sacks's anxious anticipation of the unbandaging of his "dead" leg in the casting room after surgery: "The rumbling of the stretcher-trolley seemed monstrously loud, and kept suggesting to me the roll of tumbrels, the sense of being taken to my death—or something worse than death: to the realization of an abominable nightmare, where all my fantasies of the uncanny, the unalive, the unreal, would turn out true" (121).

An even more significant formal manifestation of his self-protective distancing from disability is his use of the conversion paradigm with its radically dichotomous states. Thus his account of his mysterious recovery suggests that it is, quite literally, miraculous: "I was present, it is true, but only as an observer—a mere spectator at a primordial event, or 'Big Bang,' which was the start of inner space, the microcosm, in me. . . . A true miracle was being enacted before me, within me. Out of nothingness, out of chaos, measure was being made. . . . My soul was transfixed in a rapture of wonder" (140–41). Suddenly, somehow, he "remembers" how to walk, and the activity returns from conscious to unconscious control: "There was an abrupt and absolute leap at this moment—not a process, not a transition, but a transilience—from the awkward, artificial, mechanical walking, of which every step had to be consciously counted, projected, and undertaken—to an unconscious, natural-graceful, musical movement" (145).

Sacks uses explicitly religious terms to describe the return of this facility and the accompanying sense of corporeal integrity and wholeness:

The reality of my leg, and the power to stand and walk again, had been given to me, had descended upon me like grace. Now, re-united with my leg—with a part of myself that had been excommunicated, in Limbo—I found myself full of tender regard for it, and stroked the cast. (147)

What came, what announced itself, so palpably, so gloriously, was a full-bodied vital feeling and action, originating from an aboriginal, commanding, will-

ing, "I." . . . Grace entered, as Grace enters, at the very center of things, at its
hidden innermost inaccessible center, and instantly coordinated, subordinated,
all phenomena to itself. It made the next move obvious, certain, natural. . . .
Solvitur ambulando: the solution to the problem of walking is—walking. (150)

Thus his mediation of his experience reinscribes, rather than erases, the
line between disability and nondisability that he so precipitously
crossed and so mysteriously recrossed. Ultimately, then, his book subtly reinforces what photographer Hevey refers to as the "enfreakment"
of disability (1992).

A related professional transformation follows Sacks's personal and
corporeal conversion experience. Sacks believes his accident has put
him literally in a position to correct the scotoma—blind spot—at the
heart of neurology, its ignorance of the patient's experience, its willed
and sometimes callous objectivity.

Now I *knew*, for I had experienced myself. And now I could truly begin to understand my patients, the many hundreds of patients with profound distur-
bances of body-image and body-ego, whom I saw over the years. . . . I came to
realize, as did my patients, that there is an absolute and categorical difference
between a doctor who *knows* and one who does not, and that this knowing can
only be obtained by a personal experience of the organic, by descending to the
very depths of disease and dissolution. (202–203)

Passages like this raise the question, however, of how much compre-
hension his limited experience entitles him to claim, for there is an element of self-congratulation, if not self-promotion, here. The danger of
such a personal and professional conversion is precisely that it will em-
bolden him to fill in gaps in patients' experience, to presume that their
experience can be understood under the same cultural rubrics that appeal to him: biblical narrative paradigms, classical music metaphors,
Gothic conventions, and so on.

Sacks's exuberant sense of personal and professional rebirth is sincere, but it depends largely on his mysterious recovery from disability.
And his quick reversion to privileging lack of disability compromises
his claims to superior knowledge and compassion. His book appropri-
ates the language and the plot of the conversion narrative for what is in
effect his recovery, with full religious resonance, of what he considers
full selfhood, a rehabilitation in the moral and spiritual sense. How
much more difficult is the predicament of the chronically disabled autobiographer, whose experience may fail to conform to such a comic
plot, and whose self, by the implications of Sacks's narrative, still remains deficient, who lives perpetually "in limbo," alienated and marginalized. Thus, although Sacks gained special and valuable insight

into the world of the "patient" by virtue of his sojourn there, his recovery removed him suddenly, dramatically, and completely from the world of the disabled; his relief is only too obvious in the language and metaphors he chooses to express his experience. His self-narrative, which conflates autopathography and spiritual autobiography, substitutes for the metaphor of the doctor as God the image of *this* doctor as one of the elect. At worst it unwittingly reinforces unfortunate biblical and Gothic paradigms of disability. At best his account is complicit in the marginalization of the disabled, who inhabit what he characterizes as a world of unreality—who, most significantly, lack grace, not merely physically but spiritually.

Leonard Kriegel also links disability with falling in his autobiographical volume *Falling into Life* (1991), especially its title essay, but he does so in order to revise the trope of disability as a fall from grace. At first glance Kriegel's use of the metaphor of the fall appears to be homologous with Sacks's. Thus, under treatment for the polio that paralyzed his legs when he was eleven, "I would close my eyes and focus not, as my therapist urged, on bringing dead legs back to life but on my strange fall from the childhood grace of the physical" (4). Here Kriegel associates his prepolio past with life and grace, his postpolio present with their opposites. He also couches the hope of recovery in biblical terms:

Any recovery of muscle use in a polio patient usually took place within three months of the disease's onset. We all knew that. But as time passed, every boy in the ward learned to recite stories of those who, like Lazarus, had witnessed their own bodily resurrection. Having fallen from physical grace, we also chose to fall away from the reality in front of us. Our therapists were skilled and dedicated, but they weren't wonder-working saints. . . . We would not admit to ourselves, or to them, that we were permanently crippled. (5–6)

Unlike Sacks, Kriegel did not recover the use of his legs; in the absence of such recovery his discourse would seem to condemn him to a "fallen" state. But even within this passage Kriegel has begun to wrest the metaphor of falling from its biblical context, in which it is linked with sin, death, and damnation, and to turn it to his own purposes.

At the core of the essay is the literal use of the term to refer to that part of his rehabilitation which involved collapsing onto a mat; to be able to walk in braces the boy needed to know how to fall properly and how to pick himself up afterward. To his embarrassment and humiliation Kriegel repeatedly froze and could not complete the exercise, thus "failing" to be rehabilitated: "The prospect of letting go was precisely what terrified me. That the other boys in the ward had no trouble in falling added to my shame and terror. . . . I knew there was virtually no chance of injury when I fell, but that knowledge simply made me more ashamed of a cowardice that was as monumental as it was unexplainable" (10–11). What therapists presented to him as a means to an end—practical preparation for life as a cripple—somehow took on greater significance—as an acknowledgment of incapacity and vulnerability, of lack of control. It meant a surrender of will and submission to the forces of gravity and disease.

Eventually—suddenly and mysteriously—Kriegel got over his inability to fall: "This time it was as if something beyond my control or understanding had decided to let my body's fall from grace take me down for good. . . . It was over. . . . The truth was I had simply been worn down into letting go. . . . I found myself quite suddenly faced with a necessary fall—a fall into life" (12–13). The fall is both anticlimactic—predictably uneventful—and redemptive. Kriegel's narrative slows it down for effect, and his alternation of positive and negative, ordinary and dramatic verbs suggests its paradoxical quality: "I dropped. I did not crash. I dropped. I did not collapse. I dropped. I did not plummet. I felt myself enveloped by a curiously gentle moment in my life. In that sliver of time before I hit the mat, I was kissed by space. . . . Even as I fell through the air, I could sense the shame and fear drain from my soul, and I knew that my sense of my own cowardice would soon follow. In falling, I had given myself a new start, a new life" (13). Kriegel insists that "falling into life was not a metaphor; it was real, a process learned only through doing, the way a baby learns to crawl, to stand, and then to walk" (8). But at the same time, it takes on significance as part of a new trope, one that decisively revises the biblical construction of disability and embodiment.

His inability, or refusal, to fall had amounted to a denial of his condition, a refusal to acknowledge that larger forces dictated his life script; paradoxically, however, the longer he sustained his mute resistance, the longer the virus would control him and the more effectively it would immobilize him. The virus held captive mind and body alike. To move out of the rehabilitation hospital he had to let go—of his impulse to protect his body and of his image of himself as intact and unimpaired. That this is not merely an incremental step in a long process but a moment of profound psychic conversion is evident in the reference to the removal of negative emotions from Kriegel's soul. But the psychic conversion coincides here with a subtle but significant reconstruction of the meaning of falling. *This* fall is an autonomous motion, one Kriegel finally allows to happen; it is thus a fall forward, a form of locomotion. Grace is not the recovery of his former bodily state—not a cure, like Sacks's conversion—but rather the acceptance of his body's new condition; by moving beyond denial he can move beyond self-pity. His willingness to fall paradoxically means resuming some control over his body, his identity, his life script. In a kind of verbal judo Kriegel converts falling from a negative act, linked to damnation, to a positive one, linked to the new life into which it delivers him.

He comes to take a certain pleasure and pride in his ability to fall:

However perverse it may seem, I felt a certain pleasure when, as I walked with a friend, I felt a crutch slip out of my grasp. Watching the thrust of concern darken his features, I felt myself in control of my own capacity. For falling had become the way my body sought out its proper home. It was an earthbound body, and mine would be an earthbound life. My quest would be for the solid ground beneath me. Falling with confidence, I fell away from terror and fear. (14)

Falling is a survival skill; rather than reenacting and reinforcing his incapacity, each fall minimizes it by demonstrating his resilience. Kriegel makes a virtue of the necessity of being earthbound. His writing is earthbound too, in the sense that it refuses allegorical constructions of disability as involving judgment, punishment, or moral failure. But it is not prosaic. Only by creative use of metaphor can Kriegel deconstruct and neutralize a powerfully invalidating trope.

Despite his invocation of a turning point, Kriegel does not claim to have adjusted to his paralysis once and for all after the fall. On the contrary, he remained, and remains, plagued by a sense of unjust deprivation—of having lost a life along with the use of his legs. Still, being crippled made him a writer and gave him his subject; indeed, it made him an autobiographer: "In writing about what [polio] had done to me, I discovered purpose as a writer. If I could put my sentences down, understanding that what had happened to me at eleven now stood at the heart of those sentences, then I somehow had reclaimed responsibility for my life from the virus" (90). One might say that his paralysis made him an essayist as well. For Kriegel paralysis was not something, as it was for Sacks, to be put behind him in a single story but something to contend with constantly. His characteristic form, significantly, is not narrative (much less conversion narrative, with its confident linear progress) but the essay, a tentative form that approaches its subject obliquely. Distinctive traits of his writing are its reiteration of his anger at his fate and his tendency to revisit the advent of his paralysis in essay after essay, book after book. All this is to suggest how profoundly paralysis has pervaded his life—his sense of his identity and his trajectory in the world, his point of view.

Writing autobiography became his way of doing what in his view all cripples must do—"attempt to establish the terms and the boundaries of their existence" (68)—which may make them daunting, even threatening, examples to "normals." Kriegel's advice and example to other cripples is not to adjust to disability but rather to "affirm their existence and claim selfhood by pushing beyond those structures and categories their condition has created" (62)—that is, to rewrite the discourse that defines them: "We can serve the world as victim or demon, the object of its charity or its terror. But the only thing we can be certain of is that the world would prefer to turn a blind eye and a deaf ear to our real selves—and that it will do precisely that until we impose those selves on the world" (65).

Writing autobiography, then, is Kriegel's way—but also one he implicitly recommends for others—of imposing one's self on the world.

Wholeness vs. Holiness: Reynolds Price, *A Whole New Life: An Illness and a Healing* (1994)

Whether it results suddenly from accident or gradually from illness, paraplegia is such a radical and permanent dysfunction that it cries out for strong compensatory narrative paradigms. Unlike Kriegel, Reynolds Price was a writer long before he was crippled (by a malignant spinal tumor at the age of fifty). But like Kriegel, Price found his disability a stimulant rather than an obstacle to his writing. Indeed, his illness and disability licensed ventures into new genres. His first autobiographical volume, *Clear Pictures: First Loves, First Guides* (1989), was the indirect by-product of therapy for chronic pain: hypnosis stimulated vivid childhood memories. His second autobiographical volume, *A Whole New Life* (1994), took his illness experience as its explicit subject. Although the continuation, or resumption, of his writing after his cancer suggests that his postparalysis life was not wholly new, the autobiographical by-products are quite literally new "lives."

For Sacks the conversion trope was an obvious narrative formula for a case of seemingly miraculous recovery. With Price we have a significant variation on that formula: spiritual assurance without physical recovery—miraculous survival, perhaps, but certainly not miraculous cure. As both the title and subtitle imply, the narrative has an unambiguously comic plot on several levels; although his paralysis is permanent, Price's spinal tumor was arrested and stabilized by surgeries and radiation therapy, his pain relieved by biofeedback and hypnosis, and his life renewed by a reordering of priorities.

Attaining relief from pain after several years of suffering no doubt contributes to Price's concluding assessment that he's fine despite his paralysis. While denying that he's a saint or a martyr, he insists, against "common sense," that he is decidedly better off after his paralysis:

So *disaster* then, yes, for me for a while—great chunks of four years. *Catastrophe* surely, a literally upended life with all parts strewn and some of the most ur-

gent parts lost for good, within and without. But if I were called on to value
honestly my present life beside my past—the years from 1933 till '84 against the
years after—I'd have to say that, despite an enjoyable fifty-year start, these recent years since full catastrophe have gone still better. They've brought more in
and sent more out—more love and care, more knowledge and patience, more
work in less time. (179)

Indeed, Price builds his account on the biblical paradigm of resurrection: "Your chance of rescue from any despair lies, if it lies anywhere,
in your eventual decision to abandon the death watch by the corpse of
your old self and to search out a new inhabitable body" (188). Thus the
narrative has an overt religious, even mystical, dimension. Early on, for
example, Price has a vision of being baptized by Jesus on the shores of
the Sea of Galilee. Told his sins are forgiven, Price has the nerve to ask,
"Am I cured?" Jesus replies, "That too" (43).

Unlike many spiritual autobiographers, however, Price questions the
status of his vision: "Was it a dream I gave myself in the midst of a cat-
nap, thinking I was awake? Was it a vision of the sort accorded from a
maybe external source to mystics of differing degrees of sanity through
human history? From the moment my mind was back in my own room,
no more than seconds after I'd left it, I've believed that the event was
an external gift, however brief, of an alternate time and space in which
to live through a crucial act" (44). Though the experience is never repeated, and the rest of the narrative is more earthbound, the episode
gives Price a lasting, reassuring sense that he is being watched over and
listened to. The effect is that of a sense of election rather than of conversion; because this unbidden spiritual episode involves no dark night
of the soul, no self-abasement, the narrative does not conform to the
formula of the conversion narrative. And because the religious dimension is only intermittently manifest, the book is not a conventional spiritual autobiography. Price rejects any equation between disability and
sin; rather than a fall from grace, his illness, pain, and paralysis represent a personal crisis in which he desperately needs, and receives, reassurance from a familiar source.

Price's narrative does, however, explicitly and consistently privilege
mind over body. At first this gesture functions largely as part of his denial or transcendence of chronic pain. Eventually, after four years of un-
interrupted suffering, Price finds some relief from his pain in biofeedback and hypnosis: "The pain was still unquestionably in me; but . . . it
seemed contained and watched from a distance by my new self-pos-
sessed mind and eased body" (155–56). According to Price, his mind
had "needed to hear and believe that the unending stream of neural
alarm meant nothing now. The need had been filled. Now my mind un-

derstood that *The harm is done. It cannot be repaired; pain signifies nothing. Begin to ignore it.* The pain needs to be treated as an alarm that you can't turn off but you can mute. And you can't do that until and unless you've accepted that the damage is irreparable" (159). One key to controlling pain had to do with interpreting the signals his body was sending his brain. Relief comes only when the mind accepts that the body will not "get better."

One benefit of his skill as a writer is his ability to describe pain convincingly, which is notoriously difficult to do. Indeed, for Price writing does what biofeedback and, more effectively, hypnosis do: it insulates him from his internal bodily sensations, locating him not beyond his pain but at its outer reaches.

I think I can say that almost any degree of physical pain can be borne. And not only borne but literally displaced from the actual center of a human life and then ignored. I can make that claim because I'm convinced that all pain has one huge design on us—to rule our minds—and therefore that the secret of living with pain is wanting hard to throw it out of central control, then finding the sane means to work that steady mental combination of distancing and coexistence. (160)

In addition to functioning to deny pain, Price's privileging of mind over matter is crucial to the achievement of a comic plot. Like most men in his situation, Price is concerned about the emasculating implications of his paralysis; thus he is careful to point out that his postparalysis life is not lacking in eros:

Then the slow migration of a sleepless and welcome sexuality from the center of my life to the cooler edge has contributed hugely to the increased speed and volume of my work, not to speak of the gradual resolution of hungers that— however precious to mind and body—had seemed past feeding. It's the sex that's moved, in fact, not the eros. The sense of some others as radiant and magnetic bodies, bodies that promise pleasure and good, is if anything larger in my life than before. (190)

Libido, then, is sublimated into other forms of interpersonal contact and into his writing.[11] Although this is a significant acknowledgment of how profoundly bodily dysfunction has dictated his life narrative and altered his identity, the overall tendency of the narrative is to suggest the ascendancy of the mind over the body. Ultimately, Price's sober assessment is that what paraplegia cost him—the control of his lower body—mattered less to him than what paraplegia enhanced and enriched—the use of his "higher" faculties.

Throughout the book Price hedges on the issue of remission, remarking periodically that, so far, his pain has not recurred (80, 88, 132).

Though his recovery (from cancer, not paralysis) is miraculous, he stops short of claiming credit for it, nor does he credit God, which might be another way of claiming to have earned it. In concluding, Price qualifies his resurrection trope, perhaps fearful of tempting fate with excessive confidence. Although he does express his conviction that his experience will have transcendent and useful meaning—that "the path ahead, seen from a tall enough height, will form at least a compelling figure, a clear intentional design, of use to others" (176–77)—he explicitly denies certainty about the outcome of his illness. In the end he claims only that he is whole, not healed, and not holy—not chosen for martyrdom. At the same time, in his association of his paralysis with his sense of election he does tend to mystify his disability. In the final analysis he comes closer to reversing Sacks's paradigm—associating his paralysis, rather than recovery, with spiritual assurance—than to rejecting it altogether. In addition, Price subscribes to, or inscribes, the individual model of disability insofar as his emphasis is on overcoming his impairment—the way his injury affects his ego and his work— rather than with battling disability—marginalization in an "ableist" society.[12] To put it differently, he takes on the burden of proving his continued worth by resuming his career as a writer and even surpassing his precancer productivity.

Metaphorical Crippling, Figural Conversion: John Callahan, *Don't Worry, He Won't Get Far on Foot* (1989)

In *Don't Worry, He Won't Get Far on Foot* the cartoonist John Callahan uses a conversion narrative paradigm—but with two significant twists. First, his narrative is devoid of conventional religious references; second, the automobile accident that left him a quadriplegic does not function as the turning point. Rather, in the context of his full-life narrative Callahan presents quadriplegia as the least crippling of three conditions that concern him; far more devastating were his abandonment as a child by his birth mother, who gave him up for adoption, and his alcoholism, which began in early adolescence and got progressively worse. Disruptive as his paralysis was of his projected life narrative—and it came at a crucial juncture, when he was attempting to establish his independence from his adoptive family—its role in his retrospective written narrative is to unmask earlier problems and deeper dependencies. Once he has exposed these and addressed them, Callahan manages to adjust to his physical limitations and live a productive, more or less independent, life. In his case, then, disability is (merely) a catalyst for an overdue anagnorisis (enlightenment) and peripeteia (reversal of fortune).

Unlike the typical paralyzed autobiographer, then, Callahan does not see disability as bisecting his life. Rather, Callahan makes his turning point a moment of postparalysis insight concerning his abuse of alcohol. The crucial moment comes when he drops an unopened bottle of wine while unattended and cannot reach it. His physical inability to recover the dropped bottle exposes his utter dependency to him, and he explodes in rage at the universe. A kind of emotional floodgate opens; after crying cathartically, he feels himself being comforted by an invisible hand and is suffused by a sense of calm and resolution: "I knew with utter certainty that my problem was not quadriplegia, it was alcoholism; that I was powerless to do anything about it by myself; and that I would never drink again" (109).

Though his rehabilitation requires a great deal of agonizing emotional work as he struggles to follow A.A.'s twelve steps, this moment proves to be the beginning of his sober life, and his book is divided exactly in two by his instantaneous conversion from alcoholism through some mysterious transcendent power. What becomes clear at this point in the narrative is that before his accident Callahan had been anesthetizing himself with alcohol against emotional pain. He been a kind of emotional cripple—unable to feel much. The most obvious source of his pain was his knowledge that he was an illegitimate child given up at birth for adoption. His sense of betrayal by his birth mother and of alienation from his adoptive family, which included five "natural" children conceived after his adoption, had run deep; his feelings of anger and shame had manifested themselves in aggressive, hostile, and self-destructive behavior. Thus the opening chapter, which culminates in the accident that paralyzed him, is also in retrospect the portrait of an individual already impaired by a powerful addiction; his every move is part of a complex strategy of denying and managing his craving. The accident that paralyzed him, which resulted from his drinking, did not end his addiction in the way one might expect—by obstructing his drinking; on the contrary, it gave him another excuse to drink, and procuring alcohol in various institutions proved easy. It did, however, subject him to a condition that finally awakened him to the real threat to his autonomy.

Once Callahan renounced alcohol, he endured a period of painful retrospection and reassessment of his life, during which he suffered acute sensitivity; he felt, paradoxically, like a flayed, rather than a paralyzed, body. Ironically, then, his loss of physical sensation led to an excruciating recovery of emotional sensation, a repairing of various relationships, and thus a reconstruction of identity. Lapsing only occasionally into the clichés of self-help literature, Callahan, like Benjamin Franklin, gives a brief account of his self-reform, which involves making amends for earlier errors.

The effect of Callahan's conversion paradigm is not to deny the powerful and negative effect of paralysis on his life. Indeed, few such narratives are as vivid in their depictions of the physical and logistical complications paralysis entails; Callahan is candid, graphic, sometimes raunchy, and often funny about taboo topics like urinary, bowel, and sexual functions. But his narrative does put paralysis in perspective—as a hindrance rather than an insurmountable obstacle—by claiming as the catalyst of his conversion not his serious physical impairment but other, more amenable, personal problems. Callahan's main strategy in presenting his disability, then, is to depict quadriplegia as a relatively minor problem—not a reason for feeling estranged or marginalized (like abandonment at birth) nor as harmful as the emotional paralysis of alcoholism. His sober view of his quadriplegia is that it is not the source of his feelings of alienation and illegitimacy but a condition that can be lived with and worked around.

As a whole, Callahan's narrative retraces his trajectory from the situation depicted in one of his drawings to that depicted in another, though he presents neither as a literal self-portrait. The first image, which he exhibited in a show of art by patients at a care facility, he describes as "a small pen-and-ink of a beaten and dead baby, smudged. I signed it backward" (154). This image corresponds to his conception of himself as an infant—hurt and abandoned, with his identity obscured or spoiled (the backward patronymic—*Nahallac*—as signature); in its self-pity it is also an expression of his emotional infancy (he was still drinking when he drew it). The other image, the final one in the book, is Callahan's witty twist on a formulaic expression of humility. A man standing at a lectern and holding a trophy says, "I'd like to thank all those who made it possible for me to be here tonight" (219); behind him is a parade of progressively higher forms of life, from the aquatic to the terrestrial (a dinosaur and a cave man), of which he is the evident culmination. On one level Callahan is characterizing dependency as a function of humanity rather than of disability (the speaker is not disabled). On another he is depicting himself as the product of an evolutionary process (the twelve steps), a higher form of life than the emotional child who narcotized—indeed, virtually embalmed—himself with alcohol.

Despite Callahan's insistence on the complications attendant on paralysis, such as his frustrating dependency on hired aides who are marginal individuals, the overall plot is comic; his narrative presents an individual who manages to live a productive and fulfilling life although severely and permanently paralyzed. Of the narratives discussed so far, Callahan's is the most straightforward and demystifying in its treatment of paralysis, which it presents as a matter of logistical and medical problems rather than of emotional trauma or spiritual crisis. Of course, by identifying himself primarily as an alcoholic Callahan trades in one stigmatic "master status" (quadriplegia) for another equally, perhaps more, stigmatic. The latter, however, is one from which he can be converted to the status of "recovering alcoholic." (It is also an identity to which autobiographical self-disclosure is critical.) Thus, without denying his disability, his "confession" serves to deflect and dissipate its stigma, in a way. As a whole, his conversion narrative works to minimize, if not to "normalize," quadriplegia, presenting it as inconsiderable in comparison to alcoholism, a *truly*—morally and emotionally—disabling condition. By constructing his conversion narrative around his really disabling condition, his addiction to alcohol, Callahan redraws the boundary between nondisabled and disabled, valid and invalid.

One question raised by these narratives, as in the case of narratives of stigmatic illnesses like AIDS, is whether they undermine the stigma of particular conditions or merely exempt the narrator from it. I have argued that, as self-presentation, *auto*biography has inherent counter-discursive potential; the medium conveys the message of autonomy, which is inconsistent with the stereotype of the physically impaired as dependent and passive. Yet it must also be acknowledged that autobiography's intrinsic individualism may work against its counterhegemonic potential insofar as it focuses on the single person rather than on the body politic. Insofar as disability autobiography takes the form of the narrative of triumph over bodily impairment, it subtly inscribes the individual model, rather than the social model, of disability; it reinforces the cultural construction as a catastrophe that renders individuals either pathetic—if they succumb to it—or heroic—if they somehow overcome it. There is a strong temptation—fed both by the needs of the ego and by the literary marketplace, which prefers such narratives—to adopt the hegemonic narrative paradigm of transcendence over bodily injury rather than to challenge its cultural construction. Indeed, all the narratives discussed so far, including Callahan's, do this to some extent. All display a male pattern of concern with individual autonomy and freedom; all in various ways base their comic plots on some sort of intellectual, emotional, or spiritual compensation for the loss of physical mobility. None of the narratives examined thus far, then, goes out of its way to affirm solidarity with a marginalized group or to question the cultural ideals of individualism and independence; each autobiographer comes to terms with disability—denying, transcending, or sidestepping stigmatization—on his own.

Callahan's Cartoons: Caricature or Critique?

Callahan's book is distinguished from the others by its inclusion of many cartoons and graphic images. Some are illustrations of the autobiographical narrative; others are samples of his work. Because both sets of images represent disability in a nonverbal medium, the question arises as to their role in the discourse of disability. Callahan's cartoons often use the stock situation of the crippled beggar on the sidewalk, and he sometimes draws characters with simple hooks for hands—or even for feet. Do such images perpetuate the "enfreakment" of disability even as his narrative exempts him from it? Is he a self-hating cripple who exploits stereotypes to vent his repressed anger at his condition?

An unequivocal answer to these questions risks oversimplification, I think. True, Callahan's self-portraits are generally less grotesque than his drawings of anonymous figures. And Callahan's images of minorities, including people with disabilities, are often in deliberately bad taste—not politically correct; he is evidently willing, if not eager, to offend. But if we consider his images in the context of the surrounding narrative, trying to reconcile the cartoonist's eye with the narrative *I*, his cartoons are less cruel than they may seem at first glance.

By his own account his talent (or weakness) for caricature emerged in childhood, well before his accident; if it reflects hostility and anger, the source is not his paralysis but probably his sense of abandonment. The implicit target of the satirical drawings in the book is generally not the disabled figure, however crudely portrayed; usually, it is the attitudes and behaviors of people who are not disabled. This is at least true of the drawings that illustrate his story, as opposed to the freestanding cartoons that are included in it. The illustrations feature an autobiographical character in a wheelchair; although it is a caricature of the author, the figure is sympathetically drawn. More important, perhaps, he is usually portrayed as the victim of insensitivity at the hands of others—such as the well-meaning couple who hand him "the latest in adaptive equipment" (according to the caption)—a beggar's cup and a sign reading *Paralyzed*. (Among other things, this image puts begging by disabled people in a different light—as a form of "adaptive" behavior in an ableist culture that consigns them to economic marginality.) In contrast, the illustrations of him as an alcoholic are quite unsparing—in one the prostrate drunk victim of a car crash, surrounded by liquor bottles, asks an attending police officer to buy him a case of beer. The evident divide between sympathetic and scathing self-representation is the difference between the paralyzed self and the alcoholic former self.

His depictions of anonymous disabled characters are more problematic. Callahan's use of the stock image of the disabled beggar on the street corner might seem to perpetuate a destructive and stigmatizing stereotype—that of the cripple who makes a life and a living by flaunting his impairment and his dependency. Yet stereotypes and conventional situations are the stock-in-trade of all cartoonists, and they may be used to subvert their usual messages. Such is the case with at least some of Callahan's images. One cartoon wittily combines the stock figure of the Martian with that of the crippled beggar; a three-legged Martian tosses a coin into a cup held out by a *two*-legged Martian in a wheelchair (168). The message here is not that impaired individuals are grotesque and unproductive—much less alien—but that disability is defined contextually; in the land of the three-legged, a two-legged individual would be stigmatized and, thus disabled, might (have to) beg for a living. To portray a two-legged being (even a Martian) as a cripple is to redraw the boundary of disability to include most of those who consider themselves not disabled.

The relativity of disability is perhaps also the message of a more shocking cartoon, which pictures two bodiless heads mounted on skid carts flanked by beggar's cups; one character says to the other, who wears an eye patch: "People like you are an inspiration to me" (188). The image is crude—but perhaps only superficially so. For one thing, it graphically portrays a sensation apparently common to quadriplegics; because they have little if any sensation below the neck, they sometimes feel like disembodied heads.[13] Viewed this way, in relation to the text, the image does not objectify but *subjectifies*; however grotesque it seems, it may communicate what is otherwise a difficult sensation for a non-disabled person to understand.

A crucial link between the two sets of images, the illustrations of the story and the independently conceived cartoons that punctuate or comment on it, is the image in which Callahan shows himself being given a sign and a beggar's cup. This vividly portrays his sense of how paralysis entailed stigmatization (the acquisition of a literal label) and economic dependency equivalent to, if not identical with, begging. (It also stands synecdochically for the plight of others with disabilities.) His frequent reworking of the stock situation of the crippled beggar is not just a revision—or exploitation—of a standard stereotype, I think; it is a way of keeping a nightmare at bay. Unlike most of the other paralyzed authors discussed here, Callahan had relatively few resources—social or financial—to fall back on at the time of his accident. The circumstances of his life immediately after his "rehabilitation"—in and out of institutions—are grim. His book gives a gritty picture of what life is like for a quadriplegic who has to rely on the assistance of poorly paid, and even more poorly trained, strangers. At times he came perilously close to skid row; indeed, even when he reached a certain level of professional accomplishment and economic self-sufficiency as a cartoonist, Callahan lived literally but also metaphorically not far from skid row in Portland, Oregon. Loss of his ability to draw—or a downturn in his fortunes as a freelance cartoonist—could result in sudden downward mobility. Of the autobiographers here, Callahan is among the youngest, and he lives the most precarious life. His cartoons remind us that even a supposedly civilized society may require its less privileged impaired individuals to make their disability their occupation and livelihood. Indeed, Callahan's blatant use of images of disabled derelicts represents an unfortunately common result of physical disability and reminds us how class bound and privileged is the experience of the typical paralyzed autobiographer.

Support for this interpretation comes from a late chapter in which Callahan details the red tape in which he finds himself entangled *because* of the income that promises to makes him economically independent. In general, Callahan seems without political consciousness or much sense of solidarity with other individuals with disabilities. But in this chapter he powerfully indicts the official treatment of the disabled—at least, of those able and willing to work—by exposing the inconsistency and self-contradiction of welfare policies. The sometimes suspicious and hostile treatment he receives at the hands of bureaucrats calls into question his moral legitimacy—the bureaucratic suspicion is that his economic independence must be an illusion or a fraud—and thus touches upon what is for him an especially basic and painful issue of his identity, threatening to undo the resolution he painfully reached about his birth and adoption. Here, perhaps incidentally, Callahan suggests to what degree a disabled person's sense of invalidity results from social attitudes and policies rather than from impairment itself.

The penultimate chapter is a series of cartoons entitled "How to Relate to Handicapped People," which serves both as an example of his professional accomplishment and as a supplement to his narrative. A certain amount of residual hostility and anger may be evident in the fact that, despite the captions, most drawings illustrate how *not* to relate, and some offer mixed messages. For example, one panel advises, "Don't be afraid to ask questions," but it portrays a Callahan figure in a wheelchair beset by children asking tactless questions. The lack of help in Callahan's handbook is symptomatic, I think, of his vision. Wary of "self-righteous assholes who presume to defend the disabled" (161), he is essentially a satirist and caricaturist, temperamentally unwilling—perhaps unable—to depict positive images. At the same time, underlying the inconsistency and hostility of some of his images may be anger at the need for guidelines and suspicion of relations that are not spontaneous but scripted by formal or politically correct guidelines. As with much satire, the implicit vision may be utopian; what Callahan seems to want is a world in which impairment would not be the occasion for stigmatization in the first place.

Roll Modeling: John Hockenberry, *Moving Violations: War Zones, Wheelchairs, and Declarations of Independence* (1995)

In *Moving Violations* John Hockenberry is at pains to demonstrate that the boundary between nondisability and disability is culturally determined—contingent and arbitrary—and thus movable and permeable. His fundamental strategy, however, as his title suggests, is to emphasize his mobility and independence. As a story of his life after he was paralyzed in a car crash at nineteen, the book is most prominently an account of breaking through the barriers faced by disabled people. Although he never completed college, he not only chose a "real job" (journalism) rather than a "crip job," he also sought assignments seemingly unsuitable for a paraplegic: in search of the story Hockenberry often went where wheelchairs normally would not go: "I could feel . . . the smallness of that wheelchair-accessible world. It was a tiny fraction of the world at large. . . . Real freedom was in not needing the parking spaces, elevators, curb ramps, and bathrooms. It meant going places where there would be none of those, to face what was really possible in life rather than what was permitted" (180).

For the most part a straightforward memoir of his career, his book traces his stellar rise as a journalist from a small informal National Public Radio station in Oregon to *All Things Considered* at NPR headquarters in Washington, D.C., and from there to the greater salary and visibility of network TV. (At the outset of his career no one at NPR headquarters knew he was disabled. His reliance on a wheelchair was exposed only when the usually reliable reporter missed a filing deadline because the only available phone was in a booth.) Unique among the autobiographies considered here, then, Hockenberry's takes the form of a personal success story.

Hockenberry's powerful drive to succeed leads his father to remark, memorably, that his son uses his wheelchair "as a crutch"; that is, he relies on it to motivate himself to go places he might otherwise not reach. Sometimes, Hockenberry acknowledges, he uses the chair to get an edge on competing journalists; he exploits both its high visibility, which occasionally singles him out for special treatment among a mob of journalists, and its invisibility, which sometimes enables him to pass undetected where journalists are officially excluded (as when, in Israel, he smuggles videotape past checkpoint guards who look right through him). He shrewdly exploits his disability to achieve notable mobility both horizontally, in his extensive and improbable travels, and vertically, in his career. Hockenberry acknowledges that his career takes him out into a world where he has little contact with other "crips," but in making it on his own Hockenberry assumes he is also a "roll model" (a term he uses for a chapter title) for others.

Confounding stereotypes by living and writing a life beyond presumed limitations is a time-honored phenomenon in narratives of disability. (Indeed, Helen Keller's memoir achieved its classic status in part because her achievements so far exceeded her apparent limitations.) Such narratives do serve to encourage defiance of expectations and limits and to suggest how much is possible for people with disabilities. Yet the narrative formula of "overcoming" impairment—rather than challenging disability (though the two are not always easy to distinguish)—has its drawbacks. A high-achieving individual with an obvious impairment is always in danger of becoming a Supercrip, an Inspirational Disabled Person who overcomes impairment through pluck and willpower. According to Joseph Shapiro, this model is

deeply moving to most nondisabled Americans and widely regarded as oppressive by most disabled ones. The disability rights movement discards the notion that people with disabilities should be courageous or heroic superachievers, since most disabled people are trying simply to lead normal lives, not inspire anyone. . . .

The "supercrip" is the flip side of the pitiable poster child. It is just as hurtful . . . because it implies that a disabled person is presumed deserving of pity—instead of respect—until he or she proves capable of overcoming a physical or mental limitation through extraordinary feats. Today, these "supercrips" remain among our most glorified disabled role models, lavishly lauded in the press and on television. (16)

Of all autobiographical formulas, the success story, which attributes achievement to individual merit, is the most likely to reinforce this image of disability. As is the case with other marginalized minorities, the rare success of the extraordinary individual may reinforce the status quo by shoring up the comfortable belief that members of minorities do not face significant obstacles, whether tangible (like stairs) or intangible (like stigma).

The well-known disdain for supercrips in the disabled community puts people like Hockenberry in an awkward position. He clearly does not wish his success to be used to indict others less successful than he, but neither does he wish to downplay his accomplishments, like his risky forays into war zones. Apparently aware of the danger of reinforcing an oppressive stereotype, Hockenberry offsets the supercrip image with earthy details. Hence his frankness about his bowel and urinary functions: he candidly confesses that his excretory functions are not always in his control and suggests that the American concern for hygiene is itself unhealthy. Hence too his inclusion of frank and sometimes funny stories of his sex life. Partly, such stories are meant to establish that he is still a potent man capable of an active sex life; still, they represent significant and deliberate deviations from ideal scenarios. His counterdiscursive strategy here is to use humor to deflect disgust and to expose the shallowness of the American obsession with idealized bodies. Furthermore, he offsets what might seem a too-rosy picture of life in a wheelchair with accounts of the everyday hardships of life in New York City, where, thanks to inaccessible subway stations and uncooperative taxi and bus drivers, getting to work can be the hardest part of his job.

Another of his strategies for downplaying his distinction takes advantage of his journalistic travels. He represents life in the developing countries as in some ways less psychologically threatening, though perhaps more physically dangerous, than life in the States. He observes cultural differences in attitudes toward disability—for example, between Arabs and Jews in the Middle East and between urban whites and blacks in America. He also suggests, more broadly, that his experience of disability is not so different from the common conditions of life for a large number of people worldwide:

In the Middle East, day-to-day life was close to the experience of living in a wheelchair. . . . It was to go through life with the presumption that things were not going to go your way, an experience relatively rare in America and the industrialized world, but extremely common almost everywhere else. The presumption of physical adversity was widespread among Israelis and Palestinians faced with their relentless conflicts. (264)

The book's most successful disruption of the discourse of disability, however, has to do with his exploration of the differing responses to two previous disabilities in his family: his paternal grandfather's matter-of-fact compensation for an arm lost to a work accident; his maternal grandparents' consignment of a retarded son, at age six, to an institution and the boy's near-banishment from the family's oral and photographic history. Reconstructing this decision, Hockenberry tries not to judge his grandparents too severely. "I long to believe that there was no other way, that my uncle had to be sent away, his circumstances so unique, compelling, and clear-cut that my family can be absolved of his banishment, a life sentence for a nonexistent crime" (336). Nevertheless, the author sees it as the consequence of an impossible requirement imposed on his uncle: that he acknowledge and return his family's love even as his illness (phenylketonuria) dragged him into profound retardation. Hockenberry also suspects that the banishment of his uncle reflected an irrational fear of contagion—stigma by association. It is this response that most angers and threatens him: "The forces that put my uncle away would also place me in a category from which there is no escape. Inside me is the engine that thrashes about never stopping, always mindful that someday those same forces could decide my fate, claim that I am really helpless, that my life is not worth living, give me a label, and send me away to a place for all those like me" (337).

He sees his uncle as having been amputated from his family, cast off as diseased and virtually contagious. Hockenberry's most important autobiographical gesture, then, may be his biographical one, which reclaims his long-lost uncle's life. Hockenberry's visit to his long-lost uncle is both climactic and unfulfilling: his uncle does not know him and cannot be made to understand who this rare visitor is. Recognition is not mutual; the emotion is apparently all on one side. There is no question of undoing his uncle's banishment, releasing him from the prison of the institution and restoring to him his former name and identity. (In the absence of family visits to reinforce his identity as Petey, his uncle has become known to his present caretakers by his real first name, Charlie.) Under any name he is now incapable of recrossing the border into the outside world; the best Hockenberry can do is to write his uncle back into the family history. Though founded in a family relationship, Hockenberry's sense of loyalty to his rediscovered uncle impels him, for the first time in his narrative, to assert his solidarity with the community of people with disabilities—here embodied in someone whose severe disability makes him a virtual nonperson. This gesture is powerfully at odds with the dominant focus in Hockenberry's memoir on his exemption from marginalization. And it suggests the need to attack the basis of stigma as well as to escape it through demonstration of one's "ability"—to assert freedom collectively as well as individually.

The Political Paradigm: Autoethnography—Robert Murphy, *The Body Silent* (1987); Irving Zola, *Missing Pieces: A Chronicle of Living with a Disability* (1982)

Perhaps the strongest similarity among the various narratives discussed thus far has been the claim of compensation. Each disabled autobiographer claims to have made up for the physical deficits of his condition with some professional, intellectual, or spiritual gains. (Sacks claims to have made up his physical deficits as well.) As with illness, then, autobiographical accounts of disability tend to be best-case scenarios; those who undertake autobiography tend to be intellectuals, whose major sources of self-esteem—and income—are less likely to be damaged by physical disability. Such privileged individuals have a relatively easy time shrugging off the notion of "spoiled" identity. This is true also of the next two figures to be discussed, both social scientists.

But in contrast to the accounts already discussed, whose reliance on the paradigms of conversion narrative or success story tends in one way or another to isolate the individual, theirs more explicitly embrace the social or "minority model," in which disability is less a matter of individual anatomical dysfunction than of prejudice defining whole groups of people. Such a paradigm removes the onus from the individual and suggests the potential for oppositional cultural work—even for pride in one's identity; hence the "political paradigm."

Because anthropological fieldwork typically demands physical as well as geographical mobility, paralysis is a serious impairment for a professional anthropologist. When a spinal tumor slowly paralyzed Robert Murphy, an anthropology professor at Columbia University, his resourceful response—to make the community of paralytics his new specialty—turned a professional liability into an asset (and made him a pioneer in disability studies). It also led him to write an account of his paralysis that is framed as the record of a metaphorical anthropological expedition rather than a conventional chronological autobiography: "This book was conceived in the realization that my long illness with a disease of the spinal cord has been a kind of extended anthropological field trip, for through it I have sojourned in a social world no less strange to me at first than those of the Amazon forests. And since it is the duty of all anthropologists to report on their travels . . . this is my accounting" (ix).

Indeed, his book may be a groundbreaking but unacknowledged example of what Françoise Lionnet has referred to as "autoethnography"—"that is, the defining of one's subjective ethnicity as mediated through language, history, and ethnographical analysis; in short . . . a kind of 'figural anthropology' of the self" (99).[14] Unlike marginalizing conditions like ethnicity and race (but like sexual orientation), disability is generally not shared with family members; as a result, minority consciousness is harder to achieve, and disability has only recently begun to be conceived of in terms of the minority model.

The necessary duplexity of the autobiographer, who is always both subject and narrator, is refigured here in terms of a fundamental convention of ethnography. Serving in this book as both ethnographer and informant, Murphy becomes nearly self-sufficient as an anthropologist—an imaginative way of taking advantage of his impairment. Facing progressive paralysis with no hope of relief or remission, Murphy is irrevocably committed to the position of disability—and to solidarity with other individuals with disabilities. Such a position equips him uniquely to challenge hegemonic cultural constructions. For all the vaunted cultural relativism of anthropology, ethnography has recently come under fire for its affinity with imperialism: the Western ethnographer assumes, or presumes, the authority to write the culture of the Other. But in Murphy's case the ethnographer has been reassigned permanently to the category of Other; writing as a member of the marginalized group, he has the opportunity to validate its perspective in a transformational way. Indeed, the social world he now finds as strange as "those of Amazon forests" is not the world of the disabled; rather, it is the world he had taken for granted for so long, defamiliarized by his impairment.

As I have already suggested, in many cases disability does not impose a plot on life narrative—or supply one. Murphy's progressive paralysis is an exception. This is evident in his dreams, which reenact his crippling as an epitome of his life narrative (105); they invariably have the same tragic plot: at first he can walk, but eventually, invariably, he relapses. Murphy's condition not only plots his life narrative, however; it also truncates it: "My history is no longer smooth and linear, but bisected and polarized. And my long-range future does not really exist" (26). With his prognosis of early death Murphy had nothing to gain by organizing his narrative as a chronological account of his condition. The inexorable growth of his tumor would seem to preclude a comic plot. Even to structure his account chronologically would be to dwell on the negative, on the ever-bleaker future—a prospect that Murphy acknowledges is not savory. In response to this predicament Murphy constructs the book not as a single linear narrative but as a series of personal and professional reflections on the condition in which he finds himself.

To be sure, the first of the three sections does recount the first phase of his paralysis—from a series of apparently minor symptoms through diagnosis of a benign spinal tumor, hospitalization, surgery, partial recovery, relapse, rehabilitation, and return to a more or less normal life as a university professor.[15] The nature of his malady, however, is such that he cannot sustain or extend this resolution. Thus the last two sections are not chronological. In part, Murphy's shunning of chronology reflects a conscious decision to live in the present: "I gradually learned to live day by day, to block from my consciousness any thought about the final outcome of the illness, to repress from awareness any vision of the unthinkable. I have maintained this perspective for the past ten years" (25).

It is not a matter of denial, however; he candidly acknowledges the reasons for his narratorial choices, and in doing so he manages to speak the unspeakable: "Some fears and sentiments are better left unstated, and those that I harbored as I entered the hospital in 1976 were among them. What I refused to contemplate was the progressive and total destruction of my body, the reduction of all volition to quietude, the entombment of my mind in inert protoplasm" (29). However tersely, he voices a vision of his future here, in effect expressing what he claims he is repressing. He acknowledges that, more than most autobiographers, he knows what lies in store for him; at the same time, he reminds us that we all repress awareness of the deterioration that may await us.

He attributes the composure with which he faces his condition—in life and by implication in writing—neither to denial nor to courage but to his temperament and to the stress of his condition: "It is, however, neither courage nor bluff, only self-anesthesis of emotion and stream of consciousness, a long and carefully inculcated gift for foreclosing tomorrow and repressing today. . . . This wasn't bravery, just an early manifestation of the Disembodied Self, which would reassert itself strongly in the coming years of disability. This technique was not just my own personal dodge, but a common reaction of people under severe stress" (25). He acknowledges the odd, sometimes unsettling, impersonality of his book, ascribing it in part to his creeping paralysis: "I have . . . become rather emotionally detached from my body, often referring to one of my limbs as *the* leg or *the* arm. . . . The paralytic becomes accustomed to being lifted, rolled, pushed, pulled, and twisted, and he survives this treatment by putting emotional distance between himself and his body. . . . My solution to this dilemma is a radical disassociation from the body, a kind of etherealization of identity" (100–101). Murphy encourages us to read the pervasive intellectuality of his book not as a denial but as a consequence, and thus a formal expression, of his bodily condition. The first section's narrative, then, explains and justifies the abandonment of narrative discourse and the shift to a more analytical and reflective mode in what follows.

Murphy acknowledges that the malfunctioning of his body made him suddenly and uncharacteristically self-conscious—a precondition to the writing of autobiography; at the same time, his condition also engaged his professional interest in a way that enabled him, even required him, to see himself in anthropological perspective. Thus, although the book contains some confessional elements, such as his acknowledgment of his earlier alcoholism and of his profound dependence on his wife, the stance of autoethnographer rather than autobiographer elicits a relatively impersonal and analytical account of paralysis rather than a confidential narrative. It helps him deflect attention from the personal implications of paralysis to its social implications, for Murphy insists that disability is a "social disease." His book is not merely a generalization from his experience, however; rather, it uses his case as a focus for the distillation of his reading and research into disability.

As a paralyzed anthropologist, Murphy becomes acutely aware of the marginalization of people with disabilities. In the middle section (whose epigraph is from Kafka's "Metamorphosis"), Murphy candidly explores the consequences of disability for self-image and identity, mixing social science language with allusions to popular and high culture:

The four most far-reaching changes in the consciousness of the disabled are: lowered self-esteem; the invasion and occupation of thought by physical deficits; a strong undercurrent of anger; and the acquisition of a new, total, and undesirable identity. I can only liken the situation to a curious kind of "invasion of the body snatchers," in which the alien intruder and the old occupant coexist in mutual hostility in the same body. It is also a metamorphosis in the exact sense. (108)

Murphy acknowledges that his deepening paralysis decisively and negatively changed his self-perception: "In only a few months, I had moved subtly from the center of my society to its perimeter. I had acquired a new identity that was contingent on my defects and that either compromised or radically altered my prior claims to personhood. In my middle age, I had become a changeling, the lot of all disabled people. . . . They have become aliens, even exiles, in their own lands" (110–11).

On the whole, however, Murphy's book does not reflect lowered self-esteem, obsess about physical deficits, express anger, or represent his identity as undesirable. As I have suggested, one reason for this is that Murphy was somewhat insulated from these consequences because of class or professional standing. Thus, when Murphy reaches the point in his narrative when he is able to resume working, he declares that he did not consider himself really "disabled." The point of this assertion is not to deny his impairment, much less to distance himself from others with disabilities. Rather, it is to call attention to his good fortune as an intellectual, to be able to continue to do what counts in his world as "work." (He notes, ironically, "All I can do now is read, write, and talk—which is what academics call 'work'" [192].) For many others Murphy's disability would have been economically devastating. His impulse here is not to exempt himself from stigma but to illuminate the ways in which income and profession may grant some limited immunity to disability, to expose the rather arbitrary ways in which physical impairment becomes economically disabling.

Murphy's anthropological research also brought him into contact with the disability rights movement, which provided him with a sense of communal consciousness and collective interests that was therapeutic: "The most lasting benefits of any struggle against perceived oppression are not the tangible gains but the transformations of consciousness of the combatants. The disabled renewed and repaired their damaged egos, and they saw themselves even more clearly as a common interest group, with shared goals. . . . The disability movement is one of the best available forms of rehabilitation" (157–58). If, as Murphy asserts, "all anthropological research involves a process of self-discovery" (126), this middle section summarizing his research can be seen as covert autobiography that implies, rather than narrates, the process by which Murphy came to terms with his estrangement. Evidently, Murphy's professional status did not protect him entirely from the sort of ego damage he describes as characteristic of disability, but it did provide him with a therapeutic perspective on his transformation.

Considered as autobiography, then, the non-narrative middle section of his book suggests how he managed to come to terms with his new and disorienting condition—through recourse to his discipline. Profoundly estranged by his disability from his body, his former self, and his culture, Murphy used his anthropological training to investigate and demystify his marginalization. And in laying bare the reasons for his sense of stigmatization, he found a significant measure of relief. Furthermore, by probing the politics of identity construction, destruction, and reconstruction, the middle section brings his fieldwork and anthropological theorizing to bear on the condition of all people with disabilities. By acknowledging cultural commonality with those others, his autoethnography takes on a political dimension not present in more conventional narratives.

In the third part of his memoir Murphy takes a decidedly different tack in challenging the boundary between the "normal" and the "abnormal"; he argues that disability is a "metaphor for the human condition" (5) or "an allegory of all life in society" (ix). Here his impulse is less ethnographic than prophetic; his thesis is that the particular condition singled out and marginalized as disability represents an ignored or overlooked aspect of all human existence. This strategy of normalization through universalization, however well intentioned, has dangers that Murphy does not always succeed in avoiding. Nor is he always clear and consistent in developing his thesis. At times he seems to overgeneralize his progressive and life-threatening condition:

The paralytic's inertia is symbolic of death itself; he is life's negativity. He . . . is a living reminder of the body's frailty. It is a powerful metaphor, and a very large number of disabled people have surrendered and live permanently under its deep shadow. This is a kind of premature death in life, but it is a realm also inhabited by legions of people whose only disability is that they have given up too soon.

The forces of life . . . are strong, however, and there are millions of people in various stages of physical decrepitude who have fought off the shackles of dependency and the gravity of despair to fight their way into societies that have suspended judgment on their very humanness. They reject the limitations imposed upon them and the constructions placed on their identities. (229)

His characterization of paralysis as a moribund inertia—even if some heroically resist it—threatens to remystify disability in Gothic terms with its suggestion of a premature burial.

But this is balanced by his suggestion that the bodily immobility of paralysis may serve as an emblem of a more common and more insidious stasis:

The paralytic is, quite literally, a prisoner of the flesh, but most humans are convicts of sorts. We live within walls of our own making, staring out at life through bars thrown up by culture and annealed by our fears. This kind of thralldom to culture turned rigidified and fetishized is more onerous than my own somatic straightjacket, for it induces a mental paralysis, a stilling of thought. The captive mind misses the great opportunity given to us by the chaos of today's rapid social change. This is to free oneself of the restraints of culture, to stand somewhat aloof from our milieu, and to re-find a sense of what and where we are. It is in this way that the paralytic—and all of us—will find freedom within the contours of the mind and in the transports of the imagination. (230–31)

The paradox here, that the estrangement of marginalization may be liberating, is useful; the stigmatized, at least when their consciousnesses are raised, may be granted liberating insight into ways in which culture unfairly defines and confines us all. By redefining paralysis to include mental stagnation, Murphy redraws the boundary between disability and nondisability. Murphy's most powerful and revisionist gesture, however, remains his adoption and advocation, in the middle section, of the minority model. Insofar as he shows that disability is a "social disease," a culturally produced phenomenon rather than a universal entropic tendency, Murphy suggests that it is amenable to change.

Like Murphy, Irving Zola was a social scientist who investigated disability partly because of his impairment: as a result of teenage polio and a subsequent car accident, he walked with a leg brace, back support, and a cane. Like Murphy too, he saw his disability through the lens of his discipline (sociology), and his book also takes the form of a report on a field trip rather than an autobiography in the conventional sense. Some differences between their autoethnographies are notable, however. First, Zola's field trip was a literal one—a prearranged research sojourn in Het Dorp, a Dutch village designed for and occupied exclusively by disabled adults. Zola crosses boundaries between "normality" and "disability" that are literal as well as metaphorical. Second, although Zola was disabled, his sojourn at Het Dorp was a voluntary and short-term departure from his less restricted daily life. Third, an element of personal trial was involved in Zola's experiment: in order to facilitate his relationships with residents Zola, who had already visited the village to do research, chose to use a wheelchair for the duration of his weeklong stay, giving up his braces to experience the situation of a paraplegic. Significantly, it is the element of self-conscious role-playing that induces the transformation that furnishes the narrative's plot.

Despite careful prearrangement, upon his arrival Zola found the nondisabled administrators slow to provide him with a room and a wheelchair; at best they were uncomprehending, at worst suspicious of his motives. Because of his decision to renounce walking, he presented them with a kind of category problem: was he a member of the community of invalids or a professional like themselves? By choosing to cross the reassuring border between residents and staff, he called into question its validity and import. Ultimately, however, his decision proved as unsettling to him as it was to others. Indeed, as soon as he began to use a wheelchair, he experienced a surprising metamorphosis in his sense of himself—a change entirely the result of others' perception of him rather than of any actual impairment:

The next half hour was weird. Partly it was my getting used to being in a wheelchair after almost a twenty-year absence. But it was much more than that. Subtly, but all too quickly, I was being transformed. As soon as I sat in the wheelchair I was no longer seen as a person who could fend for himself. Although Metz had known me well for nine months, and had never before done anything physical for me without asking, now he took over without permission. Suddenly in his eyes I was no longer able to carry things, reach for objects, or even push myself around. (52)

Even more surprising, perhaps, was the way in which his own behavior and self-perception changed: "Most frightening was my own compliance, my alienation from myself and from the process" (52). He catches a sense of his invalidity from others, quickly internalizing the status his wheelchair signifies to them.

There was gain as well as loss in this metamorphosis, however: crossing this interior boundary—however temporarily—put him literally on the same level as the permanent residents and made possible a rapport researchers rarely achieve with their informants. The level of confidence he attained with the permanent residents was gratifying, if sometimes frightening. Like Oliver Sacks, Zola discovers, when institutionalized, how precarious and contingent is his sense of professional authority and autonomy. When he is discharged from the institution, however, he does not, like Sacks, revert to and celebrate his original status. Unlike Sacks, Zola is permanently disabled, marked for life. More important, however, at Het Dorp he comes to identify with other disabled people in a way he previously had not.

One thing he comes to realize at Het Dorp is that, despite his disability, he had lived a life of nearly complete assimilation into mainstream society; without attempting to pass as nondisabled he had socialized largely with nondisabled individuals and in effect had identified as "normal." As advantageous and healthy as this might be, he began to suspect that it might reflect unconscious prejudice; his assimilation had enabled him to underestimate the stigmatization to which some are subjected. Indeed, he discovered prejudice even at Het Dorp—not just on the part of well-meaning but somewhat paternalistic administrators toward their clients but also on the part of some residents towards others, on the basis of the type or degree of impairment. (Those with stable conditions distanced themselves from those with degenerative conditions.)

For various reasons, during his residence at Het Dorp Zola in effect re(dis)covered his disability; he came to identify with other impaired individuals, and he emerged a changed man, taking with him a deeper sense of connection with and commitment to those he left behind (most of whom would probably never leave Het Dorp). As it happens, Zola's account of his discovery of connectedness with a minority community is a variant on a return-to-roots paradigm more common in fiction, in which an assimilated member of some ethnic or racial minority returns to a place inhabited exclusively by such people and, often through some ritual or ceremony, is initiated into that community. (Examples would include Paule Marshall's *Praisesong for the Widow* [1983] and Leslie Marmon Silko's *Ceremony* [1977].) The status lost when Zola surrendered his crutches—and the compensatory gain of the confidence of the community—reconfigured his sense of his identity and of his loyalties. The challenge for Zola was to remain in and of the community, emotionally and psychologically, even as he stood up and walked out of it physically (to the waves and clenched fists of the permanent residents); the test was to be, on the outside, the champion and messenger those on the inside expected him to be. This passage may have an element of self-dramatization, but the publication of his account of this short episode in his life almost ten years later suggests the permanence of his sense of commitment and connection.

Zola's final perspective is almost wholly political rather than conventionally sociological or therapeutic; having experienced the segregation of the disabled under the most benign conditions, he comes away convinced of the necessity for the impaired to make their presence known to society. He cites Talcott Parsons on the way in which society, through its creation of the "sick role," prevents group solidarity and claims of legitimacy among the ill, and Zola calls explicitly for the formation of collectivity, self-assertion and self-representation by the disabled, and political and economic analysis of the social construction of disability. But he calls also for personal testimony, because it challenges the invisibility that segregation reifies. He acknowledges that stories of disability are hard to tell but insists that not to tell them is to accept invalidity. His account of his self-(re)discovery at Het Dorp, the reclamation of what he had repressed with society's encouragement, enacts or exemplifies the sort of testimony he calls for. Crossing the border *into* the community of disability, Zola comes to realize that in some sense he had always lived outside it; in his departure from Het Dorp Zola retraces an earlier, gradual, and unconscious journey and gives it a different significance. This time he crosses the border only figuratively; he vows to remain a citizen of the disabled community—and its representative; his book is the evidence that he has done so. Having connected his repression of his sense of impairment with the social oppression of those with disabilities, he is able to avow that he belongs in both worlds, that the border between them is an artificial one.

Breaking Out in Autobiography

In a study of stigma that builds on the 1963 work of Goffman, Edward E. Jones and colleagues use the term *mark* for *stigma* (perhaps unnecessarily literalizing the concept). Both their language and their approach typify sociology's tendency to categorize and objectify, but the sociological view of the restraints on self-presentation by disabled individuals may supply a helpful context for our discussion of disability autobiography. For one way of appreciating the collective achievement of these narratives of disability as self-representation is to consider them in relation to the strategies of self-presentation to which people with disabilities are supposedly restricted in everyday life:

Among the available strategies are *withdrawal*, including association with other markable persons; *concealment*, in either the strong form of passing or in the weaker form of reducing the mark's salience; *role acceptance*, which may spill over into exploitation through either supplication or intimidation or some combination of both; and *confrontation* animated by the hope of establishing normally gratifying relationships. (234; italics added)

Not all these strategies for everyday interaction are pertinent to autobiography. Thus by definition withdrawal (self-segregation) would seem to be inconsistent with the self-display involved in autobiography. So would concealment; a narrative in which an individual successfully hides an impairment is neither a disability autobiography nor a narrative of passing. Similarly, the strategies of "supplication" and "intimidation" are not likely, because autobiographers do not seek to manipulate readers in the same way that individuals manipulate each other in face-to-face encounters.

However, some significant overlap occurs between self-presentational strategies in everyday life and in writing. Thus firsthand accounts of disability may attempt in one way or another to reduce or minimize the stigma of disability. For example, Callahan deflects the stigma of disability in part by embracing that of alcoholism. Labeling that strategy *concealment*, however, may inaccurately suggest embarrassment or shame as motives. Disability autobiography can use variations of *confrontation*, such as "self-promotion and exemplification, both of which emphasize the limitations imposed by the mark in order to claim admirable talent or moral strength" (Jones et al. 234). According to Jones, "The self-promoter tries to elicit respect or even awe by convincing others of his unusual competence in some domain" (211). This is one way of describing Hockenberry's memoir of his journalistic exploits; it applies more generally to the adoption of the paradigm of the success story. In contrast, the strategy of exemplification "may often take a religious twist in that the disabled person appears convinced that it is God's will working in mysterious but acceptable ways, perhaps to test and confirm the marked person's moral strength" (213). This describes an important dimension of Price's narrative, which documents a kind of religious revival; more generally, it describes the adoption of the paradigm of the spiritual autobiography. Still, these are common autobiographical strategies, hardly distinctive of narratives of disability.

The sociologists' model of everyday strategies of interaction does shed some light on autobiographical strategies, I think, but the application of the model to these books ultimately reveals both the complexity of autobiographical practice and the poverty of the schema. Thus, although books like Zola's and Murphy's clearly enact "association with other markable persons," their strategy is hardly one of withdrawal. Quite the contrary: in the era of the disability rights movement association with other stigmatized people is more likely to represent advocacy and transgression than retreat.

Jones's theory comes closest to acknowledging the goals of most disabled people today in its discussion of confrontation:

Perhaps the most mature and adaptive goal of the markable person who adopts a confrontational strategy is to "break through" into normal interaction patterns. That refers to the successful avoidance, disruption, or reversal of the labeling process so that the potentially stigmatizing mark is kept in its place as a manageable physical inconvenience or an interesting, but no longer relevant, bit of personal history. Thus, the interaction process is normalized, and the markable person no longer feels that the marker is preoccupied with his disabling condition and no longer fears that he confuses the specific effects of the conditions with irrelevant deviant or low-power scripts. (219)

Ideally, there will come a time when disabled people, like members of other marginalized minorities, will be able to interact "normally,"

without regard to their "mark." To that end, society needs to acknowledge the existence of stigma and contest its genesis and construction.
Jones's theory may be adequate for transitory face-to-face interactions,
which lend themselves to opportunistic or pragmatic strategies of negotiation. In everyday life, where the object may be to conduct some
particular transaction with the least distraction, ready-made strategies
may be enabling. As a deliberate and considered medium, autobiography, however, may be more concerned with long-term goals such as
self-definition and renegotiating the basis of relationships between disabled and nondisabled people. Autobiography cries out for new strategies, particularly transgressive ones that disrupt or reverse stigma. (As
a result, my discussion of textual self-presentation has been concerned
with *differences* between strategies that Jones lumps together: avoidance, disruption, and reversal of stigma.)

Although I do not wish to deny the usefulness of the sociological approach, I do want to emphasize its limitations, especially as a paradigm
for analysis of autobiographical self-presentation. When applied to written narratives, it lends itself to pigeon-holing. Although Goffman's discussion of stigma, on which Jones's is built, strikes me as shrewd, Jones's
discussion of strategies tends to limit "markable" individuals to a small
number of rather predictable and often manipulative behaviors in response to their predicament, most of which carry negative connota-
tions—withdrawal,concealment, exploitation, supplication, intimidation, and self-promotion. Aside from its all-too-brief reference to the
possibility of avoiding, disrupting, or reversing the labeling process,
Jones's analysis tends to reify the low status of people with disabilities.

In contrast, discourse theory grants to individuals—disabled or not—
the ability to subject language—terms, tropes, conventional scripts—to
scrutiny and revision. Written self-representation may appeal especially
to disabled people precisely because, by shifting the grounds of interaction, it offers an alternative to what the sociologists revealingly call
the "low-power" scripts of everyday interaction. What I have tried to
suggest in this chapter, then, is *that* and *how* individuals with disabilities may use autobiography to escape, extend, or redraw the boundaries within which they are usually confined.

The sociological model does help to remind us that the condition of
being disabled is prescribed in subtle but significant ways. The condition of having a disability is a "master status" that can invoke particular
"master plots," and even the books discussed here have not always succeeded in rewriting the old scripts. (Nor have, as yet, many disabling
conditions been adequately represented; as we have seen, the literature
of disability to date has focused on a few paradigmatic conditions and
has been written largely by men.) But perhaps the most significant ten-

dency in the disability movement today is the impulse to insist on the mark as an honorific rather than a pejorative master status. (This is most obvious today, perhaps, in the Deaf community.) We are just beginning to reap the results of this construction of disability in life writing. Like people marked by illness, people with disabilities are tired of the closet; they are breaking out of it by way of the living room of autobiography.

Notes

1. I draw on Shapiro's introductory chapter for the entire opening section of this chapter.

2. Perhaps the most important and inexorable factor behind the increasing numbers of disabled people in the United States is demographic: the aging of the population. Another less obvious factor has to do with the definition of what counts as a disability; for various reasons legal and administrative definitions have tended to become more inclusive over the years. On the expansion of the categories of disability, see Stone, pp. 161–68.

3. By many estimates the number of disabled people in the United States— on the order of forty million—makes it the largest minority group, outnumbering African Americans.

4. In a kind of backlash against well-meaning but fatuous euphemisms some disabled writers, including Leonard Kriegel (1991) and Nancy Mairs (1986), have embraced the taboo term *cripple*.

5. In this connection photographs of authors of the books discussed in this chapter are particularly interesting. The dust-jacket photos of Murphy and Leonard Kriegel are such that their subjects might well not be disabled; no wheelchairs or other apparatus are visible. The photo of John Callahan on the cover of the paperback edition of his 1989 book shows him in his wheelchair. John Hockenberry's 1995 book displays, on the front of its dust jacket, a photo of the author doing a wheelie on the pedestrian walkway of the Brooklyn Bridge. Typical of his generation, far from hiding his wheelchair, he flaunts his mastery of it.

6. As a print medium autobiography presents disability, as it does illness, in a summarized, somewhat sanitized, form. The very medium in which the story is presented may be inaccessible to its creator. Thus the accessibility of print to most people insulates them from some conditions it purports to represent (visual impairments, for example). In such cases the writer-reader relationship may be particularly asymmetrical; the ease of reading may lead nondisabled individuals to underestimate the impairment represented in the book in hand.

7. A glimpse of the sort of disabled lives that usually elude life writing can be found in *I Raise My Eyes to Say Yes* by Ruth Sienkiewicz-Mercer and Steven B. Kaplan (1989). Sienkiewicz-Mercer was born with severe cerebral palsy that prevented her from being able to walk, feed herself, or talk. After spending

some time in rehabilitative hospitals, she was sent for economic reasons to a state hospital in Massachusetts, where she was warehoused among mentally retarded people. (Indeed, she was [mis]diagnosed as retarded.) Eventually, her abilities were recognized, and she benefited from a new approach to disability, deinstitutionalization. She moved into an apartment and married.

Unable to talk or write, she produced her story in collaboration with Steven Kaplan, a lawyer and advocate for people with disabilities; by a cumbersome method of pointing to customized word boards, she was able to compose brief telegraphic statements in a cryptic shorthand, which Kaplan then expanded into an account of her life narrated from her point of view. (He relied on interviews with others to complement and contextualize her testimony.)

The book tells a compelling story of a kind of imprisonment. Indeed, it is quite analogous in several regards to slave narrative. The narrator looks back on a condition of oppression based on stigmatic bodily difference. Having escaped the oppressive institution, the narrator calls for the emancipation of those left behind; thus the message is reformist, almost abolitionist, in its fervor. Also, because the narrator and witness relies on a collaborator to get her testimony written and published, the narrative, like slave narrative, raises questions of authority and authenticity. Though Kaplan seems to have been scrupulous in checking his narrative's accuracy with Sienkiewicz-Mercer, the voice of the narrative cannot be regarded as hers: the vocabulary and syntax of the prose are inconsistent with her limited verbal skills. (The issue of the linguistic medium is not quite the same as that of representing Deaf lives; it is not that Sienkiewicz-Mercer is fluent in a language other than English but rather that her disabilities have prevented her from achieving the level of verbal facility that would usually accompany her intelligence.)

More than most narratives of disability, this one relies for comic resolution not on any amelioration of her impairments nor on spiritual or intellectual compensation for bodily dysfunction but on the lessening or easing of disability—the social and cultural obstacles to her integration into society. Once recognized behind the mask of her impairment, her subjectivity can flourish through communication. Perhaps the most important aspect of this narrative is that it represents a hidden population; her account, which came to be written only through rare and labor-intensive collaboration, may stand for the many lives that do not get represented because of the effects of impairment and disability.

8. Goffman notes that those anointed to represent people with disabilities tend to be unrepresentative because of their special qualities (they tend to be more articulate and literate) and their circumstances (their selection as representatives gives them access to other social worlds) (27).

I acknowledge that this chapter is less thorough in its exploration of its topic than those on breast cancer, HIV/AIDS, and deafness; as noted earlier, disability is a far more various condition than any of these others. Nevertheless, I think the books surveyed here do raise some issues common to much disability autobiography.

9. Although Christopher Reeve's severe injury left him with medical bills that would ruin most individuals, his fame has compensated somewhat. Random House has promised him a $3 million advance for an account of his recovery, and he has booked a series of appearances as a motivational speaker for fees of $50,000 or more (Gabriel A5). He also intends to continue working as an actor and director.

10. Daniel J. Wilson, who has surveyed fifty autobiographical accounts of polio, reports that many rely on religious themes and paradigms—especially "covenants of work and grace" (23).

11. This aspect of Price's book is particularly interesting with regard to one of the book's subtexts, the issue of his homosexuality. Although it rarely breaks the surface of the narrative, when it does, one sees that Price's benign view of his fate may be influenced by relief that his illness is not AIDS. (His condition seems to have greatly reduced his risk of AIDS early in the epidemic.) One effect of his paraplegia is thus to allow him to write of eros without writing of sex, to acknowledge his homosexuality in a minimally confessional manner.

Even so, for a previous reader of my library copy of the book the book's homosexual subtext was sharply at odds with its religious dimension. This reader neatly crossed out all of Price's references to sexual desire and in the margin expressed revulsion at Price's claiming Jesus's help because Price's sexuality was clearly against God's teaching. Evidently, for this reader Price's book *ought* to have been a conversion narrative replete with a renunciation of guilty desire.

12. In the years since the publication of his book, however, he has on occasion addressed issues of disability rights in his commentaries for National Public Radio.

13. Thus Callahan reports, "I felt like a floating head" (60). Murphy expresses a similar feeling: "As my condition has deteriorated, I have come increasingly to look upon my body as a faulty life-support system, the only function of which is to sustain my head" (101). Finally, Arnold Beisser, a quadriplegic physician, has written,

Since my head continued to be familiar, and it was the only part that seemed to merit respect, I had fantasies, or perhaps they were hallucinations, of a surgical procedure that would separate the head so that it would be unencumbered by the body. Perhaps it could be reattached to another body, or simply kept alive by a machine. Such ideas now seem bizarre, but they seemed quite reasonable in the light of the confused understanding I had about what was me and what was not, which was my private space and which belonged to someone else. (19–20)

14. Lionnet's example is Zora Neale Hurston's *Dust Tracks on a Road* (1942). Michael Fischer has discussed a similar kind of autobiography, offering as examples Maxine Hong Kingston's *Woman Warrior* (1976), Michael Arlen's *Passage to Ararat* (1975), and Marita Golden's *Migrations of the Heart* (1983).

15. The irony of the term *benign*, which simply means noncancerous, increases throughout his account of declining mobility.

Like Sacks, Murphy describes his recovery after surgery in religious terms: "I had been born again, returned to the world a new person. The decomposition of my identity by illness was healed. I was whole again in body and mind." But his relapse exposes this sense of resurrection as "a bright delusion" (45). As a mere reprieve, it proves a false conversion and does not provide him with his final perspective on paralysis. Still, his diction demonstrates the powerful appeal of the conversion and resurrection paradigms.

6

Signs of Life

Deafness and Personal Narrative

Deaf history may be characterized as a struggle for Deaf individuals to "speak" for themselves rather than to be spoken about in medical and educational discourses.
　　　　　　　　　　—H-Dirksen L. Bauman, "'Voicing' Deaf Identity," p. 47.

Coming to Terms: Deafness and the Discourse of Disability

The relationship between disability and deafness has recently become particularly fraught and controversial. For reasons to be discussed later, many Deaf ("culturally deaf") people do not accept the label of disabled for themselves, preferring to think of themselves as a linguistic and cultural minority (Davis 3). That position makes the inclusion of a chapter on deafness in a book on life writing about illness and disability somewhat problematic. Its inclusion is justified, I think, on the grounds that contemporary narratives of deafness, whether by hearing, deaf, or Deaf authors, all grapple with the dominant construction of deafness as a pathology and a disability. This chapter does not assume or argue that deafness is a disability; rather, it addresses the role of life writing in the developing discourse, and counterdiscourse, of deafness. Thus, among other matters, the chapter is concerned with the stance various life writers have taken on this issue—implicitly as well as explicitly—in their representation of hearing-impaired people. To omit such a chapter would be to pretend that these matters have been effectively settled; clearly, they have not. And life writing can play a significant role in changing public attitudes about deafness.

A way into these controversies is to begin with the vexed questions of terminology. As I suggested in Chapter 5, discursive reform has been critical to the movement for disability rights; in the case of deafness, ter-

minology is equally crucial but more complex. Although many laypeople use the terms *deaf, hard of hearing,* and *hearing impaired* more or less
interchangeably, audiologists and people with hearing impairments
use them more carefully. Terms that seem innocent to the uninitiated
carry subtle inflections to the wise; as with issues of race and gender recent attempts to redefine the natural or biological as culturally constructed have given familiar terms new political implications. As we saw
in the discussion of disability in Chapter 5, the current project of discursive reform with regard to disability is to replace the individual or
medical model with a social or political paradigm. The critical gesture
has been to remove the locus of disability from individual bodies, such
as those of amputees and paraplegics, to the social and cultural contexts that impede them; the reformers make a key distinction between
impairment (the incapacity or dysfunction of the body) and *disability*
(the disadvantage created by social and cultural exclusion or restriction
of people with certain kinds of impairments). In the case of hearing, impairment would have to do with the lack of audiologically normal hearing; disability would have to do with the lack of assistive devices and
services in public places.

But some theorists have gone a step further to suggest that because
some deaf people have developed their own language and culture, they
are not disabled but rather a cultural minority analogous to other ethnic
and linguistic minorities. Rather than defining deafness as an audiological deficit, then, theorists like Lennard J. Davis suggest that "the deaf
can be thought of as a population whose different ability is the necessary use of a language system that does not require oral/aural communication" (1995, 77). What has been termed a *communication disorder* is
entirely a matter of culture: deafness is a "disorder" only when the deaf
are trying to communicate with the hearing, not when they communicate among themselves using sign language. The current moment in history, then, is one in which the construction of deafness as a pathology,
a lack, an absence, is being aggressively challenged by deaf activists,
whose construction of deafness as a cultural phenomenon rooted in a
linguistic difference requires fundamental changes in discourse.[1]

Even a binary audiological division between *hearing* and *deaf* over-
looks the fact that hearing loss varies greatly in degree, kind, cause, and
time of onset. Moreover, these distinctions are harder to measure reli-
ably and consistently than one would think.[2] The nature of the impairment and when it was incurred often matter more than its degree. People with moderate postlingual hearing loss—the vast majority of
Americans with hearing loss (about fifteen million, as opposed to approximately 250,000 who are congenitally deaf [Sacks 4, 7])—are often
at pains to distinguish themselves from profoundly deaf people—and

vice versa. For various reasons hard-of-hearing people tend to be interested in assistive devices and corrective procedures that restore hearing and enable oral/aural communication, whereas profoundly deaf people are more interested in modifying the environment to accommodate their manual mode of communication—providing closed captions for TV, signers for speakers, and so on. Thus hard-of-hearing people tend to locate, and seek to correct, the problem in the individual's lack of normal hearing, whereas Deaf people tend to locate, and seek to correct, the problem in society's lack of understanding and accommodation of their distinctive culture. People with moderate hearing loss, then, align themselves with and rely on what Harlan Lane (*Mask*) contemptuously refers to as the "audist" establishment, whereas Deaf people tend to oppose it, relying instead on activism and political organization to further their goals.

Indeed, these political differences have given rise to the use of the term *Deaf* (with a capital *d*) for "a cultural identity (deaf people, that is, who use American Sign Language, share certain attitudes and beliefs about themselves and their relation to the hearing world, and self-consciously think of themselves as part of a separate Deaf culture)" (Baynton 238).[3] Not all deaf people, then, are Deaf. The distinction between deaf and Deaf is not a function necessarily of the degree of hearing loss nor even when the loss was incurred; rather, it may be a function of heritage and education—whether the individual's parents were deaf or hearing and whether, if hearing, they encouraged their child to use sign language and associate with deaf or hearing children, and so on. Ultimately, the key factor is self-identification (Padden 2). If fluent in sign language and immersed in the Deaf community, hearing children of Deaf parents sometimes consider themselves to be in some significant sense Deaf; it may be possible, then, to be Deaf without being deaf.

Although I consider in this chapter narratives concerning a variety of kinds of hearing loss, I should note here that Deaf people take pride in their distinctive culture and see their condition and their destiny as unrelated to those with adventitious, late-acquired, or relatively minor hearing loss. Perhaps the most crucial factor in hearing loss is the timing of its onset in relation to language acquisition. Individuals with congenital or prelingual hearing loss can find developing intelligible speech quite difficult; such individuals also have a hard time learning to read and write a language they have not first acquired orally. In contrast, those individuals who lose their hearing after having learned to speak are often able to continue to function orally, even with a substantial hearing loss. Thus a distinction is commonly made between those who are pre- and those who are postlingually deaf. Deaf theorists have rightly pointed out, however, that the terminology inscribes a hearing norm. It assumes that language is literally lingual—spoken. (In doing so they expose the bias of the dead metaphor of *tongue* for language. Ruth Sidransky, the hearing daughter of deaf parents, pointedly refers to her native language as the "tongue of hands"; perhaps it would be even more appropriate to speak of her "native hand.") Prelingually deaf children of deaf parents, whose first language is American Sign Language (hereafter ASL or Sign), do not suffer the same delay in acquiring language skills as deaf children of hearing parents, who may not be diagnosed as deaf until they lag in learning to speak. (One apparent consequence is that deaf children of deaf parents are typically high achievers in schools for the deaf.)

People with substantial hearing losses who retain or develop oral skills may function as hard of hearing in an oral-dominated culture. The desire of some deaf individuals to pass as hard of hearing, if not as hearing, suggests the continuing power of the stigma attached to deafness, which has traditionally been considered a disability and often assumed to cause, or be accompanied by, mental or intellectual deficiency. (As Oliver Sacks has pointed out, if the intellectual maturation of congenitally deaf people lags, it is because they have not learned language, whether spoken or signed, early in life. The same would be true of a hearing individual who did not learn a language very young. It is not deafness per se, but the lack of language, that creates cognitive retardation [Sacks 105, 110–11, 117].)

The Deaf community, of course, resents and rejects the stigma; indeed, *it* may censure those who try to pass. Deaf people define deviance from a different center; from a Deaf perspective the more others can hear, the more different—abnormal—they are. Among Deaf people, the use of the sign-term *hard of hearing* reflects a positive construction of deafness in two ways. First, the term is used to distinguish, and reproach, those who associate with and assimilate into hearing society (Padden 50). Second, the modifying phrase is qualified in a way diametrically opposed to the way the hearing majority uses it. Thus people who have a relatively severe hearing loss are referred to in American Sign Language as "a little hard of hearing," whereas those with a minor loss are referred to as "very hard of hearing" (Padden 41). Another good illustration of the way in which Deaf discourse challenges hegemonic assumptions is that the sign-terms *oral* and *think-hearing* are insults connoting a kind of betrayal of the community (52); think-hearing refers to people who are not oral but who accept hearing norms. An obvious parallel would be the term *Uncle Tom* in the African American community.

At present the disagreements over the construction of deafness are necessarily so passionate and political that it is difficult even to summarize the issues without having one's terminology prejudge issues or align one with a political position. As much as possible, however, I want to deploy terms without pejoration; my concern is to explore how life writing takes up, in narrative representation, some of the issues that have made the discourse of deafness so politically fraught. To what degree and how do the extant personal narratives of deafness rewrite the discourse of disability? Indeed, to what degree and how do they manage to represent the experience of deafness at all?

Signing Names: The Problematic Nature of Deaf Autobiography

> There isn't a large body of literature about the deaf by the deaf. A good deal more has been produced by the educators of the deaf, parents of the deaf, and offspring of the deaf. Much of it is valuable but tinged by secondhandedness. . . . Little has been written by the deaf themselves. Their handicap has kept most—especially those born deaf—from achieving the necessary command of English.
> —Henry Kisor, *What's That Pig Outdoors?*, 1990, p. 3.

In an incisive 1996 analysis H-Dirksen L. Bauman has addressed the problems inherent in constructing Deaf identity in everyday life in an oral-dominated culture. For the most part in their formal dealings with the hearing establishment—courts, physicians, social workers, and so on—Deaf people rely on the service of interpreters who know Sign. But, as Bauman points out,

> Signing through an interpreter . . . still precludes the Deaf "I," as such, from being received in the hearing world, for once it is spoken by the interpreter, the "I" is no longer autobiographical but, rather, a biographical rendition spoken by the interpreter in the first-person singular. As the narrative transfers from sign to orality, from narrating body to interpreting body, the autobiographical "I" undergoes a type of discursive mitosis, dividing into a new textual form that is to get a life all its own. . . . As this traveling "I" gains enunciation, one wonders how well it can "speak" for itself through the voice of an other—especially as the Deaf person to whom it belongs is unable to follow its auditory journey (49–50)

As Bauman shows, such transactions are not matters of linguistic translation alone; rather, unable to transcend the social hierarchies in which they are located, they mediate the Deaf *I* in ways that are usually overlooked: "the collaboration between Deaf narrator and sign-language interpreter in everyday situations . . . usually entails the meeting of complex power relations along gender, ethnic, racial, sexual, moral, class, and generational divides—and, perhaps most important, along the divides of hearing/Deaf and the dominance of speech/oppression of signing" (50).

In exploring remedies or alternatives to the constraints on Deaf people in their everyday "autobiographical" construction, Bauman suggests that writing may give them greater authority over their self-presentation by eliminating the need for translation and cross-cultural mediation. As Bauman realizes, in everyday encounters this is not always convenient or even possible. It might seem, however, that writing autobiography would give Deaf individuals complete control over their self-presentation. But as we shall see, this is not necessarily the case. Deaf autobiography is both rarer and more problematic than we might think.

Despite the Deaf Pride and Deaf Power movements, which began in the 1970s and gained national media attention during the Deaf President Now uprising at Gallaudet University in 1988, despite the recent Deaf renaissance (which might be dated from the publication in 1960 of William C. Stokoe's *Sign Language Structure*, which legitimated sign languages), and despite a series of significant books about deafness and deaf individuals, there has been no great outpouring of autobiographies by deaf Americans.[4] Perhaps this should not be surprising, for a number of factors militate against deaf autobiography and (especially) Deaf autobiography, making them unlikely and rare entities, if not contradictions in terms.

Only in the worst-case scenario, perhaps—in which a congenitally deaf individual never acquires language, whether spoken or signed—would "deaf autobiography" necessarily be a self-contradiction. Oliver Sacks illuminates the root of the problem in such cases in his remarks on the relations among deafness, language acquisition, and the achievement of full selfhood and humanity. In reference to a congenitally deaf and virtually languageless eleven-year-old, Sacks observes, "There was a strange lack of historical sense, the feeling of a life that lacked autobiographical and historical dimension, the feeling of a life that only existed in the moment, in the present" (40).[5]

In more benign scenarios, however, subtler factors may also impede or occlude written deaf autobiography. Beyond the fundamental question of the acquisition of language are other issues of language and literacy. In his 1995 book Lennard J. Davis argues that deafness and literacy are not inherently contradictory; after all, the acts of reading and writing are themselves silent, mute (59). To challenge hegemonic notions of literacy he also points out that although language seems to be instinctual in humans ("hard-wired"), writing is not—illiteracy is the norm in most of the world—and suggests that, considered as a kind of writing in space, Sign is closer to writing than speech is (19–20). In practice, however, it has proved especially difficult for those born deaf to acquire fluency in oral/aural/written languages, and no one has devised a standard notational code for Sign that is conducive to the print medium. Thus Lane, a champion of Deaf people, points out that learning English is difficult for deaf individuals because their first language is in another mode entirely (*Mask* 177). In Lane's blunt judgment, "thanks to the misbegotten educational programs operated by the audist establishment, deaf people are mostly illiterate" (70). This lack of literacy in English is one obvious obstacle to truly self-written (rather than collaborative) autobiography and helps to explain the relative dearth of recent deaf autobiographies.

One truism of autobiography studies today is that autobiography is confined to particular cultures—it is not a universal human endeavor. Such cultures are characterized by literacy, individuality, and the valorization of particular life scripts (such as religious conversion). Such factors explain why written autobiography has arisen in some cultures and not others and why autobiography is unevenly distributed among social classes, genders, and races within those cultures. If emphasis on individualism is a cultural prerequisite for the flowering of autobiography, the form might be slow to emerge from Deaf culture, which places a higher premium on interdependence and cooperation than on individualism and autonomy: "An emphasis on the group rather than the individual underlines a key feature of the Deaf experience: loyalty to deaf friends and the Deaf community. . . . When one compares Deaf and Hearing cultures, the different emphases on group solidarity versus individual autonomy are values second only to their contrasting views on communication" (Preston 86).

Socioeconomic factors also tend to work against the production of Deaf autobiography. Because of patterns of language skills, occupational training, and job discrimination, Deaf people tend to be underemployed, clustered in the lower income brackets, not the population that typically indulges in autobiographical self-display.[6] If, as Lane suggests, "we imagine two kinds of deafness"—one associated with poverty and one with middle-class culture (*Mask* 8)—we are more likely to have narratives of the latter than of the former. Furthermore, the Deaf community traditionally has been socially segregated; its cohesion has at once reflected and reinforced its marginalization. A somewhat insular community, the Deaf have not been much concerned with presenting themselves to the hearing world in mainstream media or genres. And within that community autobiography assumes different, less durable, forms.

In addition to the question of the presence of the broad cultural values conducive to autobiography, there is the matter of the genre's relation to specific cultural practices of communication and self-expression. Here too Deaf culture may differ significantly from hearing culture. According to Paul Preston, the "deaf way" of communicating is not entirely, or necessarily, a matter of using sign language; rather, it involves relational identification (presenting oneself by reference to one's parents and often one's school), informality and interactivity, and "drawing from a rich history of oral traditions" (10). All these aspects of deaf communication put it at odds with the conventions of autobiography, which until recently was an essentially monological, individualistic genre. (At least, it was assumed to be so: gender studies and poststructuralism have greatly broadened our sense of the forms autobiography can take, and the current ascendance of relational life writing may bode well for the future of Deaf life writing.)

Significantly, then, the Deaf community shares cultural values with traditional oral communities, in which autobiography is not an indigenous genre; rather, histories—individual and communal—are passed on in face-to-face communication within the group, not written down for consumption by outsiders. For similar reasons Deaf people and Native American communities have been vulnerable to domination and colonization by "historical" cultures. (Thus the suppression of sign language in oral schools for the deaf has its parallel in the suppression of indigenous languages at boarding schools for Native Americans.) Such groups begin to be represented in life writing, or autobiography, as a result of contact with, or acculturation into, dominant groups. Thus Deaf autobiography is problematic in ways that parallel the situation for Native American autobiography.

Arnold Krupat has helpfully distinguished between "the Indian autobiography" and the "autobiography by an Indian." According to Krupat, the Indian autobiography is "jointly produced by some white who translates, transcribes, compiles, edits, interprets, polishes, and ultimately determines the form of the text in writing, and by an Indian who is its subject and whose life becomes the content of the 'autobiography' whose title may bear his name" (Krupat, *For Those* 30). In contrast, the autobiography by an Indian is an entirely self-written life by a Native American sufficiently acculturated to undertake autobiography without assistance (Krupat, "Native" 179–80).

Because Deaf culture is to some extent at odds with autobiography as traditionally understood, Deaf individuals are most likely to generate autobiography when they are approached, coaxed, and collaborated with—on the model of Indian autobiography—or when they are acculturated into hearing culture—on the model of the autobiography by an Indian. In either scenario Deaf culture would be mediated through hearing culture. It is quite possible for a Deaf individual who is literate in English to initiate and undertake an autobiographical project entirely on his or her own, but the textual medium would presumably not render Deaf experience without significant omission or distortion. (I will explore the problems of the linguistic medium in greater detail later in this chapter.)

As we have seen, the Deaf Power movement has been accompanied by the advocacy of a cultural rather than a pathological model of deafness—the idea that the Deaf community represents an oppressed cultural and linguistic minority rather than a group suffering a physical infirmity.[7] This assertion is rooted in the legitimation of sign languages such as American Sign Language as true languages with their own lexicons, grammars, and syntax. Thus the Deaf renaissance has involved the use of Sign as a medium for dramatic performance as well as for everyday communication. At the same time, ASL is not widely understood outside the Deaf community and, as a nonwritten language, ASL is not entirely well suited to communicate the ideas and desires of the Deaf community to the hearing majority. As is the case with the languages of oral cultures, ASL seems incapable of serving as a literary language insofar as literature is assumed to be written and thus publishable in print—as is generally the case with autobiography. (Hence the thematization of literacy in early African American and Native American autobiography.)

If sign language is the native language of the Deaf community, it is not clear what form truly Deaf autobiography would take; autobiography written in English may in some sense misrepresent Deaf identity and life in the Deaf community. Like indigenous oral languages, sign language is not a medium for writing one's life, as the term is narrowly construed. One problem faced by Deaf culture in seeking recognition is that its indigenous language is a minority language, and a visual/manual, rather than oral/written one, at that. Like members of oral cultures, deaf individuals are inherently at a disadvantage in representing themselves in a majority culture oriented to print. Print culture is not hospitable to sign's graphic and temporal dimension nor to its orientation to a live audience. Sign's inherent qualities of visuality and performance in space and time make video a more promising medium than print for preservation and dissemination; subtitled video may be the ideal medium for Deaf autobiography. But the use of subtitles returns us again to the problem of language and cultural translation.

An obstacle to Deaf autobiography of a different order is that people who are born deaf or are deafened in early childhood are sometimes given false accounts of the cause of their deafness because greater stigma has been attached to congenital deafness than to that caused by accident or illness. Thus Paul Preston notes that his mother had been told as a child that her deafness was a result of a fall from her baby carriage, only to learn late in life that she had a deaf aunt and cousin, each of whom had been kept ignorant of the others. (Such a pattern of family deafness points to hereditary genesis, which is presumably why it was denied or covered up [238]). Thus the stigma of deafness is such that it may induce the altering, or falsifying, of life stories, beginning with its genesis; in the case of Preston's mother a defining event in her life narrative was unexpectedly exposed as a fabrication. Ruth Sidransky, the author of *In Silence: Growing Up Hearing in a Deaf World* (1990), is similarly unsettled to discover that her deaf mother, who never learned Hebrew, does not really understand the story behind the Passover seder (223). In this case ignorance of communal history, caused in part by deafness, affects a woman's sense of her heritage; her Deaf identity may diminish her sense of her Jewish identity.

The obstacles to literary self-expression by the deaf create the danger that the discourse of deafness will continue to be that of disability, the monological expression of what Lane calls audism.

> The audist narrative of what it like is to be deaf, captured in the literature of the "psychology of the deaf" and in other hearing fiction, is the acceptable one. The deaf narrative, rarely committed to paper, is not acceptable; it can be published, but its rebuttal of the hearing narrative carries no weight. What literary critic Edward Said has observed about anthropology applies with equal force to the family of disciplines constituting audism. The native point of view is not only ethnographic fact, he wrote, "it is a continuing, sustained adversarial resistance to the discipline and the praxis of anthropology (as representative of 'outside' power) itself, anthropology not as textuality but as an often direct agent of political dominance." Similarly, deaf leaders here and abroad have been resisting the alinguistic, acultural model of their minority culture and the undeaf methods of studying deaf people that give rise to it, not merely as ignorant ravings of dangerously powerful people but as the intellectual underpinning of hearing intervention, in forcibly imposed educational isolation, in institutionalization, in ear surgery, and all the forms that audist imposition takes. (44–45)

One significant issue in contemporary deaf life writing, then, has to do with whether it represents deafness through a biomedical model, as a pathology; through a social model, as an impairment made into a disability by an indifferent or hostile hearing culture; or through a cultural model, as a legitimate way of living and being. As Lane argues, "To portray a group is to engage in a political activity" (*Mask* 69). Most contemporary accounts of deaf people, though not by any means unanimous in their politics, display awareness that representation is a political act; most, indeed, offer themselves as counterdiscourse that is doing the important work of disabling stereotypes of disability.

One important element in contemporary life writing about deafness, then, is how deafness is constructed. Clearly, Deaf people have their view of deafness, which they are beginning to express in ways that challenge the dominant construction of deafness as an absence, a deprivation, a tragedy, a lack. But the situation is complicated by the division between Deaf people and deaf people. Those who are have a stake in Deaf culture are a minority of a minority; the vast majority of people with hearing impairment have no desire to be Deaf. And so they have no stake in the cultural model; indeed, they may be interested not only in disability rights but correction of their impairment. For them deafness is a personal, not a cultural, condition—a disadvantage, even a disaster. Their narratives may be oriented very differently from those of Deaf people.

Playing by Ear: Autobiography and Moderate Hearing Loss— Frances Warfield, *Keep Listening* (1957); Hannah Merker, *Listening* (1994)

Keep Listening, by Frances Warfield, may serve as a useful point of departure for discussing contemporary life writing and deafness, as much because of what it is not—Deaf autobiography—as because of what it is—a highly crafted and self-conscious narrative whose purpose is to challenge the stereotyping of people with hearing impairments and other disabilities. After recounting her lifelong struggle with her impairment—and its subtle but unmistakable effects on her self-image, marriage, and career—she ends with a prophecy of a millennial America in which there will no longer be two kinds of people, those with and those without "handicaps," but rather "just people . . . of different capacities, at different stages of physical, emotional and mental development—all in the process of becoming whole" (158).

In her attempt to disable the stigma of disability, she transfers the notion of impairment from body to character, redefining it as a moral deficit: "The only really handicapped person will be the one who—because of some blindness, deafness, malformation, or crippling malfunction of spirit—believes that there is nothing wrong with him. . . . The tongue-tied, emotionally handcuffed non-human being who thinks that it is possible to live without giving and receiving help" (158). Though this move is somewhat facile, there is something appealing in this vision of a utopia—where, to paraphrase Martin Luther King Jr., people would be judged not by the capabilities of their bodies but by the content of their character. At the same time, it is obvious that this utopia, as envisioned by Warfield in 1957, has not materialized. And in the context of the narrative this optimistic vision proves not to be altogether convincing—or earned. In her attempt to break down boundaries Warfield sometimes reinforces them; her book, however well intentioned, is confined within some of the very boundaries it seeks to erase.

The eleven-chapter narrative falls into two major parts. The first movement is in effect a narrative of coming out: a young woman gradually comes to acknowledge that she is hearing impaired and takes steps to compensate for her impairment—first surreptitiously studying lipreading, later acquiring and wearing a hearing aid. Passing as "normal" had its rewards—avoiding stigma—but it also had its costs. It was while Warfield still denied her hearing impairment that she was most socially impaired—condemned either to avoid conversation or to disrupt it with her blunders. Ultimately, she finds the closet intolerably confining and inauthentic; only by acknowledging her impairment, at first only to herself, can she begin to overcome it: "What if I was handicapped? I wanted to say so. What if deaf was a four-letter word? I wanted to say it—'I'm deaf'—good and loud. I wanted to hear it, get free of my fear of it. I wanted out of tact and consideration and fond, well-meaning protection. It wasn't protection. It was isolation, solitary confinement. I was going to get free—even if it meant taking myself and my whole world apart" (26–27).

Coming out of the closet, however, also cost her dearly; the decisive shift in her self-image and self-identification undermined her marriage: "Getting a hearing aid was my symbolic death. It meant the end of clever Miss Warfield . . . the person Jack fell in love with and married. Our marriage was happy, but how could it go on—when Miss Warfield didn't live there anymore?" (44–45). Wearing wires was tantamount to a symbolic suicide: "My mind was made up. I would kill off clever Miss Warfield. And I would wire hard-of-hearing Mrs. Hackett for sound" (48). Gender is a factor here; once she has confronted her impairment, she no longer requires the protection of her husband. Literally and symbolically, her hearing aid comes between her and her husband, displacing him from his role: "My new life as an independent, self-assured woman depended on this new, live companion—literally—of my bosom" (59). (Born in 1901, Warfield published an earlier account of her life, *Cotton in My Ears*, in 1948; that narrative concludes with her marriage.)

The climax of the narrative of coming out comes two-thirds of the way through the book, with the declaration of the author's rehabilitation: "I knew now that I could hold my own—socially, economically, professionally—without bluffing, guessing, and pretending" (109). Just as she announces her "rehabilitation," however, she announces that she wanted more; just when she can acknowledge casually, even proudly, that she is hard of hearing, and even as she is building a career of service to hearing-impaired people, she realizes she may not *have* to be deaf and that she doesn't want to be if she doesn't have to be. As well-adjusted as she is, she still desires to hear, still aspires to be normal. She realizes that just as she was a kind of "humbug" when she chose to pass as hearing, she is in danger of becoming another kind of humbug if she continues to capitalize on a handicap she doesn't need, or want, to have (114).

The cause of the author's impairment, otosclerosis, is crucial to her construction of hearing impairment, and it makes possible a decisive shift in direction at this point in the narrative. Otosclerosis, which causes only a small percentage of hearing losses, is the stiffening or immobilization of the stapes, the last in the chain of inner ear bones that transmit vibrations from the eardrum to the auditory nerve by way of an oval window in the bone. Because it is caused by otosclerosis, the author's auditory deficit proved susceptible to surgical correction in the early 1950s—first in one ear, by "fenestration" (the opening of an alternate window in the bone), then in the other, by mobilization of the frozen stapes. The consequence of her benefiting (in midlife) from advances in surgical techniques is that what starts out as a story of acknowledgment of and adjustment to an impairment turns into a narrative of her eradication of it. So the narrative carries Warfield not only out of her closet but, in the end, out of the category of the impaired altogether. Running counter to her vision of the dissolving of the stigma of "handicap" is the narrative's second movement, which removes the impairment—and thus its stigma—from her. Indeed, at the moment she speaks so confidently of the integration of the "handicapped" and the "normal," she is a fully hearing individual.

Like a significant number of narratives of impairment or illness, then, this one derives its basic plot from the conversion narrative, with its sudden and profound change in the status of the narrator. In this entirely secular narrative the change is a physical one; "grace" is provided not by a transcendent being but by a godlike physician. Indeed, a distinctive feature of the book (and of its era) is its unquestioning embrace of a pathological model of deafness and the author's complete identification with medical authority. This is evident throughout, from the book's dedication—"To all otologists"—to the point at which its title appears in context, where the author exalts the relentless march of science in the conquest of hearing impairment; there, the author's admonition to "keep listening" means "keep believing in the promise of science to vanquish disability of all kinds" (150).

To be sure, the book is careful to distinguish between moderate hearing loss and profound deafness. In distinguishing between the two conditions Warfield draws the line between those who can function orally in a hearing world and those who can't—and especially between those whose impairment is correctable—prosthetically or surgically—and those whose impairment isn't. In making the distinction, however, she effectively writes the deaf out of her narrative: "These are, of course, two entirely different handicaps. The deaf are individuals who are born without hearing or who acquire complete or nearly total deafness before the acquirement of speech. . . . With few exceptions, they live, necessarily, in a segregated world. The hard of hearing are those who acquired deafness after having heard normally and therefore acquired speech in the normal way" (77). The prelingually deaf are consigned to a netherworld, and their status in the inclusive vision of her conclusion is not entirely clear.

Indeed, she seems to imply that the progress of the hard of hearing depends on their distinction from the deaf, who are evidently beyond redemption. Thus she cites as a turning point in the rehabilitation of the hard of hearing the 1942 decision of the League for the Hard of Hearing "to excise the word deaf from their conversation, their correspondence and other writing, their teaching, and their speeches in public. It worked. New York doctors, teachers, newspaper reporters, and the public in general gradually began to use the new vocabulary. Straight thinking was on the way" (78). The rehabilitation of the hard of hearing, then, involves the continued marginalization, if not the stigmatization, of the profoundly deaf.

Although her desire for normal hearing is not surprising, aspects of the narrative suggest it has a pathological dimension, which may have to do with the subtext of death in the narrative. The narrator was orphaned in her youth when her father, a prominent banker, shot himself, and her sister died young, apparently also a suicide. Warfield wryly introduces the morbid subtext in the book's first paragraphs: "Many people who are hard of hearing would rather die than admit it. I know, because I was one of them. I used to spend a great deal of time thinking of ways to die, and once in my early thirties I got as far as drowning myself experimentally in the bath tub. After that, I dried my hair, had my wave reset and sneaked surreptitiously to the Nitchie School of Lip-Reading. I didn't wear dark glasses and a thick black veil, though I thought of it" (7).

What starts out as a joke on her inability to distinguish similar-sounding words, *deaf* and *dead* (14), turns serious. As the narrative progresses, it becomes clear that Warfield does see deafness as a kind of deadness: in her world, or worldview, to be deaf is to suffer at least a social death. She expresses this notion in a passage concerning her recovery from ear surgery: "I told myself, at last I would feel fully alive—in a way and to a degree that I had never felt alive before. One of the chief functions of sound in people's lives is the creation of moods and the excitation of feelings. Deprived of sound, one feels deadened, emotionally flat. Especially in the middle of the night" (126). The larger implications of her conflation of deafness and deadness are evident when, returning to doctor for a checkup and postoperative treatment, she regresses to a state of dependence on a male authority figure for validation: "I suppose that, emotionally, I was four years old again, waiting for Papa, my first great lord of creation. If so, it was not surprising. A doctor is a symbolic father. And to me, just as the words deaf and dead were equated, hearing always had symbolized life. . . . Thanks to Dr. Lempert, I was reborn and reanimated" (134–35). Without subjecting Warfield to psychoanalysis we can see how the cultural stigma of deafness has underwritten her association of her parents' premature deaths with her potentially isolating physical impairment. Once her deafness is surgically corrected, then, she thinks of herself as resurrected, returned to a state of vitality and grace. Warfield's oralist bias, though not surprising, given her generation (remember, the book came out in 1957), is evident in her final pages, when she proudly recounts quite literally reclaiming her tongue once she has full hearing in both ears, using tongue exercises to refine her speaking skills and bring them into coordination with her hearing ability (157).

She announces at the outset that hers is not a story of conquest but of revolution (10), but she might better have said *salvation* or *conversion*, because *revolution* has political overtones that seem irrelevant here. Indeed, her personal conversion effectively removes her from the larger revolution (in public attitudes or ideology) she celebrates at the end of her narrative. The stigma of handicap is not removed by surgery; quite the contrary, the desire for the surgery is driven as much by cultural and psychological needs as by physical aberration. If hearing impairment could always be corrected, like hers, there might be no need for the revolution she describes; there might be no "handicapped" and "unhandicapped." Today cochlear implants bid to do for profoundly deaf people what fenestration and mobilization did for her. But as Deaf activists point out, the idea that deafness requires correction—or that deaf people will universally welcome it—reflects hearing bias. From a Deaf perspective the surgical correction of all hearing impairment would be a catastrophe, a kind of cultural genocide.

Warfield, however, sees deafness as a kind of death or imprisonment—a life sentence to solitary confinement. And her vision of it inscribes rather than erases the boundary between remediable hearing loss and "true" deafness:

It is so easy to say, "Oh, there are worse things than deafness. After all, nobody dies of deafness." But people do die of deafness—a hundred little deaths a day. It is perfectly true that impaired hearing makes no physical inroads upon the body. But it can make deep psychological inroads. Impaired hearing can invade the dignity, undermine the personality, and damage the living spirit. . . . It can bring tension, anxiety, fear. Fear of failure, fear of ridicule, fear of people; fear of new situations, chance encounters, sudden noises, imagined sounds—these are only a handful of the fears that haunt the waking and even the sleeping hours of a deafened person. Small wonder that he may feel as if he were in an invisible prison, alone in silence, unable to hear the rest of the world and perhaps—a frightening thought indeed—unable to make the rest of the world hear him. (95)

Although her narrative is engaging, candid, and well written, it suggests what profoundly deaf people—especially the Deaf—are up against. It is the very assumptions that Warfield so casually makes—the common sense of deafness—that today's deaf activists are seeking to deconstruct.

Hannah Merker's *Listening* (1994) presents a very different view of hearing loss. Merker's hearing loss, though severe and sudden, came in midlife (the result of a skiing accident at thirty-nine); thus it did not affect her formative years or her English language skills. She lipreads well—so well that she sometimes has trouble convincing others of her impairment. Although she retains enough hearing to benefit from hearing aids, her loss is significant enough that she also relies on a hearing-ear dog. Thus she is hard of hearing, not deaf, let alone Deaf (she does not know Sign and does not affiliate herself with the Deaf community). She thinks like and identifies as a hearing person: she misses her lost hearing and remains hungry for sound. Thus her book largely ignores the predicament of profoundly and/or prelingually deaf people; she expresses little interest in sign language or the controversies over the different systems of communication. She addresses herself, then, not to the predicament of the relatively small number of Deaf people but rather to the much larger segment of the population that has lost, or will lose, a significant degree of hearing.

For the most part her book avoids narrative, which tends to foreground changes in condition, either loss or recovery; rather, it is a kind of wide-ranging meditation on listening by someone who has suffered a significant hearing loss. Her basic strategy is to redraw the boundary between the "hearing" and the "hard of hearing" by redefining key terms. In particular, she exploits the disjunction between the related terms *hearing* and *listening*. In one way of distinguishing between them, listening is a kind of indifferent attentiveness, which does not guarantee the reception of a message or the consummation of an attempt to communicate: for example, "he listened but didn't really hear what I was saying." More commonly, hearing refers to a mere passive physical ability, whereas listening denotes moral or existential qualities—interest, attention, and receptiveness: for example, "he can hear, but he doesn't really *listen*." The latter distinction, in which listening is valorized over hearing, lies at the heart of the book.

When we are really listening . . . we are not just hearing. Hearing, after all, is merely receiving, the brain's recognition of sound, something that will happen without personal will, unless our hearing mechanism is defective or temporarily denied access by earplugs, by sorrow, by some acute concentration that shuts off our sensibilities. Listening happens when we become attentive, when we choose responsibly to receive *and* understand an earth message of some kind. Listening is a conscious act. (28)

Hearing is an ability of the ear or the brain; listening, of the mind or the person.

Obviously, the valorization of listening at the expense of hearing tends to minimize hearing loss. Unlike some attempts to minimize disability, it is not a transparently euphemistic renaming but rather a rethinking of what it means to hear and not to hear, to listen and not to listen. Merker thus attempts to disrupt the way in which hegemonic discourse of disability maps intellectual and moral distinctions onto physical ones (making the deaf "dumb," for example). Without denying her impairment, nor its cost in convenience, pleasure, and awareness, she defines the operative and morally relevant distinction as the one between listening and not listening (for which we sometimes use the term *deaf* metaphorically). By definition the hard of hearing cannot hear normally, but they can listen superbly.

To listen means to be aware, to watch, to wait patiently for the next communication clue. And, as anyone with a speech or hearing disability can tell you, listening is not always auditory communication.

How then do we redefine the word "listening" to include all the interacting phenomena that occur when a deaf or hearing impaired person is talking to a friend, walking alone on a beach, occupying his spot in the world on any particular day? The ears of such a one miss much. The wonder that is the human body seems willing to soar over the gap. When earth's auditory energy is received as a whisper, or perhaps not at all, other senses become sharpened, grasping communicative clues we have forgotten, in the rush of life, are there. Listening becomes visual, tactile, intuitive.

Listening . . . perhaps . . . is just a mind aware. (17)

Although Merker is, as I have noted, somewhat inattentive to the particular predicament of those who have never heard, her discourse serves all those with impaired hearing insofar as it erodes the authority of audiology; the arbiter of hearing norms has no authority over listening. The overall intent of her discourse, then, is to destigmatize lack or loss of hearing. Indeed, Merker singles out for indictment as "listening-impaired" those medical practitioners who either address her husband over her presumably deaf-and-dumb body or who insist on talking behind her even after she has made clear the nature of her impairment:

Something happens when I tell someone I am severely hearing impaired— when I say, please look at me directly so that I can see what you are saying.

Something happens and I know what it is, a canceling out of the words I have said simply because I have said them. I have spoken in a clear voice, my speech understandable. My ability to speak well masks an unalterable fact—delivery of articulate speech does not mean that receiving another's spoken thoughts takes place. To comprehend conversation, I need to be stared at. (144)

Her lipreading skills are so good that she sometimes has trouble convincing people of her impairment.

Merker's thesis is in a sense banal: not all who can hear can or do listen. But at times her exploration of a relatively obvious idea assumes quite interesting and subtle forms. The book, though short, surveys a number of kinds of listening that transcend, exceed, or otherwise do not coincide with our usual sense of hearing. Drawn to nature, she spends a good deal of time exploring the auditory capabilities of species that lack ears—including fish, insects, and other lower forms of life. She is interested in prenatal hearing in humans and in the ability of other species to hear what humans can't, ultra- or infrasonic frequencies. Here she redraws the boundary between "normal" and "impaired hearing": when compared to other species', the "normal" hearing of humans is limited to a narrow range of frequencies. In rest of the animal kingdom "hearing" may be a function not of the ear but of the entire organism. Some of the book, then, is about hearing rather than listening, perhaps, but the point is to expand our sense of it beyond our limited projection of human norms. These parts of the book also exemplify a kind of listening *to* other species, attending to their capacities and the different ways in which they apprehend the universe.

She investigates a useful distinction, borrowed from natural history, between a creature's environment and its perceptual world (how it perceives its environment, which data its nervous system attends to, and so on). Part of her book's intent is to admit readers to her perceptual world and by doing so to enlarge theirs. Thus, although her hearing loss means that she cannot hear things some readers can, the chapters on nature demonstrate her extraordinary ability to attend to the world around her. The larger point is that our perceptual worlds are not determined by our senses but by our orientation and values; they are profoundly cultural and personal constructions. And to some extent they are functions of will and desire.

Another assumption Merker challenges is that listening is what a single organism does; for her, listening, as opposed to hearing, is often a collaborative act. Hearing aids are the most familiar, most technologically advanced, but in some ways the least interesting and sophisticated way to supplement or augment impaired hearing. Thus, for example, she can listen through collaboration with an animal—her hearing-ear dog—or with a friend. Collaboration with a friend is not a matter of dependency but of interdependency—mutuality and synergism. The friend who tries to hear for and with Merker will find herself listening to sounds she usually ignores. Similarly, if Merker uses visual cues to try to describe what she thinks her friend can hear, both become more attentive to ambient noise and to the way in which each constructs out of raw material a highly subjective perceptual world. Both will come away from such sessions with heightened awareness.

It is notoriously difficult for people who are not disabled to imagine the situation of disabled people because the former take so much for granted—their senses, their physical mobility, and so on. One challenge of writing about disability, even for people with disabilities, is to convey what impairment is like without reinforcing the boundary between "normal" and "disabled." Merker takes advantage of having once been able to hear well—and of being a skillful writer—to describe for the hearing what they would lose if they lost their hearing. Thus the book opens with Merker's description of sounds she is not hearing.

How can you know that the world around me is quiet—that I do not hear your step behind me, or hear you call my name from a distance? The silence around me is invisible. How can you know that the songs of new birds in spring, the crunch of old leaves, the soft sigh of the west wind, all subtle sounds that color the day for you, are not there for me? The whir of a car, the pounding feet of a runner behind us as we walk, the slap of rain on a roof are so elementary a part of your perceptions you cannot imagine that for a person at your side they may not exist. How can you know unless I tell you?

And how can I tell you about something that is not there, if part of my mind is asleep, no longer associates sound with a particular circumstance?

So, then, we must talk to each other, listening in our own ways. . . . We have *both* forgotten these sounds are there.

And so this book is about listening . . . about new ways of listening for the hearing and the hearing impaired. (1–2)

Although this passage undeniably privileges (and perhaps romanticizes) hearing, it may serve to combat complacency in the hearing. For, in addition to giving the reader a vivid sense of the absence of sound—what Merker is missing—it will remind most readers that their ears are disengaged—deaf—much of the time. Reading the book also becomes an act of collaborative listening in which, paradoxically, a hearing-impaired woman listens *for* her readers and instructs them in how to listen; her (hearing) loss is their gain. As a listening aid for the hearing, her book helps to reconfigure the relation between hearing and hearing impairment, between nondisability and disability.

Falling on Deaf Ears: Parental Memoirs of Deaf Children— Paul West, *Words for a Deaf Daughter* (1970); Thomas S. Spradley and James P. Spradley, *Deaf Like Me* (1985)

Although deaf people have increasingly been the subjects of life writing in recent decades—especially the 1990s—these narratives are much more frequently written about than by deaf individuals, for reasons already suggested. (In this they have much in common with narratives of HIV/AIDS.) Thus, although deaf autobiography does exist, it is still quite rare; more frequently, deaf lives are written by hearing family members. Usually, the life writer is not a sibling but a parent or child, as though narrative requires the distance of a generation's remove. The differences between a parent's and a child's perspective are such that I will devote the next two sections of this chapter to parental and filial memoirs, respectively.

Helen Keller is often quoted as saying that blindness cuts people off from things, whereas deafness isolates people from other people. Implicit in this distinction is a hearing norm, for deafness does not cut Deaf people off from each other the way it cuts them off from hearing people. (Sign language can remedy the "communication disorder" of deafness in a way that nothing seems to repair the perceptual deficit of blindness.) With this qualification in mind we can see that when deafness impedes communication with nonsigning people, it impairs relations with them more generally. This may help to explain the prevalence of relational life writing about deafness, for when deafness comes between parents and children, it obstructs relations that our culture makes primary. Hearing relatives of deaf people have turned to life writing as a medium for repairing or compensating for strained or obstructed relations. Although there is some danger that communication with readers may thus displace communication with the deaf family member, the act of writing is usually a way of honoring the relationship even while acknowledging its limitations.

The parental memoir of the ill or impaired child is a fairly well established subgenre. The politics of life writing, particularly where there is cultural cleavage or inequity between subject and author (for example, racial or gender difference), has been scrutinized recently in terms of the degree to which the author has access to the subject's life and the question of who controls the narrative. Obviously, the parent-child relationship is inherently asymmetrical; parents have knowledge of and power over young children in a way that is generally not reversible—except in cases of parental regression, for example, as a result of illness or old age. Parental biography is usually unauthorized in the sense that parents rarely bother to obtain their children's consent for a memoir; at the same time, however, parental biographers usually have the sort of privileged access to their subjects' lives that we associate with authorized biography. (Indeed, they may have access to records and incidents that are unavailable to the subjects themselves; parents know things about their children that the children don't know or can't remember. Parental memoir can thus involve a kind of double subjection of children to parental authority.)

In the case of impaired children the disparity in power and authority is in some ways greater than usual. At the same time, as with impaired children generally, parents of deaf children often feel at a loss, even powerless (Sacks 118). Indeed, one motif (and motivator) of memoirs by such parents is their sense of exclusion from their deaf child's world. In many cases what parents do not witness their deaf children cannot relate to them easily, if at all. Thus the narrative can never be a fully rounded one. One major concern in such narratives is how to break the sound barrier, how to be in a position to know one's child intimately, as parents feel they should.

Typically, parental biographies are monological—dominated, even monopolized, by the parental voice; rarely, if ever, do they give the children a voice. The impairment of the child makes it all the more difficult to recruit the child as collaborator or conarrator. One acute concern of the parental memoir of a deaf child is the child's ability to communicate in some fashion, not necessarily orally. One danger built into the genre, however, is the reification of the image of the deaf *as* children, unable to speak for themselves, having to be represented by others. This happens when the dichotomy between the narrating parent and the voiceless child is mapped onto the hearing/deaf dichotomy.

Two memoirs of deaf children, both daughters, deserve mention here because of the way in which they broach these issues. Inclusion of the first, Paul West's *Words for a Deaf Daughter* (1970), is somewhat problematic because West's daughter Mandy is not "simply" deaf. That is, her hearing loss, which is profound, is linked to evident brain damage, which at the time of writing had not been definitively diagnosed. Her impairment is sufficiently severe that at the age of seven she was unable to communicate effectively in words and still not completely toilet trained; in addition, her behavior was somewhat erratic and impulsive. The danger is that the title's identification of her as deaf will misrepresent not only her but deaf people generally. That is, her other disabilities may be conflated with her deafness, which has too often been associated with cultural or intellectual deficiency.

Like many parents in similar circumstances, West does not press for authoritative diagnosis, perhaps out of a sense that diagnoses of disabilities can become self-fulfilling; rather, "in the semi-dark of not knowing, we go ahead and treat you as only deaf and encourage you to progress at a speed that doesn't compound your difficulties" (9). Whether this represents benign optimism or unhealthy denial is a matter on which readers will differ. What is important to acknowledge is that West's "words for a deaf daughter" are, to begin with, a shield against other words for her, diagnostic labels that might explain her condition but also limit her development. The book, then, is a counterdiscursive response to tests that can only reveal her deficiencies against some more or less arbitrary norm; one thing the book does compellingly is to give a sense of the ways in which she exceeds norms, for better or worse; her energy, for example, though rarely focused, seems boundless.

Much more than the usual parental memoirist, West is limited to his own observations by Mandy's inability to pass along accounts of scenes at which he was not present. Nevertheless, West makes a conscious effort to enter her world imaginatively. While acknowledging the ways in which his world is closed to her, West makes a point of noting how his attempts to give her access to that world also heightened his perception of it: "Until I knew I had to bring the world to you, I don't think I knew or saw the world at all" (154). (In Merker's terms, having a deaf daughter taught West to listen.) The process of teaching Mandy, then, brought reflexive benefits; having to take into account her particular angle of vision heightened his powers of observation: "The mind that would keep company with you must be big enough to make itself limp a little; in so doing, it might notice things it might otherwise have missed" (164). Her reliance on senses other than sound—taste, for example—sharpens his senses: "Tasting—testing—with you, I have found new ways into the world. You discover what you discover because you have lost what you've lost" (27).

Here he knowingly runs the risk of romanticizing impairment:

How, indeed, if at all, can the life of you handicapped people be put into words? Presumably you have special aptitudes that to some extent compensate for what you are short of: say, a non-verbal although perhaps intricate intimacy with animals or plants . . . or, by the same token, with things man-made that most people in their full-facultied haste ignore or overlook—the texture of a blanket, the taste of a spoon. Attentiveness for its own sake could well be what the mentally handicapped person has as his own special gift. Intent not on reporting what he perceives but on perceiving itself, he comes closer perhaps than so-called competent people to seeing infinity in a grain of sand (although he won't think of it that way). He might even see the *finiteness* of a grain of sand, thus heeding its excellence within its limitations. (162–63)

He insists that her disability must have epistemological consequences. Because Mandy evidently does not inhabit the same world he does, his charge is to try to imagine what her world must be like. To that end, the book is deliberately and delightfully defamiliarizing.

The book's most significant and distinctive formal feature is that it is addressed to its subject. Because Mandy is nearly mute, it is necessarily a monologue, but it is framed hopefully as the initiation of, or at least the preparation for, a genuine dialogue—"their first real conversation" (27). (The one actual dialogue the book represents is short, and Mandy's contribution is limited to single-word exclamations that only a parent would be able to decipher.) Its chapters are more topical than narrative in organization. Part of its ostensible purpose is to make a record of the early, essentially prelingual, years of her life on the assumption that her lack of language has compromised, if not occluded, her memory of it. Thus the book is a gift—an act of vicarious or surrogate memory (or a memory supplement, like family snapshots). Her father writes out of an urge common to many parents, to preserve his child's childhood; her impairment makes the enterprise all the more urgent and poignant.

The book is words *for* her in the sense that the words are, at least in theory, intended for her later consumption. They are also words for her in the sense that they express what she as yet cannot; she is unable to put words to this sort of use. The words are meant to be in her interest—on her behalf—like everything else he and her mother do for her. But ultimately the book is words *about* her because she is unlikely ever to be able to read and internalize the memories West puts down on paper.[8] Hence the book's pathos. As readers we sympathize with West's optimistic project of creating a record to share with his daughter, to recreate the past that her consciousness will apparently not retain; still, we are acutely aware that she is unlikely to read the words we do. (And we are aware that because we are, after all, reading a published account, it was not composed solely for Mandy.)

As if to prevent the book from being sheer parental monologue, however, West devotes an entire chapter to Mandy's words. The chapter takes the form of an annotated dictionary of the few words she knows—spelled (phonetically), defined, explicated, and contextualized. The lexicon is infantile in its size and its pronunciation; it inevitably and decisively reveals her limitations. At the same time, insofar as it gives a sense of the essential constituents, human and otherwise, of Mandy's world, it gives a sense of her uniqueness and of what Merker would call her "perceptual world." It also gives voice to Mandy in some significant way; uniquely among the books surveyed here, this one's phonetic spellings give the reader some sense of what its deaf subject sounds like. Thus the book, at least in this chapter, literally incorporates and is built around her words.

Another of the book's distinctive formal qualities is its extravagant—

sometimes Joycean—use of language. In a sense this too is a gift: the hyperverbal father puts his power at his daughter's disposal, using his extraordinary talent to compensate for his daughter's deficit and to introduce her to people beyond her immediate knowledge, "people who'd want to know you" (9). Unable to converse with her in person, he pours out bottled-up words on paper in an effort to bridge the gap between them—or in anticipation of the narrowing of the gap. At the same time, the highly inventive and crafted quality of the writing heightens our sense of the gulf between father and daughter. In the end the book's writerliness may strike some readers as overcompensation by a highly verbal father unable to communicate with his linguistically impaired child.

According to its author, *Words for a Deaf Daughter* "has become a teaching text and a manual for parents" (*Gala* ix), a good example, perhaps, of parental discourse first challenging, then being adopted by, hegemonic discourse. As such it should be supplemented by *Deaf Like Me* (1978), by Thomas S. Spradley and James P. Spradley. *Deaf Like Me* is in many ways the opposite of West's book; it is sober and workmanlike rather than verbally extravagant, doggedly chronological rather than topical. And whereas *Words for a Deaf Daughter*, written for its subject, eventually became a parents' manual, *Deaf Like Me*, written with other parents in mind, was eventually read by its subject. Most important, *Deaf Like Me* challenges the implicit audism and oralism of West's book.

Deaf Like Me is the account, coauthored by Thomas Spradley and his brother James Spradley, an anthropologist, of the early life and education of Thomas Spradley's daughter Lynn, who was born deaf. A remarkable and moving book, it takes the point of view of two extremely conscientious and well-meaning parents who at first accepted oralist orthodoxy without question. This understated narrative may more convincingly expose the insidiousness of oralist dogma than Lane's polemical indictment of audism because it shows how oralism plays upon the hopes, fears, and guilt of hearing parents of deaf children. Lynn Spradley is bright and eager to communicate, and she makes just enough slow progress with oral methods to reinforce her parents' efforts in that mode; at every turn the experts assure her parents that in time their efforts will pay off. If they show signs of discouragement or dissent, they are told that any deviation from pure oralism could irretrievably damage Lynn's prospects of living a "normal" life. Their belief in oralism is at times more a matter of resignation than of resolve: "the oral approach offered the only adequate solution. There was nothing else to do. We couldn't just give up. We couldn't consign Lynn to a world of silence, loneliness and dependence" (183). If only they maintain an exclusively oral environment, if only they work hard enough with (which is to say, *on*) Lynn, she will learn to speak intelligibly. They eventually see through this but not for quite a long time. The period of their passive acquiescence constitutes almost the entire narrative, which covers only the first several (but crucial) years of Lynn's life.

Oralist orthodoxy is delivered to them in person by teachers, administrators, and physicians; in seemingly authoritative pamphlets and books, complete with scholarly apparatus; and in curricular materials and home study courses that presume to script their lives (86). Among these media is autobiography, in the form of short narratives in oralist magazines by successful products of oral schools (113, 183). What these narratives don't always acknowledge is how rare or atypical their authors might be, at what stage of their development they had become deaf, or the degree of their impairment. Only after a number of years of oral schooling do the Spradleys hear a teacher acknowledge how few of her students she expects to succeed at oralism and how long—sometimes a decade—oralist methods are pushed on children who are extremely unlikely ever to learn to speak clearly.

The audist establishment, then, provides this couple with a kind of script that they attempt to follow, a prescription for "treating" their daughter. That narrative is based on a hegemonic model of deafness as pathology that is never argued for, examined, or allowed to be questioned. In effect, oralism presents them with propositions that cannot be disproved. If Lynn does not learn to speak, the implication is that they have not worked hard enough, not maintained a pure enough environment, not made enough sacrifices.

None of this would be credible if it didn't exploit the stereotype of deaf people as dumb, ill behaved, poor, dependent, isolated in ghettos. Sign language is dismissed as "primitive gestures"—not really language or culture at all but a kind of subhuman form of communication. (At the same time, in visiting an oral school the parents are distressed to find students making "strange," "unnatural," animal-like noises. Deaf children are apparently damned if they do and damned if they don't try to talk.) These schools see manual communication as a last resort—only for those who fail utterly to become oral; furthermore, the schools associate sign language with manual labor, the low-paying trades that are taught in residential manual schools (146). Thus the schools also map oral/manual, normal/abnormal dichotomies onto an invidious socioeconomic hierarchy; oralism is middle class, manualism blue collar. (This is particularly ironic because this dichotomy may be in part a function of the failure of oral methods.) It is only after the Spradleys have stumbled onto signing that they realize that Lynn's "retarded" development may owe more to inappropriate methods of instruction than to her deafness. Once introduced to sign language, she acquires it speedily, quickly outstripping the rest of the family, constantly asking questions to which they know, but cannot express, the answers.

The parents' persistence in oral methods is understandable, as it reflects their desire for their daughter to grow up in what they think of as their world, to be like them, whereas manualism is seen as leading to a ghettoized existence among the invisible, inaudible deaf population—a life of isolation among savages (analogous to Indian captivity as seen by the Puritans): "the alternatives conjured up animalistic, nonhuman images in my mind. I feared to think of them. I didn't want to investigate them as a possibility for Lynn" (207).

Like West's narrative, like all parental narratives of impaired children, *Deaf Like Me* arouses in the reader a powerful urge for a happy ending— a breakthrough or triumph over impairment, like the one that surgery provides in Warfield's narrative. But its eventual resolution instead is to contradict the oralism that both Warfield's and West's books endorse or reinforce. Like Warfield's book, it is shaped as a conversion narrative, but here the parents are converted to a faith diametrically opposed to Warfield's pathological model of deafness and to West's implicit endorsement of English as the sole language for him and his daughter, her only hope of redemption and reunion with her parents. In terms of the conventional (albeit implicitly "ableist") trope the Spradleys were once "blind" (to the validity of sign language), but now they "see." For them grace is not surgical resurrection by a godlike physician; rather, it is a new vision of their daughter's condition—introduced to them by dissident deaf parents at their school—which implies an alternative "therapy": in this Sign conquer.

The central narrative formula is one shared with that classic American conversion narrative, Jonathan Edwards's *Personal Narrative* (1765): a true conversion follows a series of false assurances. A new teaching technique or technological aid repeatedly arouses the Spradleys' hopes; they see repeated "breakthroughs"—the first time Lynn recognizes (lipreads) a word (*ball*), the first time she pronounces a word or name (her brother's name). Then she lapses or backslides; hopes are dashed, salvation denied. When it finally comes, however, salvation issues from an unexpected quarter, seemingly from Satan's quarter—from those peculiar gesturing people the Spradleys have been warned may try to steal their daughter. Unlike most conventional conversions, then, the parents' true conversion involves a betrayal of the god to whom they have prayed for so long.

One powerfully counterdiscursive aspect of the narrative is the account of the parents' anagnorisis (enlightenment) and dianoia (new course of action), especially their belated attempt to learn sign language. They finally begin to grasp the enormity of the burden they have placed on Lynn. (They realize that she has no "voice" because she can't hear hers; they realize, by watching TV with the sound off, how difficult lipreading is even for individuals already familiar with English grammar and vocabulary; they come to realize that learning to speak and to lipread are highly dependent, for different reasons, on being able to hear.) The process of learning Sign is a profound role reversal in which they become students, children, marginalized outsiders: "I had the curious feeling that *we* were the ones who didn't know how to 'talk.' We were as 'deaf' to Jim and Alice's language as they were to ours. In this small group, they were obviously no more handicapped in communicating than Louise and I, perhaps even less. I had always thought that *deafness* was the handicap. Could it be, instead, their minority status? Deaf Americans dominated by a larger hearing society?" (229). The Spradleys suddenly have an uneasy, somewhat guilty, sense of what Lynn's life has been like—how frustrated she has been by being forbidden the use of her native language. Though humbling, the process is finally liberating and gratifying for them as well as for her.

Perhaps their most troubling realization is that, in being deprived of her "natural" language, Lynn has in some sense been deprived of identity, of selfhood—of the subjectivity that comes with language:

Of all the injuries that oralism had inflicted on Lynn, the most insidious had been to rob her of a name. We had unwittingly told her, "You are not a person until you can see 'Lynn' on our lips, until you can say 'Lynn' with your voice. We will accept no substitutes." Lacking a name and a language to give it life, she could not say, "I *am* someone. I am *Lynn*." Without an accepted symbol for herself, her capacity for self-awareness and self-control had failed to take root and grow. She could not experience that universal feeling that says, "I can control the things around me by learning their names." (248)

She has also been deprived of the self-identification that the Deaf community can provide. Although the narrator doesn't quite say that, the title implies it, because the phrase is taken from Lynn's delighted discovery of other people who are deaf like her. The title is a particularly generous parental gesture insofar as it suggests that she has a primary identification with people other than her immediate family, none of whom is deaf.

One sharp difference between *Deaf Like Me* and West's largely monological text is that the 1985 edition of the Spradleys' book contains an epilogue by Lynn, which she wrote when she was nineteen. Eventually, then, she was able to respond in her voice to her father's book—which, unlike West's, was not written for or addressed to her. Although she had been aware her father was working on a book about her, she had been too young to appreciate it until her sixth-grade teacher at the California School for the Deaf discovered a copy and read it in class, one chapter at a time. (By her own account, the book was too difficult for her to read at that time [280].) Lynn's life as a child, "taken" without her knowledge, was thus returned to her in written form. Here we have the unusual situation of the subject of a parental memoir extending and responding to the original narrative. Like any child—but more so because of her deafness—she is not in a position to question the narrative, which fills in episodes she could hardly remember—in part because they are prelingual episodes. But she endorses it, because it rings true to her (and to her classmates, many of whom went through similar experiences). Indeed, her epilogue consists largely of a condensed sequel, which begins with her transition from home—about the time the book was finished—to a residential school for the deaf (against her parents' initial wishes) and ends with her poised to graduate from high school.

Here, then, the narrative—retrospectively and almost accidentally—begins to right the built-in imbalance between the parental and filial voices. But it is well to note that the imbalance has already been thematized with awareness of its politics, in the parents' awareness that they are "deaf" and "dumb" in a Deaf world until and unless they acculturate by learning the native language. Indeed, they eventually see that the hegemonic status of oralism had effectively silenced them; it ruled some of their ideas inexpressible. For example, their concern that Lynn would never learn to talk was a "fear we could not express out loud" (112). Oralism served as a repressive and oppressive force in their lives too.

If *Deaf Like Me* seems in retrospect somewhat programmatic and thesis driven, one of its virtues is that it conceals its propagandistic purpose until quite late. The narrator (despite its dual authorship, the narrative point of view is that of Lynn's father) shrewdly declines to superimpose his later viewpoint onto the early hopes, apparent breakthroughs, and setbacks. This is not to say that the narrative's reversal comes as a surprise. The book's republication by Gallaudet Press is one tip-off (the cover speaks approvingly of sign language), and the tone of the narrative hints at a coming change of mind. On the whole, though, this is an effective counternarrative to the innumerable oralist narratives that the Spradleys believe misled them. One of the more heartening events in all of contemporary life writing about deafness is the appearance of Lynn Spradley as author of her epilogue; the most impressive conversion of all—and perhaps the real payoff for her parents' conversion from oralism—is her conversion from character to narrator, from voiceless subject to coauthor.

Lending Ears: Filial Memoirs of Deafness—Lou Ann Walker, *A Loss*
for Words: The Story of Deafness in a Family **(1986); Ruth Sidransky,**
In Silence: Growing Up Hearing in a Deaf World **(1990); Leah Hager**
Cohen, *Train Go Sorry: Inside a Deaf World* **(1994)**

Significant memoirs of deafness have also emerged in recent years from
a complementary source, the hearing children of deaf parents. Their
situation is radically different, of course, from that of the hearing parents of deaf children.[9] For one thing, as Lou Ann Walker points out,
hearing children of deaf parents are not tempted to invest emotionally
in the correction or abatement of deafness (107). On the contrary, they
are likely to take parental deafness as normal until their experience
broadens sufficiently to make them aware that hearing is the statistical
and cultural norm. Consequently, narratives by children do not betray
the obsessive concern with "progress" toward "normality" that infuses
many parental memoirs of impaired children. Because children assume
parental deafness to be unalterable and because hearing children of
deaf parents generally grow up able to communicate with their parents,
filial narratives have little, if any, stake in the alleviation of parental
deafness or acculturation into the hearing world.

In one way, of course, the position of the hearing child of deaf parents
is more complex than that of the hearing parent of a deaf child. Although both the parents and the children of deaf people may find themselves caught between two worlds, only the children are likely to find
their identities in question. (In this they have interesting affinities with
children of racially or culturally mixed marriages and with adopted
children, particularly in cross-cultural adoption.) Thus, as we shall see,
unlike parental memoirs filial ones often thematize and enact identity
formation and affiliation.

Paul Preston's 1994 book, *Mother Father Deaf: Living Between Sound and*
Silence, an ethnography of hearing children of deaf parents, provides
much insight into the phenomenon of hearing children speaking for and
about deaf parents and the complex social status of such children. It is
common, according to Preston, for one hearing child in the family, usually a daughter, to become a kind of "designated family interpreter"
(96).[10] Though age is a factor in the designation of this role, gender is
more influential; interpreting involves the sort of selfless or relational behaviors—helping, mediating, caretaking—typically gendered as female:

Like other forms of caring, interpreting becomes inseparable from feelings of
love and ties of obligation, and this concern for others rather than self represents a defining aspect of femininity.
 Nurturing and connecting with others are not the only aspects of interpreting that evoke feminine associations. Many informants spoke of needing to be

adaptable, invisible, and even subordinate when assuming the role of interpreter. These characteristics coincide with the generally tentative or inferior status traditionally available to women and, as such, contrast with the more fixed, visible, and dominant roles available to men. (101)

At the same time, however, the role of interpreter confers a measure of power or prominence in the family not usually accorded to a child: "Although the negative associations of diminished identity and status were true for several women and men, a few other informants stressed that interpreting provided them with a much greater degree of visibility and control. . . . Rather than being a passive and objective translation, interpreting could also be understood as authoritative and dynamic cultural brokering" (102). The role of family interpreter is thus paradoxical; it demands a kind of self-abnegation even as it places a child in a position of rare responsibility. A role assigned to females because of their subordination in a patriarchy may thus serve as a platform for self-fulfillment and self-assertion. Overall, however, the role places the interpreter persistently and sometimes painfully on the border between the hearing and deaf worlds and reminds her of her indeterminate status: "It was a role that potentially robbed informants of a sense of themselves while reiterating their chimerical identity—as neither deaf nor hearing, as both deaf and hearing" (76).

Ruth Sidransky testifies to this in her 1990 memoir *In Silence: Growing Up Hearing in a Deaf World*: "I stepped between the deaf and the hearing worlds never quite fitting into either, never knowing who I was" (95).[11] If deaf people are marginalized, their children—especially those who serve as family interpreters—are constantly constructing or negotiating identity in a liminal "contact zone." In what amounts to survey of a cross-section of her peers, Sidransky outlines a variety of responses to this difficult situation, putting her personal and narrative strategies in a broader context:

There were those of us who were sucked into a silence we carried with us always. There were those of us defiantly proud of our parents yet secretly ashamed of their garish sounds. There were those of us who, as soon as we were able, left home and abandoned our parents to grow old alone in withering silence. There were those of us who ignored our deaf parents, never quite learning to sign well enough to tell them what was in our hearts and minds. There were those of us who deliberately turned our heads when our parents raised their arms and hands to speak to us. And there were those of us who loved our parents with passion. We were the ones who buried the silence within. We abandoned our dreams and took care of our deaf mothers and fathers. They were our children, and we were their parents. We, the children, were invisible. (96)

Even as she locates herself among the more compassionate members of her peer group, she hints at the price she too paid ("the silence within," invisibility).

Educated middle-class women today, of course, are likely to be painfully conscious of the gendering of their role as family interpreters; furthermore, the Deaf rights movement has made the position of interpreter all the more delicate and fraught. The results of the problematization of an already liminal position may be seen in several recent narratives by the daughters and granddaughters of deaf adults; the inherent tensions of the role are at the heart of narratives by Sidransky, Lou Ann Walker, and Leah Hager Cohen. In the cases of Sidransky and Walker, the children of deaf parents, their life writing can be seen as a voluntary extension and creative expansion of roles that were at first compulsory—a working out of these roles' inherent conflicts with the greater distance and control that writing affords. The case of Cohen, the grandchild of a deaf couple, is in some ways more complex.

Thus, although (written) autobiography remains rare among deaf individuals, the family memoir appeals to hearing children as well as hearing parents of deaf people. Having represented their deaf parents to the hearing world orally and in writing since early childhood, hearing children, especially designated interpreters, may find it natural to write about their parents in adulthood. Indeed, according to Preston, so bound up are their identities with their parents' deafness that, even when asked about themselves, hearing children of deaf parents often volunteer stories about their parents (46). Their parents' deafness is a crucial fact in the children's autobiographies, for it has crucially marked and shaped them since infancy.

The contradictions built into the status of the hearing child of deaf parents are many. Such individuals are simultaneously insiders and outsiders: birthright members of the deaf community yet seemingly destined to grow away from it; bound by family ties and loyalty to a marginalized group yet equipped to assimilate into the dominant culture; capable at once of being victim, advocate, and oppressor (Preston 60). The term that Preston borrows for his title—*Mother Father Deaf*, a sign-language identifier for hearing children of the Deaf—suggests their precarious yet intimate relation to the Deaf community. The term explains, and thus authorizes, their presence among Deaf people; at the same time, its reference to *parental* deafness acknowledges the children's difference. Although the term is used for all children of Deaf parents, it is a lifelong identifier only for hearing children, because deaf children become known as Deaf in their own right (x). (Deaf children of Deaf parents are known as "Deaf of Deaf.")

Without minimizing the paradoxes of the children's situation, Preston points out its positive potential: "Hearing children of deaf parents could provide a means of de-stigmatization through direct facilitation of encounters between the Deaf and the Hearing. By acknowledging their Deaf heritage as adults, informants could also continue this advocacy by forging new inroads into a world often impenetrable to their deaf parents" (181).[12] Of course, such inroads might take the form of sympathetic inside accounts of the Deaf minority for the hearing majority— whether in life writing or other genres. Concerned with the potential loss of family history, in particular with the ruptures and gaps caused by deafness, Ruth Sidransky's father urged her to preserve family history, deaf and hearing alike—an exhortation that may serve as authorization for her book: "Every person on earth has story. I tell story to my daughter, you Ruth tell to your children, then no life is lost and all remember all people. This is the life. Past must be to know. Help life to live, important to children who come in family later, maybe hundred years later. My father never tell me about his family. I know nothing. He is absent man of earth" (176). Here, then, a deaf man endorses oral history as an antidote to inaudibility, invisibility, and absence. Still, such acts of representation by people who are not deaf are increasingly subject to criticism on grounds of exploitation or inadvertent objectification. The rise of identity politics generally, and militant Deaf politics particularly, further complicates the liminal status of hearing children of deaf parents.

Like parental narratives, then, filial ones necessarily view deafness in an important sense from outside, and they do run the risk of unintentional reinforcement of marginalization. Having been called upon on to interpret, mediate, and manage affairs for their parents, family interpreters—precisely those most likely to write filial memoirs—run the risk of patronizing their parents and by implication all deaf people, by presenting them as incapable of functioning in a hearing world. Thus, despite their literally filial status, hearing children of deaf parents may be as prone to paternalism as hearing parents of deaf children; in this case paternalism is a function of hearing status alone rather than of generational status. Another risk is that of writing a narrative of their victimization, the story of having been deprived of a normal childhood as a result of having been pressed into service as unpaid in-house interpreters at an early age—at worst, a kind of child abuse.[13]

It should be noted here—as Paul Preston is at pains to point out— that what passes for normal childhood is not natural and universal but specific to particular cultures and that the prevailing norms of modern American family roles assume the absence of disability, especially in parents. Modern Western civilization in general and American culture in particular put a premium—at least officially—on innocence and dependency in young children. It may be unfair to judge Deaf parenting by hearing norms, as Deaf culture values cooperation more and privacy less than hearing culture (Preston 20). Preston suggests that hearing children of Deaf parents may be deprived of their childhoods in a different sense, though one still related to the issue of cultural norms: precisely because their stories are so anomalous, they are not told, not recognized, not reinforced—and so not remembered: "After listening to these men and women, I realized that some childhoods were 'lost' because these adults had no frame of reference for their experiences. They were unable to make the necessary translation from the prevailing cultural stereotypes to the specifics of their own lives" (19–20).

Without endorsing the norm of a protected childhood, however, one needs to take seriously the sense among some hearing children that the extraordinary demands placed on them may have complicated the development of their identities. Thus the themes and implicit motives of filial narratives will be quite different from those of parental ones. Whereas the Spradleys write explicitly, and West implicitly, to redeem their children's lives, to reclaim them from the objectifying discourse of medical and educational institutions, hearing children of deaf parents may write in part to recover their childhoods from the constraints that deafness placed on them—as well as to honor their parents. Such childhoods, "lost in translation," may be recovered by filial narrative.

Published in relatively quick succession, Walker's *A Loss for Words* (1986), Sidransky's *In Silence* (1990), and Leah Hager Cohen's *Train Go Sorry* (1994) suggest the outlines of an emerging subgenre of life writing. Because Cohen is two generations removed from deaf family members, I will focus first on Walker and Sidransky, both daughters of deaf parents. Their narratives, though significantly different in emphasis, tone, and ethnic inflection, share themes distinctive of such narratives. One of these has to do with the way in which having deaf parents complicates dating and mating. Both Walker and Sidransky cite relationships that were haunted or even doomed by the stigma attached to deaf relatives; the prospect of having deaf parents-in-law or deaf children or both often repelled potential mates (Sidransky 248; Walker 121–22). Both women, usually ardent defenders of their families against stigmatization, find themselves defenseless against this contamination by association.

Another common trait is what we might call the scholarship-student syndrome; like Richard Rodriguez, author of *Hunger of Memory: The Education of Richard Rodriguez* (1981), both daughters pursue academic excellence with a vengeance, as if to make up for their parents' lack of opportunity for higher education. Both develop a passion for English, compensating—perhaps overcompensating—for their parents' limited facility with it. An element of guilt necessarily accompanies these pursuits; indeed, as for Rodriguez, the writing of their memoirs may be in part an expiation for the distance that their deftness with English carries them from the deafness of their parents.

A more troubling similarity is that both Walker and Sidransky cite instances of sexual molestation that might not have happened to children of hearing parents. (Parental deafness is a factor either because the daughters were interacting with adults on behalf of absent parents or because the deafness of parents somehow prevented them from detecting the abuse or protecting their daughters against it.) Both try to blame their parents' deafness rather than their parents. Thus, rather than condemning her mother for sending her unaccompanied to the offending butcher, Sidransky wonders whether her deafness ever exposed her mother to such mistreatment (106). Sidransky realizes how hard it would be for her mother to make a credible accusation. Walker is somewhat harsher in her judgments, portraying her father as emasculated because of his inability to protect her from an obscene phone call (88) and sexual touching from a stranger (135–36). Although this topic moves their narratives toward the genre of abuse-survivor narrative, neither becomes a narrative of victimization by parents. They minimize the incidents of molestation; both narrators present them as part of the cost of deafness to them *and* their parents. Still, such instances serve to suggest the potential burdens of exposure in the role of family interpreter.

Of the two memoirists under discussion here, Walker is the more troubled by her ambiguous parent/child role. In her view her parents' deafness not only prevented them from protecting her, it required her to protect them. On the one hand, she takes pride in her competence as a mediator and in her ability to shield her vulnerable parents from thoughtless and sometimes hostile hearing people. She is candid about the quite literal "gaze" of the hearing world. (One of the several signs she explains is that for *stare*: "the fingertips of both hands almost poking into one's own face" [100].) On the other hand, she makes clear the cost of providing such protection. When she censors, rather than passes on, rude remarks from hearing people, she becomes the receptacle of animosity directed at her parents; she contains both the hostility of the hearing world and the resentment it stirs in her. So, in interpreting for her parents, she absorbs much of the friction between the worlds. One motive or function of narratives like hers, then, is to modify that gaze; whereas in childhood Walker had limited control over her parents' exposure to the public, here she has complete control. This, of course, brings new dangers and responsibilities. Thus one impulse in filial narratives—to continue to shield her parents—risks sanitizing family history. Hagiography may be preferable to accusation, but ultimately neither is desirable.

Because life writing involves representing the family before a much larger public than that already encountered in everyday life, causing pain by exposing hurt is always a danger. Apprehensive about that possibility, Walker submitted her manuscript to her parents before publication. Although they did not necessarily approve it, they consented to its publication; in that sense it is authorized biography. Significantly, their response to reading it in manuscript, as reported in the prologue, seems to typify their lack of assertiveness; after reading a manuscript in which their grown daughter at times vents her anger at her childhood role, they remarked: "We hope no feelings hurt" (3). (The uncertainty of the verb tense here makes their remark somewhat ambiguous, but their concern is for others' feelings, not their own.)

Highly and widely praised in reviews, Walker's book is, among other things, her working out of her complex relation with her parents. Though considered by many to be championing the deaf, it is certainly not hagiographic; it is not even an altogether flattering portrait of her parents or by implication of deaf people generally. To begin with, her title, *A Loss for Words*, would seem to characterize deafness as a deprivation, if not a tragedy—a sentiment that is anathema to Deaf activists today. Without denying that deafness is in some significant sense a deprivation, one can see that to equate hearing loss with a loss of words is, perhaps unwittingly, to inscribe hearing values.

Perhaps the most poignant example of lost words is the attempt of her mother's hearing father to communicate to his grown daughter for the first time his love for, and pride in, her. Immediately afterward Walker's mother had to ask Walker, who overheard him, what her father said. Walker's comment—"So much had been lost" (164)—seems to refer not only to this particular message but also to the fact that a daughter could reach middle age without ever having been told explicitly of a parent's love. As the closer of the chapter the line has special impact. Significantly, however, Walker later offsets this anecdote with a comment on her grandfather's funeral; there she makes it clear that she sees the loss as stemming as much from her grandfather's ineffectual attempts at communication as from her mother's deafness. She concludes, "I'd seen plenty of families where there was more communication and less love" (203).

Although Sidransky, like Walker, is frank about her parents' difficulty with English, she balances this acknowledgment by documenting their resourcefulness in working around it. For example, she learns that when her mother sees movies by herself, without her daughter to sign the plot and dialogue to her, she makes up plots. Here, far from impeding her enjoyment of the visual medium, being "at a loss for words" makes it a more interactive experience, with the deaf viewer cowriting the script (74–75).

As noted earlier, the role of interpreter can be stifling, insofar as one speaks always for others, never for oneself. Such a role puts Walker in a sense at a loss for her own words. Although she is, from one perspective, in a position of authority over parents who have difficulty voicing their thoughts in and to a hearing world, she is also deprived of the freedom to experiment, to cut loose in adolescence, to try out different identities—to become herself by herself. And she seems to feel that the unusual authority granted her as a child may have delayed her development and impeded self-expression.

Family memoirs are necessarily plural rather than singular in focus; inherently unstable, they oscillate between biography and autobiography. One of the most interesting features of both these family memoirs is the way in which what is purportedly a family story veers sharply toward autobiography before the authors finally curb and redirect that impulse. Neither narrative is strictly or even essentially chronological in organization. (As stories of more than one generation, they can't be, because before the narrators' parents come together, their life narratives are separate but simultaneous.) And yet, without organizing the narratives exclusively and chronologically around the plot of the narrator's self-development, both books describe the same trajectory for her, from submersion in the family, through rebellion against it, to a more distanced but still intimate relationship with it.

Walker's rebellion against her situation comes well after her adolescence, late in the book. There, in chapters called "Vanilla Fires" and "Quicksand," Walker finally unburdens herself. "Vanilla Fires" takes its title from a note used by a Deaf gang member to order a vanilla shake and French fries at a fast-food restaurant; Walker seizes upon the phrase's synaesthesia to suggest the seething emotions beneath the sometimes placid exterior of Deaf people and their hearing children. "Quicksand" refers to her sense, as a professional interpreter, that the Deaf world was a kind of quagmire in which her energetic, but always insufficient, efforts threatened to sink her. Having to interpret for a deaf woman who claims to be the Virgin Mary becomes the occasion for Walker's overt railing against her invisibility and inaudibility. She suddenly unburdens herself of a legacy of anger and hurt:

For the first time in my life, I wanted to cry out. This isn't me! It's her! I have talked and listened and heard and there is no me! I have heard and hidden the insults for so long, I have been the conduit for so long that I am disappearing!
. . . My greatest fear had always been: The more you get to know me, the less there is to know. I was a black void. On the outside I was bright and shining and cheerful. Inside I was hollow. Deafness is also a void. It is a lack of something. Not the presence of anything. How could I be angry at what wasn't even there?

Deafness had protected my parents. There were gentle souls in a harsh world, but there was a naïveté that shielded them. I'd thrown myself into that harsh world without any protective covering. And when I got bruised, it hurt. I could hear. I could speak. But I, too, was helpless. There was ultimately nothing I could do—or can do—for them. And so I was enslaved to do even more. I was a caretaker and I felt deep down inside I could never do enough for others because I could never make my mother and father whole. I didn't feel guilty because they couldn't hear and I could. It was much more complicated. I could never make them hear. And I could never make the world hear them. So what had I ever accomplished? What could I ever accomplish? (181)

Sidransky expresses similar feelings of being put upon and denied her needs: "I didn't dare hear myself. It meant breaking an unforgivable taboo; to hear myself could only diminish my capacity to hear the others who needed me. My mother said, 'I am helpless.' My father said, 'Take care of us.' I did not ask, 'Who will take care of me?' I was alone, walled in their silence and mine. Incommunicado. Blank" (153).

And yet, as I have stated already, both narrators work through or past this anger to some sense of reconciliation with their families. (Indeed, though deafness gives it special urgency here, the pattern is common to many filial memoirs.) Part of the solution lies in the power and authority of the narrative act. For the designated family interpreters are no longer bound either by filial loyalty or by the ethical code of the interpreter, which prohibits any interjection of subjectivity. Interpreters are in theory subject to those they serve in a way that autobiographers or memoirists are not. In life writing, hearing children can represent their families and their deafness without necessarily sacrificing their values, ideas, and insights—their identity.

For Sidransky her role as family memoirist is distinctly and blessedly different from that of the young girl representing her parents in court against the charges of a hostile downstairs neighbor, who characterized them as "freaks . . . not fit to live with normal people" (240). "I was cast into the role of omnipotence once more; the sense of power was overwhelming. I did not recognize that this power was an abuse of my childhood. No one was to blame for this abuse. It was simply so" (243).

In court she is cast in a powerful role, but the power is exercised on behalf of parents to whom she is obliged and against others whom she fears; she is not ready for responsibilities of this order. The narrative representation is not so overtly adversarial; most important, it is not forced on her before she is ready. In the end the result is a more balanced, nuanced, and powerful act of representation.

Sidransky traces her estrangement from the language of her parents, her excursion into purely verbal expression, oral and written English, only to return eventually to a sense that she owes much to the discourse of her parents. To "discover" her identity, she believes, she needed to move out of the enclave of the Deaf: "In glintings it came upon me. I was in possession of myself away from the deaf threshold. Transposed from silence's enclave, which demanded I move in a rhythm unnatural to me, I had a change of heart. I wandered off to my own kingdom, my own kind, listening to and interpreting my own noises. I was no longer untied, loose and alone" (285). Yet ultimately, she sees that her escape is illusory or misguided:

I dreamed of escape to foreign lands, to new languages to shield me from my mother tongue, the tongue of hands. It was to be an escape from the language of hands to the language of voice alone, where no one would ask me to speak with my fingers, where instead I could ask the meaning of new words with my own voice.

I denied my own language. My hands did express a universal language. Translation wasn't needed, superfluous. The language of hands has its own feelings, its own tone. It was and is exquisite. But I wasn't quite ready to accept its beauty. . . . It was touch that connected me to people, connected me to myself. Sign language was rich, my attempts to be rid of it futile, foolish. (286)

She comes around, then, to her father's view, which she expresses in his idiom: "'Hands everybody's language. Make to understand all people who cannot understand different language from the mouth. Not necessary to hear sound.' I saw the curve of his hand enjoin me to touch another as he had touched me. I taught Saul [her husband] sign, and we played in another language. His signs were young, awkward, almost comic. And I reached for my native language, my hands" (286). It is not enough for her to continue to read manual language; she must build her world and continue her story in the language of her parents.

For Sidransky, then, the paradigmatic story is the fairy tale of the singing maid Romaine, "who enchanted the king of the realm with her lyrical voice" (55). Admitted to his household, Romaine enjoys singing but becomes envious of the princess's beauty; when her fairy godmother grants Romaine's wish to resemble the princess, she finds she has lost her voice (the princess can't sing). Using voice as a conventional—though clearly inadequate—metaphor for language, the story carries an anti-assimilationist message: Sidransky must not fetishize oral and written language, lest she lose her distinctive idiolect and her appreciation for her native hand.

Leah Hager Cohen's *Train Go Sorry: Inside a Deaf World* (1994) is not at first glance life writing at all but rather a report on the Lexington School for the Deaf in a time of turmoil. A bastion of oralism from its founding in 1864, Lexington has been struggling since the 1970s to accommodate new signing pedagogies. As an account of the school, *Train Go Sorry* necessarily grapples with the major issues in the deaf community today; Cohen writes with astuteness and balance about controversial issues such as mainstreaming, the instructional use of sign language, and cochlear implants. As journalism, her book is lively, engaging, and responsible, one of the best recent books on life in the deaf community.

Yet the book also functions as life writing in three important ways. The first of these is its singling out of individual students for special coverage. The gesture is all the more significant because these students are from different backgrounds. One, Sofia, is a young woman whose family, Bukharan Jews, emigrated from Samarkand; the other, James, is a young African American male from a poor New York family. These cultural differences protect them from stereotyping; one can begin to sense how deafness inflects other cultural traits.

These chapters, interspersed throughout the book, provide valuable and rare accounts of the lives of the sort of deaf individuals who do not write autobiographies and are not likely to be the subjects of biographies or memoirs. James's struggle with a personal essay required for application to the National Technical Institute for the Deaf suggests the obstacles—psychological and cultural as well as linguistic—to life writing by ordinary deaf people. Although he is attracted by the requirement of a personal essay—which to him signifies institutional selectivity—he finds the process of writing such an essay quite alien to his self-conception. James has to be coached not only in the conventions of written English and of the genre but also in confident self-presentation and self-advertisement (158–59); his difficulties are such that the autobiographical requirement nearly screens him out. Thus the book enters into the historical record the lives of deaf individuals who are not usually represented there—because of their youth, ethnic or racial backgrounds, and socioeconomic status.

A second way in which the book becomes life writing is that, in establishing her deaf heritage, Cohen retells parts of her deaf grandparents' lives. Like Sidransky, she is concerned that the lives of deaf people tend to vanish without leaving historical signs. Of her grandfather, she notes, "Sam's own motions—the words of his hands, the path of his body as it worked the [basketball] court—are traceless; once realized and finished, they left no mark" (82). And of her grandmother, she observes,

Not even her memory belongs to her. The facts of her childhood jog and shift, are worn down like bits of sea glass, the real memories supplanted by stories she has been told, for a deaf girl's reality is easily manipulated by the parcelers of information. Sitting at the wooden table in my parents' kitchen, she once gave me three different accounts of how she became deaf in the space of five minutes: she was born that way; she fell off an ironing board when she was one; she developed an infection at age five. (133–34)

Thus one motive of the book is to fix the evanescent narratives of her deaf grandparents, whose stories otherwise will go unnoted or misrepresented. As in the more strictly filial memoirs the retrieval or reconstruction of family memory here is part of a conscious effort to offset a kind of culturally induced amnesia.

Third, insofar as the book's primary subject is the school, it supplies a chapter in the life of an important deaf institution. Given the particular importance of schools for the deaf (they often serve as introductory self-identifiers), such an account offers a valuable supplement to the few deaf lives that have been written. Though not a systematic ethnography like Preston's, Cohen's offers more immediate and in some cases sustained access to the lives of deaf individuals. Although Cohen tries to be comprehensive and fair in this part of the book, to a large extent the school is personified by its hearing superintendent, Oscar Cohen, who is also the author's father. Thus, even as school history, the book is inseparable from filial memoir and autobiography: Oscar's pursuit of a career "in deafness" was a function of his having been the child of deaf parents. Immersion in the deaf community similarly shaped his daughter's life: her family lived in the dormitory wing of the school when she was young. The school was thus literally her home, and the boundary between the deaf community and her hearing family was porous; in some significant sense the school was her family. This in turn bonds her loosely to its alumni, for whom school is a primary identifier of their relational selves.

Indeed, so intimately associated with the deaf world was Cohen that she not only expected but hoped to grow up deaf: "I played at signing the way other children play dress-up; part of trying on possibilities, practicing for the future, it was laden with excitement and anticipation, even aspiration. I wanted to grow up and be deaf, be a Lexington Student, with all the accouterments: hearing aids, speech lessons, fast and clever hands" (10). Having grown up hearing, she realizes how naive and romantic that expectation was; the book is in part her attempt to work out, or rework, her relationship to the world of deafness—by retracing the stories of her grandparents and by examining her father's role in administering the school in difficult times. Its subtext, however, is her exploration of her identity.

Her access to the school was presumably greatly facilitated by her privileged relation to its superintendent, a relation that also gives her a potential bias. After all, she is the hearing daughter of a hearing superintendent of a school for the deaf at time when the power, and potential prejudice, of hearing administrators is being aggressively challenged by Deaf activists. (A significant recent milestone in deaf history is the protest at Gallaudet in 1988 that replaced a hearing with a deaf president.)

As a hearing person, then, and as the director of a famous old oral school, Oscar is one of the enemies. But as the son of deaf parents and as a person who grew up signing and has spent his life living and working with deaf people, he is trusted and respected. He is framed by these dual images, regarded suspiciously by some, welcomed warmly by others.

As I grew up I was slow to realize that the deaf community I had idealized was fraught with political tensions. I was even slower to understand that my status as a hearing person would forever restrict my membership in that community. For most of my childhood, I continued to nurture a secret belief that I belonged to this special world, and it to me. (15)

Unlike Walker and Sidransky, she is two generations removed from family deafness and thus unlikely to patronize or to blame deaf family members. Indeed, she pointedly cites her father's distaste for the victimization narrative (79). At the same time, as a hearing person she is aligned with a father figure under challenge from his deaf charges—her "step-siblings"—and his deaf peers. Her position is thus different from, but perhaps equally as conflicted as, that of Sidransky and Walker.

On the intellectual level she acknowledges that she has a tangential relation to the deaf community and no real claim to Deaf identity:

For seven years I had lived among members of this minority group, witnessing bonds that transcended language. I longed for the warmth of words left unspoken and nevertheless understood.

But as I got older I had to reconcile this desire with the fact that I was not deaf. I had become a full-grown hearing person. Although I could (and did) choose to socialize and work with deaf people, I could never be a member of the deaf community. Cultural identity is fixed. No amount of tricycling up and down Lexington's halls could ever change that. (17)

And yet the process of researching and writing the book reflects her deep impulse to return to a "deaf world."

The advantage of her complicated relation to the deaf community is that her book, more than most familial memoirs, is aware of its potential complicity in a hegemonic culture that may oppress or exploit minorities even as it purports to help them. She explains succinctly how mainstreaming, which is designed to give disabled children full access to the same educational resources as "normal" ones, can isolate deaf students from the vital resources of Deaf culture, and why cochlear implants, designed to correct profound deafness, are viewed by Deaf activists as robbing deaf children of their cultural heritage.

As an adult Cohen maintains her relation to the deaf community in part by learning sign language and becoming a professional interpreter. But like Walker, she is plagued by a sense of impotence and anonymity, of being a passive instrument or medium (263); moreover, she becomes uneasy about the politics of her role.

I no longer viewed interpreters simply as agents of connection. I also saw them as members of the very group that had dictated the hierarchy of languages that positioned ASL last. Good interpreters function as cultural mediators; now I wondered how, as hearing people, they could fairly represent both cultures, when they must harbor an inevitable bias toward their own. Deaf people constitute the only minority group in the world forced to rely solely on interpreters from outside their culture. By taking part in this equation, how could I help but perpetuate this inequity? (256)

Cohen sees her role here as that of a true mediator between cultures rather than as a passive translator or unwitting oppressor. At the same time, writing offers Cohen—as it did Walker—an escape from the constraints that professional interpreting placed on her subjectivity.

Her position on political issues seems fair and balanced; only an extremist, I think, would fault her account of controversial issues. But her narrative point of view does call her objectivity into question, even when it tries hardest to embody it. This happens in two ways, both linked to her use of narratorial omniscience. In particular, her use of an omniscient point of view to reveal her father's thoughts aligns her with him despite her claims of neutrality. Her devotion of so much textual space to him and her narrative technique both betray her identification with him. Like all familial memoirs, this one oscillates between auto- and biography, but the obvious artificiality of her self-erasure from scenes involving him introduces an element of self-deception. The book is more autobiographical than it sometimes acknowledges.

Her use of omniscience can be jarring in other scenes, such as James's visits to his brother in jail. Although the nuances and details here are those of an eyewitness, she narrates as though she were not present. This technique seems uncannily and unnecessarily to reproduce the stance of the transparent interpreter; just as the ethic of interpretation prevents interjection or intervention on her part, so does her narrative technique erase her presence from the scene. Yet the use of omniscience simultaneously endows her with the ability—and assumes the prerogative—to read others' minds. On the one hand, this technique imposes on her a ghostliness akin to that which she rebelled against in interpreting. On the other, it assumes rights it hasn't earned. Although her presence must have affected the behavior she reports, her reportage erases her presence. Though this technique is widely used in journalism and even historical writing today, it seems an odd choice for someone so self-conscious about the politics of interpreting.

She candidly acknowledges that interpreting was an overdetermined career choice: "I had always thought that interpreting might be my ticket into the deaf community, the logical way in which my adult self could belong. But it wasn't my self that was engaged. As an interpreter, I'm not really being *with* deaf people. I do not think there is any way for me to recover the relationship with deaf people I felt as a child. I am a hearing adult. English is my language. I belong to hearing culture" (264). This is in part also an acknowledgment of the end of her childhood "wannabe" syndrome, her naive enthusiasm for the deaf world. Thus, as for Sidransky and Walker, the writing of her book is clearly a way of renegotiating her relation to a world to which she feels she somehow belongs but that she fears may exclude her. Like the children of the deaf, moreover, she has trouble locating her home. Writing the story of Lexington School gave her a way of exploring and developing her relationship to the deaf community, without claiming membership in it. Autobiography is the subtext here; an important dimension and function of the book is her coming to terms—in her terms—with her identity vis à vis two cultures on whose border she has lived and worked. Like Sidransky and Walker, Cohen performs a delicate balancing act, acknowledging her identity as a hearing person, on the one hand, affirming Deaf culture in defining herself in relation to the deaf community, on the other.

"deaf Autobiography" vs. "Deaf Autobiography"—Henry Kisor, *What's That Pig Outdoors? A Memoir of Deafness* (1990); Bernard Bragg, *Lessons in Laughter: The Autobiography of a Deaf Actor* (1989)

In addition to the accounts already considered, which look at deafness outside or from its periphery, there are two recent full-length autobiographies by deaf men: *What's That Pig Outdoors? A Memoir of Deafness*, by Henry Kisor, and *Lessons in Laughter: The Autobiography of a Deaf Actor*, by Bernard Bragg, as signed to Eugene Bergman. This pair of books nicely illustrates the complexity of the contemporary representation of deafness, for whereas Kisor is deaf, Bragg is Deaf. And that makes all the difference.

Deafened by illness at three, Kisor was able to learn lipreading and to relearn speech with the help of dedicated parents and innovative pedagogy. As a result, he was mainstreamed before the term was fashionable and eventually went on to graduate from Trinity College in Hartford, Connecticut. He married a hearing woman and has made a career as a journalist in the print medium. Now the book editor of the *Chicago Sun-Times*, Kisor is justifiably proud of his professional achievements and his success in the hearing world.[14] At the same time, he is acutely aware of the controversies about deafness today.

His book is an attempt to stake out a moderate position, which of course leaves him vulnerable to attack from both sides. Although he professes in his introduction that he doesn't want to take sides, he acknowledges that he may at times seem to be an advocate of oralism (9–10). And this is true; like most autobiographers—deaf, Deaf, or hearing—he tends to validate his identity and life path. For this reason his assertions in his final chapter, that his life should not serve "as a model for that of anyone else" and that "individual experience and potential varies so greatly that each case of deafness must be judged by itself," although no doubt sincere, are somewhat problematic. Kisor remarks at the outset on the dearth of writing about deafness by the deaf. Against such a background Kisor's life is liable to be taken as exemplary no matter how much he protests to the contrary. Advocates of oralism are likely to seize upon it as a narrative validating a besieged methodology. Like any success story by someone with a serious impairment—such as Hockenberry's *Moving Violations*, for example—it is liable to make its author a kind of "supercrip" whose example can be used to indict the less fortunate—unless it foresees and subverts that use of it.

Examination of his book reveals two crucial gestures in his narrative, considered as deaf autobiography. The first is normalization, a persistent and pervasive minimizing of deafness as difference. Admittedly, although Kisor can pass as hearing in some circumstances, he rarely tries to do so, and he is certainly not trying to do so as an autobiographer. But as one who lives in the hearing world, he tends to downplay his difference from those around him. His explicit insistence on the normality of his childhood typifies his implicit approach throughout: "From ages five to thirteen . . . my life was for the most part no different from that of an ordinary American youngster. . . . I was just another kid on the block" (43). One might say that his is a memoir of difference with a difference: his avowal that his distinction, his deafness, did not much matter. For Kisor deafness is a disadvantage (and a disability [261]), but in practice it is something he has been able to work around.

His narrative is emphatically a deaf autobiography, however, in the sense that at each stage of life—childhood, college, early career, love life and marriage, childrearing, profession—he attends to the role of his deafness. But his thrust is always to demonstrate how he successfully compensated for it or to defuse problems with humor. (Like Bragg, he learns obligatory lessons in laughter.) If he runs into ridicule, discrimination, or rejection, his response is to try harder, take another tack, to get where he wants to go. And in explicit response to Lou Ann Walker's picture of her childhood, he goes out of his way to assert that his children had no special responsibilities imposed on them; their childhoods were as normal as his (175). There is a delicate balance here, typical of accounts of successful assimilation by members of marginalized groups. On the one hand, as narratives of triumph over adversity they depend on periodic resistance; without conflict there is no story. On the other, the narrators' success militates against claims of systematic oppression: their achievement demonstrates that determination makes anything possible.

One measure of Kisor's success is his ability to make a career as a journalist—especially as a book editor, a role requiring high literacy. For Kisor, then, the idea of "deaf autobiography" is not at all problematic, much less oxymoronic. On the contrary, it draws on his well-developed professional skills, one of which is writing profiles of authors. Indeed, writing *auto-* rather than *bio*graphy circumvents his one serious handicap as a book editor, which is his difficulty conducting interviews. Although he maintains his oral skills through constant practice and regular therapy, writing his life is much easier than writing someone else's. His book is a linear account of how he became the person and the professional he is.

For the most part his narrative displays little anger. The exception is his bristling at standardized testing and diagnostics—which he sees as official stereotyping. In one instance he is so offended by the mandatory psychological counseling accompanying speech therapy that he later obtains his case history in order to expose and debunk its perverse assumptions about "deaf personality" (125). According to Kisor, this is "a set of traits [some deafness experts] theorize are created by the environment of deafness. Because lack of ready communication at an early age has deprived them of the opportunity to develop emotionally in many ways, the deaf sometimes are psychologically typed as immature, rigid, egocentric, impulsive, and overly trusting. And that's just for starters. [According to these same "experts"] if their emotional development has been severely thwarted, many suffer debilitating mental illness" (243–44). Kisor's resistance to linking speech therapy with psychological therapy is part of his lifelong strategy of normalization; in obtaining and taking issue with his case history, he literally goes out of his way to rebut the discourse of audism that defines him as somehow "abnormal," suffering from a defective personality if not a mental illness. (The analogous cataloging of homosexuality as a mental disorder by the American Psychiatric Association is revealing; the APA dropped this practice in 1973 [Alwood 130].) At the same time, Kisor concedes that his resentment of the advice to "accept his deafness" reflects his internalization of stereotypes of the deaf:

Nor can I take issue with Miss Jones's statement that I refused to associate with the deaf. . . . Associating with them, I feared, would diminish me in the eyes of hearing people. I did not think the limitations of the deaf in general applied to me, and I did not want the hearing to feel that they did, either. Miss Jones evidently believed that they did, or she would not be trying to dissuade me from my chosen career.

    . . . It's true that I knew very little about other deaf people and indeed subscribed to the ordinary hearing person's stereotyped notions about them, simply because I was culturally a member of the hearing world.

    Because I had always lived among the hearing, I had looked at deafness not as an existential condition to which I must submit—the view of most deaf people and professionals in the field—but as an adversary to defeat. . . . It was for an ambitious young deaf man a useful, workable idea, one that could keep him forging ahead until he had grown old enough to recognize his limitations and accept them with equanimity. (127–28)

Though he regrets its basis in prejudice, he never repudiates his "denial" of his deafness, because it serves his ambition; by not accepting his deafness, he manages to escape the conventional limits on the deaf. His stance I think illuminates the position of many members of marginalized groups: it is difficult to escape marginalization without subscribing to some attitudes that inscribe it. Kisor seems as concerned to show that his is not a "deaf personality" as to show that the idea of a "deaf personality" is a false and oppressive construct. His book thus inscribes the individual rather than a minority model of deafness; for him deafness is a physical deficit to overcome rather than a cultural identity.

    The other related, though not entirely consistent, discursive gesture is Kisor's casting of himself as the underdog. Beginning with Walker Percy's preface, Kisor is presented as a "courageous person overcoming a serious handicap" (vii). It goes without saying—and it is unobjectionable—that he is an underdog vis à vis hearing people. What is perhaps questionable is whether he is an underdog as an oralist: "I am a member of a minority within a minority: I am what is called an 'oralist'" (7). He locates himself between an audist establishment, on the one hand, that stereotypes him as a defective "deaf personality" and a Deaf community, on the other, that regards him as a defector, alienated from his true identity, a traitor to his kind, living forever in a kind of limbo.

Some people . . . assume that I am at heart forlorn and despondent, and concealing my pain. According to the ideology of many educators of the deaf—and many of the deaf themselves—I must live a melancholy life simply because I communicate wholly by speech and lipreading rather than with sign language. By insisting on doing so, they declare, I am a poor shadow of a hearing person, not a contented and fulfilled deaf person. I belong neither to the hearing world nor to the deaf community, they say; I am an outcast from both. (242–43)

Throughout his memoir he has insisted upon his uniqueness, his integrity, and his right to define himself. And it is no surprise that he resents and resists patronizing by the Deaf as much as by the hearing. (His oralism is no betrayal of a community of which he was never a part.)

But precisely because his memoir portrays him as so well acculturated to a hearing world, his claim of underdog status with regard to the Deaf establishment is problematic. As a profoundly deaf oralist he may be numerically in the minority. And the idea of Deafness as a cultural identity may be gaining credence and momentum. But from a Deaf perspective, he is a member, by virtue of his oralism, of an elite advantaged in power and prestige. His oralism gives him entree to a world inaccessible to many Deaf individuals. He is thus not among the most disadvantaged group of deaf people—the quarter of a million congenitally deaf Americans, about one-tenth of 1 percent of the total population.

The historic upheaval at Gallaudet over the appointment of a new president was stirred in part by the assertion of the chair of the board of trustees that "the deaf are not ready to function in a hearing world" (4). Kisor's memoir presents its author as living refutation of that unfortunate but telling claim. And to that extent his narrative *is* exemplary. It exemplifies the success of particular oralist pedagogies and an assimilationist philosophy. It is thus, as we have seen, implicitly invested in the individual model of disability.

Unlike Warfield, who had residual hearing, Kisor uses no hearing aid, and he is not a good candidate for an implant or corrective surgery, but like her he explicitly celebrates assistive technology. Late in the text Kisor's autobiography acknowledges the virtues of the social model of disability, which focuses on the accommodation of society to the needs of impaired people; indeed, he devotes the whole penultimate chapter to tracing the invention, development, and distribution of various assistive devices in his lifetime. Like Bragg's narrative, as we shall see, Kisor maps two parallel comic plots—one individual (the trajectory of his career), one communal (the improving condition of deaf people). But whereas Bragg finds the communal parallel to his personal success in the movement for Deaf pride, Kisor finds his in the technological developments—from TDDs and computers to cochlear implants—that have made the United States in the last two decades, by his estimate, the best place and time to be deaf (217).

Kisor acknowledges and defends his lack of interest in, and use for, Deaf culture, and the book ends by warning of the dangers of extremism among Deaf activists: for example, separatism and discouragement of research into causes and treatment of deafness. Indeed, the book concludes with an indictment of claims of the "New Orthodoxy"—that deafness is a cultural trait rather than a physiological defect, that oralism is doomed to fail with all who are born deaf or deafened in early childhood (deaf defeatism), and that assimilation into the hearing world represents "tragic self-denial" (256–57). Despite his alarm about a new orthodoxy, the critical success and sales of his oralist and assimilationist narrative reflect the residual power of the old orthodoxy, which conceives of deafness as largely a matter of audiological deficit.

Kisor's memoir illustrates a larger dilemma. His attempt to minimize his deafness is linked to his wish to be recognized for his accomplishments—the traditional distinction justifying male autobiography from Franklin on—rather than for his "handicap" (even for "overcoming" it). Thus his claim to an ordinary childhood is essential to his claim to fame. Yet his deafness also dogs him. First, it threatens to deny him success and distinction; it *is* an obstacle in his path. Then, even after he overcomes it, it threatens to overshadow his accomplishments. Kisor doesn't want to be known as "the deaf editor" of the *Chicago Sun-Times*, yet his deafness is the hook for his story. The story of his "triumph over deafness" will inevitably be as much a story of deafness as of triumph; indeed, many people will become aware of his deafness only by reading of it in his memoir. The very book that celebrates his success as an individual depends for its success on a trait he wishes to downplay.

There is no question as to Bragg's status as a Deaf individual. He was born deaf to deaf parents and educated in residential deaf schools (including Gallaudet); in everyday life he relies on Sign, not speech, and he has had a prominent career in Deaf drama. Like its author, his book has impeccable Deaf credentials. It was not written by Bragg but "signed to" Eugene Bergman, a deaf professor of English at Gallaudet who transcribed and edited Bragg's stories into an autobiography. It was published by Gallaudet University Press, and its introduction by Harlan Lane, an authority on deaf history and Deaf culture, serves to authenticate it as Deaf autobiography.

Lane asserts that Bragg's book is a Deaf autobiography both in form and substance. Concerning its form, he describes it as an "engrossing autobiographical montage of stories told in sign language"—thus drawing attention to its being a series of signed anecdotes rather than a seamless retrospective narrative. Concerning its content, Lane claims that the book expresses "recurrent themes addressed by deaf authors across the centuries, legends rooted in the deaf collective unconscious" (x):

In *Lessons in Laughter*, the reader will find such timeless themes of the deaf experience as the deaf man who is valued by his beloved mostly as an object of study, who turns his deafness to advantage on the job, who tries to pass as a hearing man, who is exploited by unethical hearing people, who resists transformation into what he is not, whose deafness disqualifies him from someone's love, who comes to see he is a member of a linguistic and cultural minority—but one different from all the others. (xi)

Here, in effect, Lane codifies the contents of Deaf autobiography (a set of standard topics) and a comic master plot (growing self-confidence and pride in Deaf identity).

Lane is careful not to present the book as narrow or insular—of interest only to the Deaf: "There is much more to this engaging work, however, than solely a lesson in deaf culture. . . . [It conveys] a fresh vision of the human condition" (xi). But his major emphasis is on the book's political implications: "*Lessons in Laughter* is a cry of outrage at the crimes of the intolerant: the unwillingness of hearing people to allow deaf people self-determination; the recasting of deaf people's difference as deviance; the fraud perpetrated by hearing people who claim to normalize deaf people; and the refusal of hearing society to acknowledge deaf language and culture" (xii). Lane makes the book sound angrier and more tendentious than it is. Indeed, his introduction mimics the apparatus of abolitionist slave narrative, wherein a "wise" outsider—Lane is hearing—offers his moral and intellectual authority to collaboratively produced testimony of triumph over oppression and puts his political interpretation on the "raw" narrative. As with slave narrative the authenticating apparatus threatens to preempt—to speak for rather than about—the author of the framed narrative. Insofar as the invocation of such external authority is a mark of minority autobiography in its incipient stages, it tends to reinscribe the marginalization that it wants to defy or deny.

In contrast to Lane's rhetoric, Bragg's preface quite matter-of-factly addresses his predicament as a Deaf storyteller and his ambivalence about committing his stories to print: "I am a storyteller. I don't write stories, I perform them. . . . But to me, stories live only when I perform them dramatically in sign and mime before an audience. They disappear into thin air after I have acted them out—except when they are transferred to print. . . . Up until now, they have vanished once the curtain has fallen, but no more. Each will live on here" (viii). The collaborative nature of his autobiography is more a function of his Deafness than of his deafness. It reflects not so much inadequacy in English as

Bragg's powerful sense that sign language, his native language, is the proper medium for his life story.

If, to revert to Krupat's distinction, Kisor's autobiography is the deaf equivalent of autobiography by an Indian, in that it represents the product of an individual sufficiently acculturated to write his life, Bragg's is closer to the paradigm of Indian autobiography, in that it is the product of collaboration with a second party. Thus, like an individual from an oral culture who functions as a repository and performer of tales with communal significance—Black Elk, for example—Bragg depends on a collaborator to make his stories available to a reading audience.

Although, like Black Elk, he collaborates with an individual who commands the hegemonic language, Bragg's collaborator, unlike Black Elk's John Neihardt, shares his culture (Eugene Bergman is also deaf). Moreover, unlike Black Elk, Bragg could presumably have written his life; his decision to sign it instead and have it translated into a language he already knows is a self-conscious, principled, politically informed choice. Finally, he is able to read it; thus, unlike Black Elk, Bragg is in a position to review the manuscript, ask for changes, and assist in the revision. (In some ways his situation with regard to his collaborator parallels that of any actor whose autobiography is "told to" a writer, but the collaborative strategy is not a matter merely of saving time and labor, or of deferral to superior narrative skills.) The politics of the collaboration, then, are quite egalitarian. There is no danger of expropriation or distortion of his story by an unwittingly ethnocentric collaborator. (And, to pursue the analogy with celebrity autobiography, there is less possibility of the exploitation of the "manual labor" of writing by the star subject; Bergman is no ghostwriter toiling invisibly in the background.)

The book thematizes the gap between hearing and Deaf culture in several ways that bear on the issue of identity. For example, Bragg recalls trying to secure a table for a group of deaf and hard-of-hearing friends at a busy restaurant; because the hostess could not understand what he was saying, he spelled his name for her, only to find that she had written it down as *P-O-I-C*. At the time he laughed and passed it off as a sign of the futility of his long years of trying to improve his speech; Bragg sees that his speech teachers may have given him too much confidence in his oral skills. But the anecdote may also stand as an example of the way in which the hearing world fails to recognize those who don't speak its language the way they do. In contrast is the anecdote in which other students, at the prompting of a teacher, gave him a "name sign" when he entered a deaf residential school. Though he missed his mother, he realized that he was still "among my own kind" (10)—because his new schoolmates, unlike his earlier playmates, were deaf like him. The collaborative act of naming endowed him with a new identity within the Deaf community; it was an informal but significant rite of passage. At the restaurant his identity gets lost in translation between cultures; at the deaf school he gains a new name that confirms his Deaf identity.

The anecdote from which the title *(Lessons in Laughter)* is derived has a double meaning. Its literal reference is to the fact that Bragg and his classmates were actually instructed in how to laugh—not when, or at what, but how to produce sounds that hearing people would recognize as laughter. The story illustrates how a behavior that seems natural and instinctive, almost reflexive, is in fact culturally shaped and how the deaf have to be taught things that hearing people learn without being taught; it is also a subtle yet striking illustration of how deaf individuals are taught to discipline their bodies according to hearing norms. The broader, more metaphorical reference in the book's title is to the many incidents that teach deaf people to laugh at hearing customs—because from a deaf perspective they seem odd, and because laughter lessens the pain of marginalization (16).

One important subject of the narrative is the role of sign language in Bragg's life and art. Though born to deaf parents and thus a native signer, Bragg was given intensive speech training when he entered the New York School for the Deaf in the mid-1930s; the effect of this oralism was that he needed to be instructed in the power and value of sign as a language and to have it validated as an artistic medium. He learned from one teacher, Mr. Panara, that "this, our native language, could be . . . a powerful vehicle for expressing the richest and subtlest feelings and conveying nuances of meaning as sophisticated as those of the most articulate English speakers and writers" (21). But only when he was exposed to a drama coach did he really grasp the true eloquence and range of ASL: "Where Panara used 'total communication,' a combination of signing with speaking, resulting in a cultured, literary, 'Englished,' sign language, Hughes's signing hewed to the different, natural structure and syntax of sign language, always concise and graceful, conveying the subtlest nuances with astounding precision. To watch him sign was to observe a high priest solemnly conjure spirits with incantatory gestures" (35). Discovering and working with Marcel Marceau was a parallel process, through which he realized the possibilities of a speechless drama; together these epiphanies made possible, even necessary, a career in a field that might seem to exclude the deaf by definition (because conventional drama consists mainly of spoken dialogue).

His reevaluation of his native language has the power and resonance of a conversion experience.

I had totally revised my concept of English after my encounter with Mr. Panara. Before Mr. Panara, I was made to feel ashamed of sign language by my teachers. I had been taught to regard it as evil, impure, a polluter of English, as something to be used on the sly with one's companions. I was not the only one to feel so; my mother used to practically order me to tear up her letters every time I was through reading them. She was simply ashamed of her poor English and always made sure I would not be contaminated by it. For many years, even in adulthood, I would read her letters with my eyes closed to her language and, without thinking, tear them up and cast them away. (81)

(This is a scene that has its analogue in the autobiographies of members of a number of marginalized minorities.)

Whereas communicating in writing induces a sense of self-consciousness and even inferiority in his mother, Bragg has sufficient faith in Sign, the medium of his art, to devote his life to it. At the same time, he realizes the advantages to deaf people of English as a print medium; "It is time for some of these stories to be immortalized in print as part of deaf culture" (76). Bragg refers here to tales of a legendary deaf prankster, which he includes and preserves along with the anecdotes of his career. Like autobiographies of oral people, then, Bragg's becomes in part a repository of communal lore—for both minority and majority audiences.

The extent to which the book is focused on Bragg's career is evident in its use of theater terms to give a topical gloss to its chronological units: "The Stage Is Set" (childhood and early education); "The Rehearsal" (education at Gallaudet); "Tryouts" (early career); "The Premiere" (Bragg's ten-year career with the National Theater of the Deaf); "Reviews" (family memories and professional anecdotes); "The World Tour" (theater work abroad); "New Scripts" (contemporary developments, including the upheaval at Gallaudet); "Denouement." Though the book is subtitled *The Autobiography of a Deaf Actor*, the later chapters tend toward memoir—the story of his career as an actor—rather than autobiography—the story of Bragg's development as an individual. Bragg establishes his (Deaf) identity quite early on, and later chapters are scenes in which he plays many roles, in life as well as on stage, without problematizing or developing his identity.

A formal feature of the book that reflects its anecdotal origins—and the extent to which it is more memoir than autobiography—is the alternation between long stretches of narrative in Roman type and shorter indented sections in italics. Generally, the difference is that between scene (Roman type) and summary (italics), between showing and telling, between presenting anecdotes and reflecting on them. The two type styles do not seem to correspond to the respective contributions of Bragg and Berman, Sign vs. English. But the device may reflect Bergman's editorial sense of the need for transitions between the anecdotes in Bragg's repertoire and for an ongoing narrative line and comprehensive retrospection. The alternation hints at the differences between the poetics of written narrative and the poetics of signed storytelling, which seem to include a minimum of evaluation and commentary.[15]

Thus, aside from the short italicized sections, there is little introspection or reflection after the first several chapters; rather, the struggles are outward—for example, with David Hays, director of the National Theater of the Deaf (NTD), over its orientation.[16] The book, then, has two major focuses. One concerns Bragg's career, from learning Sign to making Sign a vehicle for artistic expression and professional success as a mime and actor. The other concerns the life of a Deaf individual in a hearing world; in Bragg's account to be Deaf is not to be impaired but to be discriminated against—not to be deficient but to be enlisted in a battle for cultural recognition. But though the relative lack of introspection and reflection on what it is like to be deaf, or to become Deaf, may disappoint some readers, it may be a function of Bragg's security in his Deaf identity. Bragg's downplaying of his deafness is not, like Kisor's, a product of assimilation; rather, it is a matter of his taking it for granted in a way that being Deaf (and Deaf of Deaf) makes possible. Thus, without being in any way assimilationist (think-hearing), Bragg has assumed the prerogative of any well-known actor—that of writing a memoir focusing mainly on his career and accomplishments rather than an introspective autobiography. The book is notable in the extent to which its world is populated by Deaf people; in this way it is an immersive narrative.

In the end the book does return, however, to the politics of deafness—in two ways. First is the story of Bragg's recruitment for a segment on sign language in a documentary film on language. After he declines upon learning that the other segments have to do with communication among whales and chimpanzees, the studio representative returns with a revised script in which the animals have been replaced by people with mental retardation or palsy. Eventually, the producer understands why Bragg and his colleagues resent such associations. Thus the story speaks—in English—to the way in which even presumably sophisticated individuals may relegate Sign to the status of primitive preverbal communication and/or associate deafness with mental impairment.

Second is the book's conclusion, in which Bragg witnesses the Deaf President Now movement at Gallaudet, his alma mater and his employer. Here the Deaf community challenges the authority of the hearing establishment; Deaf people and sign language go on the march. The collective triumph of Deaf culture parallels and reinforces the success of Bragg's career. Though not consistently integrated, the book's two concerns converge here in the image of I. King Jordan, the newly installed deaf president of Gallaudet, conferring on Bernard Bragg an honorary doctorate. Jordan's competition with hearing rivals is mirrored in Bragg's with David Hays. Bragg does not overthrow or displace Hays as director of the National Theater of the Deaf, but he does achieve a success on his own as a performer in productions oriented toward a deaf audience.

From his perspective as a neurologist Oliver Sacks has speculated interestingly on whether the subjectivity of deaf individuals may be as different from that of hearing individuals as speech is from Sign: "'We are our language,' it is often said; but our real language, our real identity, lies in inner speech, in that ceaseless stream and generation of meaning that constitutes the individual mind. It is through inner speech that the child develops his own concepts and meanings; it is through inner speech, finally, that he constructs his own world. And the inner speech (or inner Sign) of the deaf may be very distinctive" (73). Similarly, although he expresses skepticism about the Whorf hypothesis—that language precedes and largely determines thought and reality—Sacks suggests that the different origins and mode of Sign "may determine, or at least modify, the thought processes of those who sign, and give them a unique and untranslatable, hypervisual cognitive style" (74–75n). However intriguing such speculation may be, such differences in subjectivity may not register in written autobiography. At least they do not seem to have been explored so far.

A related issue is whether Sign has a distinctive poetics. According to the linguist William C. Stokoe, (as quoted in Sacks) it does:

In a signed language . . . narrative is no longer linear and prosaic. Instead, the essence of sign language is to cut from a normal view to a close-up to a distant shot to a close-up again, and so on, even including flashback and flash-forward scenes, exactly as a movie editor works. . . . Not only is signing itself arranged more like edited film than like written narration, but also each signer is placed very much as a camera: the field of vision and angle of view are directed but variable. Not only the signer signing but also the signer watching is aware at all times of the signer's visual orientation to what is being signed about. (89)

This no doubt applies to Bragg's dramatic and narrative art, but such effects are apparently minimized in the transference of his stories to the printed page. If Deaf subjectivity is distinctive from hearing subjectivity, this difference seems to get lost in transliteration to published autobiography.

Lost in Translation: The Problem of the Linguistic Medium of Deaf Life Writing

> Like most individuals within the Deaf community, more than half of all infor-
> mants had sign names—a unique sign for that individual. Moreover, almost all
> informants' spoken names were pronounced differently by their deaf parents.
> —Paul Preston, *Mother Father Deaf*, 1994, p. 27.

In a pioneering paper on what he calls "CODA autobiography," Timothy Dow Adams has drawn attention to the issue of the linguistic
medium of deaf life writing—the disparity between the primary language of the childhoods being represented, which was American Sign
Language, and the language in which those years are represented,
which is standard English. Incongruity between the language of the
narrator-author and that of the autobiographical subject is not peculiar
to deaf life writing. Indeed, rarely, if ever, do autobiographical narrators
limit themselves to the linguistic resources of their younger selves:
memoirs of childhood are generally written in adult language. Similarly, slave narratives generally use a dialect that the narrators did not
generally command as slaves. But in both sets of narratives—memoirs
of childhood and slave narratives—linguistic maturation and/or literacy are often thematized and associated with other sorts of personal development; that is, the narrative's language makes a point about how
far the narrator has come from his or her origins. The narratives do not
question, but capitalize on, the assumed superiority of standard English over Southern black dialect, adult speech over baby talk. (In the
slave genre the ex-slaves' mastery of the masters' dialect is not only
proof of their escape from slavery but evidence of their capacity, individually and collectively, for literacy and by implication their race's
worthiness for emancipation and full civil rights.)

Because ASL is not a written language, standard English would seem
to be the indisputable dialect for narrative. But in an era in which Deaf
advocates are staking so much on the legitimacy and expressivity of
sign language, the use of standard written English by default, rather
than by choice, seems unfortunate. Narratives written in standard English of the lives of individuals who sign would seem incapable of fully
registering an important cultural difference, much less of legitimating
Sign as a language. In the case of narratives by children of deaf parents
who sign or by parents of deaf children who sign, the use of English
would tend to efface the differences between the generations, between
the hearing narrators and deaf characters.

Given the lack of an obvious alternative, English may be unavoidable
as the language of narration, but dialogue raises other issues. Although
the presence of direct dialogue in biography and autobiography is a rel-

atively recent convention, it is now a staple of scenes that are narrated in detail; for a family memoir concerning deafness to be silent in this regard—that is, without dialogue—would seem a failure of nerve at the very least. The convention is that dialogue may be reconstructed or even invented rather than remembered; no one expects verbatim transcription. Thus autobiographers have considerable latitude in presenting dialogue—prose license, as it were. As in fiction, however, dialogue is expected to sound realistic, to correspond in manner to the actual speech of the character represented. The obvious problem presented by dialogue in life writing about deaf people is how to represent dialogue that may have taken the form of sign language, a combination of speech and Sign, or "deaf English," which does not conform strictly to the syntactical or grammatical rules of standard English.

When the conversation was signed, the question is whether the translation into English should be literal or liberal, a sign-by-sign transcription or a rephrasing in standard English. Transcription is not as easy as it might seem, because in genuine sign languages, like American Sign Language, signs do not correspond to English words; sign-by-sign transcription would result in entirely unidiomatic "speech." That option has the advantage of giving a sense of the different syntax of sign language; it reminds readers that what they are reading was not originally uttered in the language presented—in fact, it was not uttered at all. It helps to place them, imaginatively, in a deaf world by conveying a sense of how differently sign is structured. However, in conveying the otherness of Sign, transcription may also unintentionally reinforce a reader's sense of its being incorrect, sub- or nonstandard. As Paul Preston points out, in explaining problems he faced in transcribing interviews with hearing children of deaf parents who sometimes reverted to Sign, "While this method [literal translation] conveys the sense of difference between sign and spoken language, it creates a false impression of sign language as an ungrammatical or disjointed language" (32).

The problem here is similar to that of the use in literature of any nonstandard dialect for dialogue; no matter how sympathetic an author may be to its utterer, any nonstandard dialect tends to look or sound ungrammatical when surrounded by narration in standard English. This is especially the case with phonetic renditions of dialect; devised to convey the sound of oral people in a print medium, phonetic spelling may have the effect of branding them as illiterate. A character who may be speaking fluently, even eloquently, in her idiom may come across on the page as failing to spell correctly, her language "shown up" by the surrounding standard English narration. Just as the print medium tends to misrepresent oral people, so is it handicapped in presenting people who sign. The syntax of their "speech" may register as faulty, deficient.

If the deaf characters are not signing but speaking, the problem of dialect remains, for often the speech will be deaf English, which sounds "broken." One issue in deaf life writing, then, is how to solve or at least finesse the problem of which linguistic register to use for deaf characters' "speech." Short of abandoning print for another medium, no simple or entirely successful solution seems to exist. (Even the abandonment of print does not entirely solve the problem. Although videotape would convey the look, grace, and nuance of sign language, it would be unintelligible to most hearing people without subtitles, and the addition of subtitles reintroduces all the problems of the written representation of signed dialogue. But at least a visual medium would foreground sign language itself.)

Despite the lack of an obvious or single solution, it may help to remember the success of writers like Mark Twain, in *The Adventures of Huckleberry Finn*, and Zora Neale Hurston, in *Their Eyes Were Watching God*, in using dialect in literary works without condescension. To oversimplify somewhat, Mark Twain's innovation was to make a nonstandard dialect the language of the narrative; he thus avoided the invidious contrast between a narrative in "proper" English and dialogue in dialect. (There remain, of course, discrepancies between Huck's narrative language and the various dialects of the other characters.) Although Hurston did not use a dialect character for a narrator, she devised a highly metaphorical style that drew on the figurative extravagance of her oral characters, thus minimizing the gap between the oral or folk and the literary voices of her book.

One important consideration in the development of deaf life writing is the handling of this issue, which is one of the subtler manifestations of the problem of hegemonic discourse. For many deaf people *English*, the hegemonic language, is a second language acquired with great difficulty, sometimes under duress. On the other hand, it is the native language of most of those who write—and read—about the deaf. One danger of life writing about deaf individuals is that it will reenact the sometimes painful subjection of the deaf to English and the cultural repression of deaf modes of communication. The issue manifests itself differently depending on the position of the narrator. In the case of Henry Kisor's memoir the issue is perhaps moot—not so much because of his lifelong oralism as because he grew up immersed in hearing culture: there is little occasion for him to render deaf dialogue. In contrast, Bernard Bragg, as a deaf child of deaf parents, was always immersed in the deaf community. Though his decision to sign his narrative, as we have seen, is both original and exemplary, it does not avoid the problem of the presentation of dialogue; in their Authors' Note, he and his collaborator explain their decision to present signed conversation in liberal translation:

The rhythm, syntax, and grammar of American Sign Language differ drastically from those of English. Therefore, any verbatim translation from American Sign Language to English often results in awkward, stilted language. In reality, a signer's story is a work of art, sparkling with witticisms and the most subtle nuances of expression. That is why we choose a free rather than literal translation of dialogue in this book. Of course, not all the dialogue is translated from sign language. Some deaf people are bilingual and use English almost as readily as they sign. (xiii)

Although the book as a whole pays unique homage to sign language, the collaborators make little effort to suggest the diversity of communication styles among its characters. By rendering all dialogue in the same register, the book ignores or erases significant differences.

In memoirs of deaf children by hearing parents the issue of language will be highly charged; the narrator's choices, however, will not always be difficult—in part because the child may be the only deaf character. Thus, as *narrator*, Thomas Spradley doesn't face much of a problem in this regard. Because he narrates only the first few years of his daughter's life, and because those years are largely prelingual, he has little deaf dialogue to represent. (Of course, from the oralist perspective from which the parents first view their daughter, that is precisely the problem, that Lynn produces no presentable speech.) Although Paul West goes a long way to rendering faithfully what his daughter Mandy can and does say, and although he honors the ways in which his daughter's speech is distinctive—especially in its lexicon—Mandy is severely limited in what she can communicate; again, there is little dialogue, and that is what troubles the narrator. Either because of the limited chronological scope of the narrative or the limited development of the deaf daughter, neither narrative does much translation; standard English is adequate to what it purports to convey.

In the case of the filial memoir issues of language parallel the issues raised in second-generation ethnic autobiography—how to present the conversation of parents (and others) in another language that the child understands but may no longer use. The parents whom the child wants to honor may speak a language the narrator has outgrown or at least grown away from. When the language of the home is translated into standard English, something distinctive may be lost. When the language of the home is reproduced as fractured English, the narrator's standard dialect may seem to patronize it. Preston notes that some hearing children of deaf parents have adopted "coda-talk"—a kind of creole or patois based on deaf English—as a medium of communication among themselves and of expressing their sense of liminality. Even among "codas," however, coda-talk is somewhat controversial. "Coda-talk was seen by proponents as a way of expressing two conflicting linguistic heritages. Many other informants—even those who were active participants in CODA—were highly critical of coda-talk as 'immature' or 'a mockery of sign language.' . . . Public usage was tantamount to a betrayal of a family and cultural trust" (223). Although some have embraced coda-talk as a medium of in-group communication, identity reinforcement, self-help, and recovery, it seems to have little potential as a medium for deaf life writing, because it is not the language used by deaf children with their parents but rather a simulation of it or even a creole that blends deaf English and child talk. But the controversy over its use within CODA suggests the complexity of the issue of the proper linguistic medium for representing life in deaf households.

In *Train Go Sorry* (1994) Leah Hager Cohen, who notes early on that "no practical written system for American Sign Language" exists, marks signed dialogue by putting it in italics (ix). Though helpful, this is of course only an indicator of the medium of the original communication, not a rendering of its distinctive qualities. On the whole she avoids deaf English and renders dialogue in the same register as the narrative voice. Sidransky and Walker both address the issues of language and literacy quite forthrightly. Walker is blunt about her parents' trouble communicating in English, their embarrassment over it, and their reliance on her editing of their writing.

Mom and Dad's sentences sounded as if a foreigner had written them, as if English weren't their native tongue at all—and of course, it wasn't really. Still, I was to find out later that their writing was far superior to most done by deaf adults—even deaf college graduates.

Back then, a proud and self-conscious third grader correcting her parents' letters, I was filled with a mixture of pleasure and embarrassment—pleasure because I was useful to my parents, embarrassment because they couldn't do what I thought all other parents did with ease. (81)

Her discussion of the issue reveals the complex gestures of her narrative. On the one hand, here she undoes her earlier editing, exposing her parents' limited command of English; on the other, she makes it clear that English was their second language and praises their command of it in relative terms.

Walker does a number of things to compensate for the fact that much of the conversation of her childhood will inevitably be lost in translation. For example, she contextualizes family communication by establishing the conventions governing it—distinguishing the times when her parents tended to use sign alone, when they used voice along with sign, and when they used only speech (when teaching a sign). When it comes to representing dialogue in the narrative, she favors liberal translation—"Promise you'll write" (12)—over more literal rendition—"They were appreciated we asked them for the marriage" (44). To remind the reader that conversation represented was not originally verbal, she occasionally pauses to describe or explain a sign her parents use. All these are ways of foregrounding the issue, if not of solving the problem.

Of signing, Oliver Sacks has said that it

has a playful quality, a style, quite different from that of speech. Signers tend to improvise, to play with signs, to bring all their humor, their imaginativeness, their personality, into their signing, so that signing is not just the manipulation of symbols according to the grammatical rules, but, irreducibly, the voice of the signer—a voice given a special force, because it utters itself, so immediately, with the body. One can have or imagine disembodied speech, but one cannot have disembodied Sign. The body and soul of the signer, his unique identity, are continually expressed in the act of signing. (119)

Of the narratives of and by the deaf surveyed in this chapter, Ruth Sidransky's comes closest to conveying some of these qualities. Like Walker, Sidransky is candid about her parents' struggle with, or deficiency in, English. Thus she describes her father's letters as mimicking his broken spoken English—"the language of the deaf transposed to written words. It was awkward. At times his language was incomprehensible to the hearing reader unaccustomed to his deaf thought process, but it was his language, striking at the essence of meaning" (174).

More consistently than Walker, Sidransky tends to specify whether dialogue was signed, spoken, or both. And because she favors literal translation, the speech of deaf characters "sounds" much like their sign language. (Aside from noting, as Walker does, her parents' distinctive pronunciation of her name, she makes little attempt to communicate the auditory quality of their speech, however.) Although Sidransky sometimes adopts the syntax of her parents (170) for her speech as a *character*, it would not be appropriate for her to use deaf English as the language of the narrative, for she is fluent in standard English. Indeed, she notes that her father would often insist that his children speak rather than sign with each other in his presence, even if that meant effectively excluding him from the conversation: "It made me uncomfortable but he took pride in watching his offspring speak. For him, it was a mark of success, an entry into another place from which he was permanently excluded" (170–71).

Like Walker, Sidransky wants to honor her parents' linguistic abilities. Her first gesture in that direction is her expression of her regret that her memoir cannot be written in their language:

If there were a way, if I could, I would write this book in sign language. I cannot. Signs do not transpose to the printed page; they are understood only in the flesh, hand to hand, face to face. And so I write in universal printed English, words to conjure the magic of my first language—words my mother taught me, words my father taught me—words told by the flick of a finger, the sweep of a hand. Sentences, liquid, rising not from the human voice but from the human body. (3)

As a child living to some degree in a world apart from that of her friends with hearing parents, Sidransky had a tendency to invent words when she didn't know the names of things (46). Her inclination to create her own lexicon continues as an adult, and the license she takes in writing her memoir is, I think, meant to be seen as the legacy of her parents' deafness—that is, of their use of a language with its own aesthetic, as well as its own grammar, syntax, and semantics. What from one point of view is insufficient is from another extravagant; Sidransky seems to suggest that her bilingual childhood has not disadvantaged but advantaged her; she is no slave to narrow rules of usage. She makes the most of her linguistic resources to give the reader a sense of her dual legacy. One of her devices is to offer transcriptions of sign or even of deaf English in which the substance of the message is so powerfully conveyed that the idiosyncrasies of its medium seem assets rather than liabilities.

For all that she is committed to the primacy of sign and to its physicality, however, Sidransky sees herself as having no alternative to English in print. She makes every effort, as in the last excerpt, to convey—with English words like *magic, flick, sweep, liquid, rising, body*—the fluency, economy, engagement, and enchantment of sign language. Insofar as she does succeed in expressing the beauty of Sign, she does so more by *de*scribing it, than by *tran*scribing it, in English. It is an act of simulation rather than imitation, the presentation in one medium of the qualities of another, which is mostly absent.

Thanks to a combination of unusual circumstances, an anomalous, perhaps unique book does exist that very nearly sidesteps the problem of a linguistic medium for deaf life writing: *"Deaf Maggie Lee Sayre": Photographs of a River Life* (1995). In 1982 anthropologists seeking to document and interpret the lives of Ohio and Tennessee river dwellers were led to a deaf woman, Maggie Lee Sayre, in a nursing home; in response to their handwritten inquiries she produced albums of photographs she had taken to document the life of her family on the river.

"Deaf Maggie Lee Sayre," edited by Tom Rankin, consists of Sayre's photos, captioned by her (in collaboration with a sign-language interpreter); a one-page account of her life that Sayre typed at Rankin's request; and his introduction.

Sayre's book is a third-person family memoir rather than a first-person autobiography. It begins, "Maggie Lee Sayre was born to Archie and May Sayre on April 4, 1920," and much of it is cast in the third-person plural. Its focus, then, is on the family and its way of life rather than on its author and her deafness. Events like the death of her sister, those of her parents, and Sayre's consignment to a nursing home are handled matter-of-factly. Similarly, the photos are a documentary of her family's life rather than an autobiography in any conventional sense. (Indeed, fish figure in these photos almost as prominently as people.) Because she took most of the photographs, Sayre hardly ever appears in them; like her written narrative, then, her photo albums are quite literally self-effacing. At same time, the albums and the book that published them represent a significant sort of life writing (in the unconventional medium of light-writing). At the very least they inscribe her distinctive point of view, because no one else in her world was inclined to take such pictures.

In addition to providing valuable insight into the life of river dwellers, the book is a rare example of self-representation by an ordinary deaf person. Sayre took up photography accidentally, but it helped compensate for her inability to express herself orally. She and her older sister Myrtle attended the residential Kentucky School for the Deaf for nine months a year, beginning when they were seven and eight, respectively. There they learned to sign and were given name-signs, but they never learned to talk. They communicated with their hearing parents through home signs and a note pad (the parents' literacy was limited [18]).

Sayre's simple camera had originally been given to Myrtle in a manufacturer's promotion; Maggie inherited it when Myrtle died in her late teens. Thus Sayre's acquisition of a new medium of communication came through the tragic loss of the only person in her immediate world with whom she could communicate in her primary medium, sign language (18). Her camera compensated not only for her inability to express herself orally but also for her sudden isolation. With her new technology and her new point of view—from attending school on shore—she became a kind of intuitive participant-observer of river life (19). Ironically, deafness brought her closer, through her education, to mainstream life; though somewhat isolated from her parents and her community by her lack of oral skills, she was in some ways less marginalized than they. Although she lived on the borders of the hearing and deaf worlds, river life and town life, her particular circumstances minimized her need to communicate with strangers. In such circumstances deafness may have been less "disabling" than it would have been in an urban or suburban environment.

Sayre's documentation of her life was thus a function of many factors—her deafness, the loss of her sister and the acquisition of a camera, her education, and her liminality in her community. The book is perhaps more a river memoir than a deaf memoir; though its subject and author is deaf and her photos are in part a response to her deafness, its subject is not deafness, much less Deafness. It is a record of an unusual life that resists categorization, one in which the disadvantage of deafness was perhaps minimized. Though the book came to be published only through the mediation of others, it does circumvent some of the apparent obstacles to deaf life writing. It thus suggests some unconventional possibilities for life writing and disability (and for self-representation by people who are otherwise unlikely or ill equipped to write their lives).[17]

We are still less than a generation into the Deaf renaissance, if we date it from the acknowledgment of the legitimacy of Sign as a language. (Stokoe's book arguing this was published in 1960, but its argument was only slowly and grudgingly accepted.) It now appears that the use of computers may offer ways of transcribing or "writing" Sign. For example, a system known as SignFont purports to capture much of the expressiveness of Sign. According to Oliver Sacks, "If SignFont, or some other form of written Sign, were adopted by the deaf, it might lead them to a written literature of their own, and serve to deepen their sense of community and culture" (78–79). Deaf autobiography might be a beneficiary of such a development—though the question of accessibility to hearing readers would remain. In the meantime, no doubt resourceful life writers will extend the experiments in life writing and language carried out by the writers surveyed here.

Signs of the Times

Since the early 1980s mainstream presses have published accounts of deaf lives that were inconceivable much earlier. The number of full-life narratives is still so small that each new text is in danger of being taken as more representative than it could be. Still, with each new "life," we have a greater sense of the various ways in which loss of hearing, in all its complex manifestations, can inflect life experience and interact with other cultural and physical factors. Although there are still relatively few memoirs and autobiographies of deafness, it would appear that the flowering of deaf life writing has begun.

Far from univocal, deaf life writing has become a significant medium for airing the controversies over deafness, communication methods, pedagogical methods, cultural values, and the very terms to be used in discussing all these. The outcome of the battle over the construction of deafness is of course yet to be determined. (Indeed, deafness is such a various phenomenon that it is unlikely that any one construction will win over all parties.) Although the lack of unanimity can be confusing to onlookers, it is evidence that momentum may have shifted away from audism, which was more or less unchallenged until relatively recently; in life writing as elsewhere, Deaf counterdiscourse seems to be on the rise. At the moment, then, the playing field is more level than it has been for years; both sides are being voiced—or signed. The advent of multiculturalism—which of course is far from uncontested—has both stimulated and created a potential audience for the cultural, as opposed to the pathological, paradigm of deafness.

Deaf life writing may remain problematic, but the developing tradition is perhaps all the richer for the obstacles it must overcome; its new self-consciousness about the politics and language of its mediation of deafness has engendered experiments that should inform life writing concerning other cultural groups. Until recently, most testimony of deaf lives has been "hearsay" in more senses than one; now, even though some testimony is still vicarious, deaf lives are being written in greater numbers. Signing individuals have been given lasting and memorable traces on paper; in one way or another, deaf life writing is full of vital signs.

Notes

1. The analogy with the gay rights movement is suggestive. Like homosexuals, deaf people are generally born to parents who do not share their culture. And like homosexuals, deaf people have worked hard to demedicalize and destigmatize their condition.

2. For a good discussion of the difficulty of defining *functioning hearing* for everyday life, see Higgins 29–34.

3. As much as possible, I will observe the use of Deaf and deaf to distinguish between cultural and audiological deafness. Useful as this orthographic distinction may be, its inaudibility privileges written over oral discourse; speech disables it. Even in writing, it is nullified at the beginnings of sentences. It should be noted too that the deaf and the Deaf are not separate populations. See Preston 12–17.

4. Some important precursors in the genre of deaf autobiography should be mentioned here. Harlan Lane made available a selection of accounts by eighteenth- and nineteenth-century Europeans in *The Deaf Experience* (1984). In

America, of course, the classic account of growing up deaf and blind is Helen Keller's (1903). Also worthy of mention is Albert Ballin's *The Deaf Mute Howls* (1930). Although it is far from a full-life narrative, this book offers intriguing glimpses of Ballin's life in support of his indictment of oralism and his plea for the widespread teaching and adoption of what he refers to as "the universal sign language."

(No sign language is a truly universal language; there are those in the Deaf community today, like Barbara Kannapell, the founder of Deaf Pride, who feel that its universal adoption—that is, by hearing as well as deaf people—would threaten, if not destroy, the Deaf world, because the use of ASL is the major element that distinguishes Deaf culture from the dominant culture [Sacks 128–29n].)

5. For a more sustained account of an individual with little language of any sort, see Susan Schaller's *A Man Without Words* (1991).

6. Lane attributes these occupational patterns not to hearing impairment but to the failure of oralism: "Since educational programs for deaf children have not succeeded in teaching them English and yet rely on English for all teaching, the programs long ago settled for instructing their deaf students in manual trades" (*Mask* 131).

7. For the definitive statement of this polemical view see Lane, *The Mask of Benevolence* (1992). A concise statement of this thesis can be found on pp. 18–21. (See also useful reviews by Melvin Konner and David J. Rothman.) Lane acknowledges, but perhaps does not fully reckon with, the fact that the Deaf are a minority within a minority: perhaps one million out of the tens of millions of Americans with hearing loss. Although he acknowledges in passing that for "adventitiously deafened hearing people . . . an infirmity model is appropriate" (206), Lane's advocacy of a cultural model downplays the situation of the large majority of hearing-impaired people who have no desire to be Deaf or learn sign language but rather to function as fully as possible orally in the hearing world.

8. In 1993 Dalkey Archive Press published a volume in which it reprinted *Words for a Deaf Daughter* along with *Gala* (1976), a kind of wish-fulfilling fictional sequel, in which a writer brings his disabled daughter to the United States for a visit. In the preface to that volume West acknowledges that his daughter's impairments prevented her from ever reading the earlier book (vii). "It has turned out to be the record of a heyday, of her finest hours" (ix). At the same time, he notes that he wrote much of it literally in her presence, which was at once distracting and stimulating, and that "she knew what was going on." In this way he makes her a kind of collaborator as well as muse.

9. It is worth noting that both groups are somewhat smaller than they might be, if not for the stigmatization of deafness. Deaf couples have historically been discouraged from having children because of the fear of passing on hereditary deafness (Preston 10). Indeed, Lou Ann Walker suspects that her father's deaf brother was talked out of having children by his hearing father (19). Moreover,

some hearing parents would abort a fetus if they knew it was to be born deaf. An interesting subtextual issue in *Deaf Like Me* is that Louise Spradley was exposed to rubella and developed a rash while pregnant in 1964; the narrative implies that, had she been diagnosed definitively, and had abortion been legal where she lived, Lynn Spradley might never have been born.

10. Such family interpreters often become professional interpreters, as was the case with Lou Ann Walker.

11. Sidransky's title seems to accept the common assumption that deaf people live in a "silent" world, unaware or ignorant of sound, but it may refer instead to ways in which she, as the child of deaf parents, felt silenced. Although it is true that, in the world of deaf people, sound is different and necessarily plays a different role than it does for the hearing, Douglas C. Baynton has pointed out that silence

is not a straightforward or unproblematic description of the experience of a deaf person. First, few deaf people hear nothing. Most have hearing losses which are not uniform across the entire range of pitch. . . . Sounds will often be quite distorted, but heard nevertheless. And second, for those who do not hear, what does the word silence signify? Unless they once heard and *became* deaf, the word is meaningless as a description of their experience. . . . Silence is experienced by the hearing as the absence of sound. For those who have never heard, deafness is not an absence. To be deaf is *not* to not hear for most profoundly deaf people, but a social relation—that is, a relation with other human beings, those called "hearing" and those called "deaf." (226)

Thus the metaphorical equation of silence with deafness too readily defines deafness as a lack. For an excellent discussion of the role of sound in the lives of deaf people see Padden, chapter 6, "The Meaning of Sound."

12. Preston uses initial capitalization with *hearing* as well as *deaf* to refer to groups rather than individuals. See his discussion of the deaf/Deaf distinction, pp. 15–17.

13. The term *CODA*, an acronym for children of deaf adults, refers both to hearing children of deaf parents (with a lower-case spelling) and to a support group addressing their presumed needs. The very idea that codas *need* support reflects the belief that they have somehow been damaged by their parents' deafness—by analogy with children of alcoholic or otherwise dysfunctional parents. Not surprisingly, then, the organization is itself controversial (Preston 23).

14. He candidly acknowledges the limitations of lipreading, however; the title of his book represents his misreading of "What's that big loud noise?"

15. A comparison of Bragg's story of his first summer job in his 1989 book with an earlier version in Leonard Lane and Ivy Pittle's *A Handful of Stories: Thirty-seven Stories by Deaf Storytellers* (1981) reinforces this sense. The stories in the anthology are "transliterated from the Deaf Storytellers Video Tape Series" produced under the auspices of Gallaudet College. The earlier version is a more minimal literal translation, whereas the latter is, as the Authors' Note remarks, "free." The early version lacks the abundant descriptive detail of the autobiography, provided presumably to compensate for the lack of visual stimulus on the printed page.

16. Although founded in 1967, early in the Deaf renaissance, the NTD did not commission and perform a play in Sign until 1973 (Sacks 145). Until then, all its productions were of plays written in English and translated into Signed English. Even after 1973 the NTD continued to orient itself to a hearing audience; this was increasingly unacceptable to Bragg.

17. I am grateful to Timothy Dow Adams for bringing this book to my attention.

7

Epilogue
The Value of Body Stories

> We have banalized the body, demystified it, displayed it to the point that there may be no more to learn about it—at least, about its exterior. We have listened to its talk, in an effort to penetrate its most reticent messages. But we still don't know the body. Its otherness from ourselves, as well as its intimacy, make it the inevitable object of an ever-renewed writing project.
> —Peter Brooks, *Body Work*, 1993, p. 286.

Although the personal literature of illness and disability is no longer neglected, it remains vulnerable to dismissal from different sides. Aesthetes may see it as entirely too concerned with the body, too mundane and utilitarian to be "literary." Political activists may see it as too sentimental to be effective counterdiscourse. (They might argue that its singling out of subjects, its investment in individual fate, limits its emancipatory potential.) I hope to counter such objections here without making extravagant claims for the books in question.

To the activist, narratives of illness and disability may be suspect because they are only words, not action. Thus gay activists might argue that personal narratives are an utterly inadequate response to the urgent threat posed by the AIDS epidemic and, moreover, that for critics to treat illness as in any way a discursive construction is to trivialize human suffering. In the face of this argument one must concede that other responses to AIDS—medical and political—are more urgent than narrative treatments of it.

But in the absence of a magic bullet people continue to live and die with AIDS, and part of their suffering is caused by ignorance and by prejudicial discourse. As Verlyn Klinkenborg has noted,

When you contract a disease, you contract the world of that disease, and that world is what threatens self-definition. In this, as in so much else, AIDS has reminded us of things that were on the verge of being forgotten. It has distanced us from the medical optimism of the nineteen-fifties and sixties and reasserted the fact that no sickness—and certainly no epidemic—comes without its myths, which can be every bit as damaging as the sickness itself. (78).

It is this gratuitous collateral damage done by disease that counterdiscourse in the form of illness narratives can address and perhaps alleviate. (Andrew Holleran has suggested that the only thing he really wants to read about AIDS is a headline announcing CURE FOUND [Murphy 315]. At the same time, Holleran's awareness of the limitations of discursive responses to the AIDS epidemic has not prevented him from writing some of the best essays about its effect on the gay community, in *Ground Zero* [1988].) In arguing for a narrative-based approach to medicine, Howard Brody has noted that "suffering results when an illness experience is perceived as meaningless or as threatening the integrity of the patient's life and relationships, and healing occurs when a more comforting meaning is assigned to the illness and the patient sees himself reconnected to his social network" (90). If this assertion is valid on the collective as well as the individual scale, published illness narratives may be in some significant sense healing. Although they may be unable to relieve the symptoms of the body, they may help to relieve the suffering of the self.

At their best narratives of illness and disability acknowledge that our bodies are not ultimately in our control. At the same time, however, they remind us that we do have considerable influence over the way our bodies, healthy or not, are viewed. A degree of stigmatization is associated with all four conditions discussed in this book; indeed, stigma is one powerful stimulant of the narratives—individually and collectively. Although a wide range of conditions has been described in illness narratives, it is no accident that the largest bodies of works have to do with conditions that raise questions of special concern in the cultural politics of fin-de-siècle America. With each of these conditions, then, the narratives tend to address larger agendas. This is most obvious in the cases of breast cancer and AIDS, in which narratives tend to be conscripted into ongoing struggles over the bodies of women and gay men. In assigning meaning to bodily dysfunction, such narratives often contest dominant cultural constructions. The narratives, "mere" words, carry out important cultural work.

Of course, the sort of cultural work that many narratives attempt may not always be consistent with literary aspiration. In a provocative 1995 piece in the *New Yorker* dance critic Arlene Croce took choreographer Bill T. Jones to task for a work entitled "Still/Here," which included taped testimony by people with terminal illnesses. Without having seen the work, Croce condemned it as manipulative "victim art . . . intolerably voyeuristic." Using Jones as a whipping boy, Croce launched a broad attack on the way in which late twentieth-century art generally represents "disease and death." According to Croce, rather than transcending or sublimating painful experiences like proper nineteenth-century geniuses, today's artists tend to use raw testimony and all-too-graphic images to extort sympathy from their audiences and to disenfranchise critics: "By working dying people into his act, Jones is putting himself beyond the reach of criticism. I think of him as literally undiscussable— the most extreme case among the distressingly many now representing themselves to the public not as artists but as victims and martyrs" (54). One thing that troubles me about Croce's piece is that its logic, applied to writing, would seem to rule out nonfictional, and especially autobiographical, narratives of illness or disability; at least, by categorizing them as "victim testimony," it would put them beneath critical notice (even as it accuses them of evading critical scrutiny). There is much to be said for transmuting experience in art, as there is much to be said for rising above adversity. But not all adversity ends in triumph, and that which does not should not arbitrarily be ruled inexpressible. (The responsibility of the critic would seem to be to judge works on their merits rather than to dismiss them categorically.)

My relation to the personal literature of illness and disability is clearly different from Croce's relation to dance. The works I address do not typically present themselves as art. I do not expect their intentions and ambitions to be simply or purely aesthetic, nor am I primarily interested in evaluating them in aesthetic terms, sorting out the literary from the subliterary. In focusing on only four conditions—breast cancer, AIDS, paralysis, and deafness—I have tried to sample a full range of testimony on each, with little initial concern for quality. Indeed, some of what I regard as the best recent writing about illness goes undiscussed in this book—because it did not have to do with the conditions selected for discussion.

Nevertheless, part of my response (and responsibility) is inevitably to evaluate; clearly, much of the work discussed here puts a critic in an awkward position. It is discomfiting to find fault with the sincere testimony of someone with a life-threatening condition or that of a grieving caregiver or relative. Nevertheless, the publication of a book invites, even demands, evaluation. The critic's responsibility is to apply standards—whether aesthetic, moral, or political—openly, consistently, and fairly; I hope I have done so. The alternative—not to judge the works— is far more patronizing. And to refuse even to consider them as potential art seems a form of denial, an arbitrary ruling out of an important, if threatening, aspect of human experience.

Croce's diatribe was revealing in its assumption that dance involving anyone of less than ideal body shape and condition could not be art worthy of critical attention: "As a dance critic, I've learned to avoid dancers with obvious problems—overweight dancers . . . old dancers, dancers with sickled feet, or dancers with physical deformities who appear nightly in roles requiring beauty of line" (55). But perhaps what was most objectionable about her piece was its dismissal of any representation of marginalization—at least in relatively unmediated forms, particularly self-representation—as "victim art": "In quite another category of undiscussability are those dancers I'm *forced* to feel sorry for because of the way they present themselves: as dissed blacks, abused women, or disfranchised homosexuals—as performers, in short, who make out of victimhood victim art" (55). Croce is here attacking not only particular kinds of art but more generally "identity politics"—the tendency to identify individuals with the racial, ethnic, or gender groups of which they are members.

In the cases of the conditions dealt with in this book, to be sure, identity politics often plays a role. In our era one constructive response of those marginalized by bodily difference has been to assert solidarity, textually or extratextually, with others who share that difference. And although identity politics risks overemphasizing certain kinds of differences and reifying those distinctions in counterproductive ways, it seems to me that the current emphasis on bodily distinctions is justified if it contributes to the reduction of stigma and marginalization. It does so, I think, by helping us to see through the body in two senses: to think *about* and *with* our bodies, to reexamine the implications, cultural and political, physical and metaphysical, of our embodiment.

One of Croce's problematic assumptions is that the work she attacks exists only to seek sympathy or pity. It doesn't seem to have occurred to Croce that it might be precisely the goal of such work to challenge the idea that marginalized people are necessarily pathetic victims. In the case of illness and disability often the foremost motive of life writing is to recover variously dysfunctional bodies from domination by others' authority and discourse, to convert the passive object into an active subject. In my experience narratives of illness and disability rarely, if ever, assert victimhood as a basis for sympathy. They are much more likely to try to *de*victimize their subjects and others like them. Indeed, one of the most powerful motives in contemporary narratives of illness and disability is the impulse to invalidate the dominant cultural tropes of "invalidity"—to demystify and destigmatize various conditions. Croce seems to want to preserve not only the stigma but the invisibility of certain conditions. This book and many of the books it analyzes seek to challenge the assumptions behind such erasure.

To claim that illness narratives are worthy of critical attention is not to claim that they are literature. Generally speaking, I would concur with Anne Hunsaker Hawkins, who concluded *Reconstructing Illness* (1993) by saying that "pathography is a genre that awaits its masterpieces" (159). Of the writing I have surveyed here, little of it may prove to have lasting value as literature in the traditional sense—books that require and reward rereading and close analysis. But these works are so new that it would be premature to attempt definitive judgments. I trust that my personal preferences are evident in the body of the book, but the purpose of my evaluative comments has not been to predict canonization for, or to convey it on, any of the works but rather to analyze the role each plays in the development of the discourse of illness and disability.

Genres are not justified only or even mainly by their production of classics. Moreover, it is well to remember that most nonfiction books that come to be considered timeless classics had rather immediate, pragmatic aims when they were composed. (Consider, for example, Frederick Douglass's *Narrative*.) Like related life-writing subgenres devoted to particular kinds of experience—captivity narratives, conversion narratives, and slave narratives, for example—narratives of illness often have specific, limited, utilitarian agendas. Partly because of the pressure under which much of it is composed, autopathography in particular may be highly conventional and even formulaic. Indeed, writing about illness may have inherent limitations that makes the production of masterpieces unlikely.

To those who dismiss illness narratives as inherently non- or subliterary, however, I respond that we should think of illness narratives as serving concentric circles of readers in different ways. In the center are those most immediately involved with the condition in question: those who are ill, those who are at risk, those who are caregivers, those who are bereaved. Written illness narratives may help these readers by providing specific sorts of information, resources, and reassurance; more generally, written accounts may help them achieve some therapeutic perspective on their predicament, to assign it redemptive meaning. For such readers one major function of illness narratives is simply to give formal public expression to their experience, to suggest that it matters.

For those less immediately involved—families and friends of those with the conditions in question—the narratives serve to communicate what those in the center are living through. Thus, for example, friends and acquaintances of people with cancer are often uncertain how to interact with them. Written narratives may help to provide a sense of what the person with cancer is going through and how to respond appropriately. One quite practical purpose of such narratives, then, whether one considers it a matter of manners, ethics, or morals, is to teach those who are well how to respond to those who are ill.

One of the most fundamental functions of illness narrative, then, is to validate the experience of illness—to put it on record, to exemplify living with bodily dysfunction, to offer lasting testimony.[1] (The same could be said of talk shows and other media attention.) Readers in these inner circles may not be fussy about what they read; indeed, they may find themselves reading voraciously in a single narrow subgenre to help them live through a crisis. Paradoxically, some of the most intimate bodily experiences may be easier to read and write about than to discuss in person; such discourse, however, ought not to be dismissed as voyeuristic. At base, narratives of illness are efforts to give meaning to, or find meaning in, bodily dysfunction and thereby to relieve suffering. People who narrate their illness or disability may be said to share their bodies with others in a kind of secular healing ritual.

For the broader public the purposes of such narratives and the effects of reading them are less well defined. With less personal interest in the condition in question and less pressing need for validation of it this circle of readers may be more oriented to aesthetic qualities—more interested in the poetics than the politics of illness narrative. They may seek out narratives that are particularly self-conscious, writerly works. Or not. Though the sample of works surveyed here is perhaps not entirely representative, personal narratives of illness and disability are in general less transgressive and formally innovative than one might expect. Though their foregrounding of bodily dysfunction may resist or oppose the Western repression of the body, they may also revert in different ways and degrees to formulas or conventions that privilege the soul (such as the conversion narrative). On the whole, though, they generally remain rooted in a familiar solid world and tell more or less straightforward stories. In some ways, then, they tend to perpetuate premodernist narrative conventions. Indeed, part of their appeal to general readers may be that they may satisfy certain appetites that much contemporary literature does not. As the novel has moved toward minimalism, on the one hand, and self-reflexive postmodernist metafiction, on the other, readers may long for old-fashioned plot, vivid characters, life-and-death crises, definitive closure—all of which many illness narratives supply. For these reasons many of these narratives are surprisingly good reads, gripping narratives with compelling topics.

In addition, illness and disability—once they have been validated as subjects for life writing—serve as pretexts for the writing of lives that would otherwise be unstoried and evanescent. As we have seen, the flourishing of illness narrative has been the occasion for the writing of the lives of individuals who until recently might have been excluded from even the democratic provinces of autobiography and memoir. The tendency of illness narrative to graft another story onto the basic plot of bodily dysfunction means that the repertoire of life writing is enriched by such narratives. Because of their initiative in such dysfunction, such narratives may serve to bring into the light topics traditionally taboo. For example, I think of Mark Doty's memorable description of his partner's body immediately following his death, as its vital warmth dissipated (29–30). To write this without voyeurism, morbidity, or embarrassment requires consummate control of language; the passage is among other things a tour de force. But its value is not so much aesthetic as more broadly cultural; it demystifies a taboo scene, casting light into a dark corner from which most of us avert our eyes. (Though not formally innovative, such writing is significantly transgressive.)

In some texts, then, the details of particular illnesses or disabilities recede in importance; the significance of embodiment more generally comes to the fore. And it is here that other forms of "body writing" may come into play. I am particularly enthusiastic about writing—not necessarily "narrative"—that takes advantage of bodily dysfunction to explore embodiment as a medium of experience. When I first undertook this study, I expected to find more of this in current illness narratives. What I found, however, was that generic illness narrative is, understandably, so invested in recovery that the achievement of closure often takes precedence over consideration of what dysfunction feels like and how it alters self-perception. The essay and the pathographic sketch, which do not depend on plot, are in some ways better suited to this than the chronological narrative. Books by Oliver Sacks (*The Man Who Mistook His Wife for a Hat* [1985]), Leonard Kriegel (*Falling into Life* [1991]), Nancy Mairs (*Carnal Acts* [1990] and *Plaintext* [1986]), Samuel Wilson Fussell (*Muscle* [1991]), John Hull (*Touching the Rock* [1991]), Lucy Grealy (*Autobiography of a Face* [1994]), Tim Brookes (*Catching My Breath* [1995]), Anatole Broyard (*Intoxicated by My Illness* [1992]), Andre Dubus (*Broken Vessels* [1991]), Mark Doty (*Heaven's Coast* [1996], especially Part I), and John Updike (*Self-Consciousness* [1989]) exemplify the range of what I would call body writing. Such writing relies less heavily on chronology and plot; it combines vividness of description, apt and detailed verbal simulation or representation of somatic experience (personal or witnessed firsthand) with speculation about the cultural, political, and epistemological implications of embodiment. (Among narrators of illness, Mark Doty is notable for the degree to which he dissolves the boundaries between himself and his partner, body and spirit, heaven and earth, grief and love, absence and presence, without subordinating either element to its counterpart.) By addressing particular and sometimes rare bodily conditions such as asthma (Brookes), facial disfigurement (Grealy), exercise bulimia (Fussell), stuttering and psoriasis (Updike), they help to take us out of our bodies and into others'; ultimately, though, they return us to our bodies with greater understanding of how they may shape and condition our identities: our bodies, our selves.

Our bodies are, after all, the medium of our experience, our individuation, our very existence—"the source of sensation and the spring of action," in Jonathan Miller's phase (14). They give us being, and (from a secular perspective, at least) they take it away. On the one hand, in an era when medical technology promises to replace vital organs and extend life, narratives of illness and disability may serve, among other things, as a kind of reality check. They remind us of the vulnerabilities of embodiment. As Anne Hunsaker Hawkins has put it, "For readers who are not themselves sick, pathography serves a preparatory function, so that when they do encounter some life-threatening illness (and most of us eventually will), this experience will inevitably be informed by what they have read" (11). On the other hand, when the same biomedical technologies tend to reduce people to patients and patients to cases, personal narratives may individually and collectively help to reclaim bodies from medical colonization, to reinvest bodily dysfunction with meaning. If the threat of meaninglessness is the most profound threat posed by illness, disability, or other bodily injury, by organizing the experience of bodily dysfunction in coherent ways narratives of illness promise to restore or shore up our sense of the integrity and value of our lives. As Arthur Frank has said, "Illness can teach us all how to live a saner, healthier life. Illness is a threat to life, but it also witnesses what is worth living" (Will 15). Finally, then, narratives of illness and disability are a medium in which the writers probe and give expression to the complex dialectic of mind, body, and culture. At best, then, illness narratives remind us of what we share with each other—living in and as bodies, with all the pleasure and pain, joy and frustration, that that entails.

When the body takes a turn for the worse, the mind often turns toward words. Thus, if illness and disability are reminders of our mortality and frailty, narratives of those conditions are testaments to our resilience and vitality. Today especially, narratives of illness and disability are helping us recover our bodies and restory our lives. But there will always be a call for stories of illness and disability; their ultimate value is, after all, to help us understand what it means to be some body.

Notes

[1] In his *Wounded Storyteller* (1995) Arthur Frank has been especially attentive to the ethical dimension of witnessing illness.

References

Index

References

1. Introduction

Ashe, Arthur, and Arnold Rampersad. *Days of Grace: A Memoir*. New York: Alfred A. Knopf, 1993.

Brookes, Tim. *Catching My Breath: An Asthmatic Explores His Illness*. New York: Vintage, 1995.

Broyard, Anatole. *Intoxicated by My Illness, and Other Writings on Life and Death*. New York: Fawcett-Columbine, 1992.

Chester, Laura. *Lupus Novice: Toward Self-Healing*. Barrytown, N.Y.: Station Hill, 1987.

Duff, Kat. *The Alchemy of Illness*. New York: Pantheon, 1993.

Frank, Arthur W. *At the Will of the Body: Reflections on Illness*. Boston: Houghton Mifflin, 1991.

Frank, Arthur W. "Reclaiming an Orphan Genre: The First-Person Narrative of Illness." *Literature and Medicine* 13.1 (spring 1994): 1–21.

Frank, Arthur W. *The Wounded Storyteller: Body, Illness, and Ethics*. Chicago: University of Chicago Press, 1995.

Gilman, Sander L. *Disease and Representation: From Madness to AIDS*. Ithaca, N.Y.: Cornell University Press, 1988.

Greene, A. C. *Taking Heart*. New York: Simon & Schuster, 1990.

Hawkins, Anne Hunsaker. *Reconstructing Illness: Studies in Pathography*. West Lafayette, Ind.: Purdue University Press, 1993.

Heller, Joseph, and Speed Vogel. *No Laughing Matter*. New York: Putnam, 1986.

Howells, William Dean. "Autobiography, A New Form of Literature." *Harper's Monthly* 119 (1909): 795–98.

Kleinman, Arthur. *The Illness Narratives: Suffering, Healing, and the Human Condition*. New York: Basic Books, 1988.

Kramer, Peter D. *Listening to Prozac*. New York: Viking, 1993.

Kramer, Peter D. "The Anatomy of Melancholy." *New York Times Book Review*, April 8, 1996, p. 27.

Lorde, Audre. *The Cancer Journals*. N.p.: Spinsters Ink, 1980.

Mattingly, Cheryl. "The Concept of Therapeutic Emplotment." *Social Sciences and Medicine* 38 (March 1994): 811–22.

McGowin, Diana Friel. *Living in the Labyrinth: A Personal Journey Through the Maze of Alzheimer's*. New York: Delacorte, 1993.

Monette, Paul. *Borrowed Time: An AIDS Memoir*. New York: Harcourt Brace, 1988.

Morris, Adalaide. "The Body Politic: Body, Language, and Power." *College English* 52 (1990): 570–78.

Parsons, Talcott, with Rene Fox. "Illness and the Role of the Physician: A Sociological Perspective." *American Journal of Orthopsychiatry* 21 (1951): 452–60.

Pray, Lawrence M., with Richard Evans, III. *Journey of a Diabetic*. New York: Simon & Schuster, 1983.

Price, Reynolds. *A Whole New Life: An Illness and a Healing*. New York: Atheneum, 1994.

Radner, Gilda. *It's Always Something*. New York: Simon & Schuster, 1989.

Rothman, Sheila M. *Living in the Shadow of Death: Tuberculosis and the Social History of Illness in American History*. New York: Basic Books, 1994.

Selzer, Richard. *Raising the Dead*. New York: Viking-Whittle, 1994.

Shorter, Edward. *Bedside Manners: The Troubled History of Doctors and Patients*. New York: Simon & Schuster, 1985.

Smith, Sidonie. "Taking It to a Limit One More Time: Autobiography and Autism," pp. 226–46. In *Getting a Life: Everyday Uses of Autobiography*. Ed. Sidonie Smith and Julia Watson. Minneapolis: University of Minnesota Press, 1996.

Sontag, Susan. *Illness as Metaphor*. New York: Farrar, Straus, & Giroux, 1978.

Styron, William. *Darkness Visible: A Memoir of Madness*. New York: Random House, 1990.

Updike, John. *Self-Consciousness: Memoirs*. New York: Alfred A. Knopf, 1989.

West, Paul. *A Stroke of Genius: Illness and Self-Discovery*. New York: Viking, 1995.

Wood, Mary Elene. *The Writing on the Wall: Women's Autobiography and the Asylum, 1868–1932*. Urbana: University of Illinois Press, 1994.

2. Medical Discourse and Subjectivity

Angier, Natalie. "Bedside Manners Improve as More Women Enter Medicine." *New York Times*, June 21, 1992, p. 18.

Brody, Howard. "My Story Is Broken: Can You Help Me Fix It? Medical Ethics and the Joint Construction of Narrative." *Literature and Medicine* 13 (spring 1991): 79–92.

Brookes, Tim. *Catching My Breath: An Asthmatic Explores His Illness*. New York: Vintage, 1995.

Cameron, Jean. *For All That Has Been: Time to Live and Time to Die*. New York: Macmillan, 1982.

Charon, Rita. "Doctor-Patient/Reader-Writer: Learning to Find the Text." *Soundings* 72 (1989): 137–52.

Churchill, Larry R., and Sandra W. Churchill. "Storytelling in Medical Arenas: The Art of Self-Determination." *Literature and Medicine* 1 (1982): 73–79.

Coombs, Robert H. *Mastering Medicine: Professional Socialization in Medical School.* New York: Free Press, 1978.

Cousins, Mark, and Athar Hussain. *Michel Foucault.* New York: St. Martin's, 1984.

Donnelly, William J. "Righting the Medical Record: Transforming Chronicle into Story." *Soundings* 72.1 (1989): 127–35.

Epstein, Julia. *Altered Conditions: Disease, Medicine, and Storytelling.* New York: Routledge, 1995.

Foucault, Michel. *The Birth of the Clinic: An Archaeology of Medical Perception.* Trans. A. M. Sheridan Smith. New York: Random House, 1973.

Freidson, Eliot. *The Profession of Medicine: A Study of the Sociology of Applied Knowledge.* New York: Dodd, Mead, 1971.

Hillyer, Barbara. *Feminism and Disability.* Norman: Oklahoma University Press, 1993.

Hunter, Kathryn Montgomery. *Doctors' Stories: The Narrative Structure of Medical Knowledge.* Princeton, N.J.: Princeton University Press, 1991.

Klass, Perri. *A Not Entirely Benign Procedure: Four Years as a Medical Student.* New York: New American Library, 1987.

Kleinman, Arthur. *The Illness Narratives: Suffering, Healing, and the Human Condition.* New York: Basic Books, 1988.

Konner, Melvin. *Becoming a Doctor: A Journey of Initiation in Medical School.* New York: Viking, 1987.

Kübler-Ross, Elisabeth. *On Death and Dying.* New York: Macmillan, 1969.

Mattingly, Cheryl. "The Concept of Therapeutic Emplotment." *Social Science and Medicine* 38 (1994): 811–22.

Mayer, Musa. *Examining Myself: One Woman's Story of Breast Cancer Treatment and Recovery.* Boston: Faber, 1993.

McCullogh, Lawrence B. "The Abstract Character and Transforming Power of Medical Language." *Soundings* 72 (1989): 111–25.

Parsons, Talcott, with Rene Fox. "Illness and the Role of the Physician: A Sociological Perspective." *American Journal of Orthopsychiatry* 21 (1951): 452–60.

Reiser, Stanley Joel. *Medicine and the Reign of Technology.* New York: Cambridge University Press, 1978.

Roberts, Helen. *The Patient Patients: Women and Their Doctors.* London: Pandora, 1985.

Sanes, Samuel. *A Physician Faces Cancer in Himself.* Albany: State University of New York Press, 1979.

Shorter, Edward. *Bedside Manners: The Troubled History of Doctors and Patients.* New York: Simon & Schuster, 1985.

Smith, John M. *Women and Doctors: A Physician's Explosive Account of Women's Medical Treatment—and Mistreatment—in America Today and What You Can Do About It.* New York: Atlantic, 1992.

Starr, Paul. *The Social Transformation of American Medicine.* New York: Basic Books, 1982.

Waitzkin, Howard. *The Politics of Medical Encounters: How Patients and Doctors Deal with Social Problems.* New Haven, Conn.: Yale University Press, 1991.

West, Candace. *Routine Complications: Troubles with Talk Between Doctors and Patients.* Bloomington: Indiana University Press, 1984.

3. Self-Reconstruction

Altman, Roberta. *Waking Up, Fighting Back: The Politics of Breast Cancer.* New York: Little, Brown, 1996.

Boston Women's Health Collective. *Women and Their Bodies: A Course.* Boston: The Collective, 1970.

Brinker, Nancy, with Catherine McEvily Harris. *The Race Is Run One Step at a Time: My Personal Struggle and Everywoman's Guide to Taking Charge of Breast Cancer.* New York: Simon & Schuster, 1990.

Burney, Fanny. "Mastectomy Letter," pp. 596–616. In *Journals and Letters of Fanny Burney (Madame D'Arblay),* vol. 6. Ed. Joyce Hemlow et al. Oxford, U.K.: Oxford University Press, 1975.

Butler, Sandra, and Barbara Rosenblum. *Cancer in Two Voices.* N.p.: Spinsters Ink, 1991.

Epstein, Julia L. "Writing the Unspeakable: Fanny Burney's Mastectomy and the Fictive Body." *Representations* 16 (fall 1986): 131–66.

Feldman, Gayle. *You Don't Have to Be Your Mother.* New York: Norton, 1994.

Gee, Elizabeth. *The Light Around the Dark.* New York: National League for Nursing Press, 1992.

Gilman, Charlotte Perkins. "The Yellow Wall-Paper," pp. 286–300. In *Major American Short Stories,* 3rd ed. Ed. A. Walton Litz. New York: Oxford University Press, 1994.

Hawkins, Anne Hunsaker. "Pathography and Modern Medicine: The Undoing of Cultural Trance." Paper presented at First-Person Singular: Autobiography Past, Present, and Future, a symposium sponsored by Hofstra University, Hempstead, N.Y., March 1994.

Herndl, Diane Price. *Invalid Women: Figuring Feminine Illness in American Fiction and Culture, 1840–1940.* Chapel Hill: University of North Carolina Press, 1993.

Ireland, Jill. *Life Wish.* Boston: Little, Brown, 1987.

Isaac, Betty. *A Breast for Life.* Hicksville, N.Y.: Exposition, 1974.

James, Alice. *The Diary of Alice James* [1894]. Ed. Leon Edel. New York: Penguin, 1987.

Kahane, Deborah Hobler. *No Less a Woman: Ten Women Shatter the Myths About Breast Cancer.* Englewood Cliffs, N.J.: Prentice-Hall, 1990.

Lorde, Audre. *A Burst of Light.* Ithaca, N.Y.: Firebrand, 1988.

Lorde, Audre. *The Cancer Journals.* Argyle, N.Y.: Spinsters Ink, 1980.

Love, Susan M., with Karen Lindsey. *Dr. Susan Love's Breast Book*, 2nd ed. Reading, Mass.: Addison-Wesley, 1995.

Lynch, Dorothea, and Eugene Richards [photos]. *Exploding into Life*. New York: Aperture, 1986.

"Mammograms—or Not—At Age 40." Editorial. *New York Times*, January 28, 1997, p. A20.

Mayer, Musa. *Examining Myself: One Woman's Story of Breast Cancer Treatment and Recovery*. Boston: Faber, 1993.

Middlebrook, Christina. *Seeing the Crab: A Memoir of Dying*. New York: Basic Books, 1996.

Rollin, Betty. *First, You Cry*. New York: New American Library, 1976.

Smith, Sidonie. *Subjectivity, Identity, and the Body: Women's Autobiographical Practices in the Twentieth Century*. Bloomington: Indiana University Press, 1993.

Sontag, Susan. *Illness as Metaphor*. New York: Farrar, Straus, & Giroux, 1978.

Spence, Jo. *Putting Myself in the Picture*. Seattle: Real Comet, 1988.

Wadler, Joyce. *My Breast: One Woman's Cancer Story*. Reading, Mass.: Addison-Wesley, 1992.

Williams, Terry Tempest. *Refuge: An Unnatural History of Family and Place*. New York: Vintage, 1991.

Wittman, Juliet. *Breast Cancer Journal: A Century of Petals*. Golden, Colo.: Fulcrum, 1993.

Young, Iris Marion. "Breasted Experience," pp. 189–209. *Throwing Like a Girl and Other Essays in Feminist Philosophy*. Bloomington: Indiana University Press, 1990.

4. HIV/AIDS and Its Stories

Alwood, Edward. *Straight News: Gays, Lesbians, and the News Media*. New York: Columbia University Press, 1996.

Arterburn, Jerry, with Steve Arterburn. *How Will I Tell My Mother?* Revised and expanded, Nashville: Oliver-Nelson, 1990.

Ascher, Barbara Lazear. *Landscape Without Gravity: A Memoir of Grief*. Harrison, N.Y.: Delphinium, 1992.

Ashe, Arthur, and Arnold Rampersad. *Days of Grace: A Memoir*. New York: Alfred A. Knopf, 1993.

Badgley, Laurence. *Choose to Live: The Four Fold Path, An AIDS Healing Companion*, 2nd ed. San Bruno, Calif.: Human Energy Press, 1987.

Badgley, Laurence. *Healing AIDS Naturally*. San Bruno, Calif.: Human Energy Press, 1986.

Bardach, Ann Louise. "The White Cloud." *New Republic*, June 5, 1995, pp. 27–28, 30–31.

Bergman, Susan. *Anonymity: The Secret Life of an American Family*. New York: Farrar, Straus, & Giroux, 1994.

Brandt, Allan M. "AIDS: From Social History to Social Policy," pp. 147–71. In

AIDS: The Burdens of History. Ed. Elizabeth Fee and Daniel M. Fox. Berkeley: University of California Press.

Brodkey, Harold. *This Wild Darkness: The Story of My Death.* New York: Henry Holt, 1996.

Brudnoy, David. *Life Is Not a Rehearsal: A Memoir.* New York: Doubleday, 1997.

Burns, Janice A. *Sarah's Song: A True Story of Love and Courage.* New York: Warner Books, 1995.

Chandler, Marilyn. "Voices from the Front: AIDS in Autobiography." *a/b: Auto/Biography Studies* 6 (1991): 54–64.

Cox, Elizabeth. *Thanksgiving: An AIDS Journal.* New York: Harper, 1990.

Crimp, Douglas. "Portraits of People with AIDS," pp. 117–33. In *Cultural Studies.* Ed. Lawrence Grossberg, Cary Nelson, and Paula A. Treichler. New York: Routledge, 1992.

Doty, Mark. *Heaven's Coast: A Memoir.* New York: HarperCollins, 1996.

Douglass, Frederick. *Narrative of the Life of Frederick Douglass, An American Slave.* 1845. Reprint, New York: New American Library, 1968.

Dreuilhe, Emmanuel. *Mortal Embrace: Living with AIDS.* Trans. Linda Coverdale. New York: Hill and Wang, 1988.

Egan, Susanna. "Encounters in Camera: Autobiography as Interaction." *Modern Fiction Studies* 40 (1994): 593–618.

Epstein, Julia. *Altered Conditions: Disease, Medicine, and Storytelling.* New York: Routledge, 1995.

Fisher, Mary. *My Name Is Mary: A Memoir.* New York: Scribner's, 1996.

Franklin, Benjamin. *The Autobiography of Benjamin Franklin.* Ed. Leonard W. Labaree et al. New Haven, Conn.: Yale University Press, 1964.

Glaser, Elizabeth, and Laura Palmer. *In the Absence of Angels: A Hollywood Family's Courageous Story.* New York: Putnam, 1991.

Greco, Stephen. "Excerpts from a Journal," pp. 114–23. In *Personal Dispatches: Writers Confront AIDS.* Ed. John Preston. New York: St. Martin's, 1989.

Harris, Daniel. "On Reading the Obituaries in the *Bay Area Reporter,*" pp. 163–68. In *Fluid Exchanges: Artists and Critics in the AIDS Crisis.* Ed. James Miller. Toronto: University of Toronto Press, 1992.

Hawkins, Anne Hunsaker. *Reconstructing Illness: Studies in Pathography.* West Lafayette, Ind.: Purdue University Press, 1993.

"Hot Type." *Chronicle of Higher Education,* May 3, 1996, p. A14.

Hudson, Rock, and Sara Davidson. *Rock Hudson: His Story.* New York: Morrow, 1986.

Johnson, Fenton. *Geography of the Heart: A Memoir.* New York: Scribner's, 1996.

Kruger, Steven F. *AIDS Narratives: Gender and Sexuality, Fiction and Science.* New York: Garland, 1996.

Lewis, C. S. *Surprised by Joy: The Shape of My Early Life.* New York: Harcourt, Brace, 1956.

Melson, James. *The Golden Boy.* New York: Harrington Park, 1992.

Melton, George R., with Wil Garcia. *Beyond AIDS: A Journey into Healing*. Beverly Hills, Calif.: Brotherhood Press, 1988.

Monette, Paul. *Becoming a Man: Half a Life Story*. New York: Harcourt, Brace, 1992.

Monette, Paul. *Borrowed Time: An AIDS Memoir*. New York: Harcourt, Brace, 1988.

Nardi, Peter M. "AIDS and Obituaries: The Perpetuation of Stigma in the Press," pp. 159–68. In *Culture and AIDS*. Ed. Douglas A. Feldman. New York: Praeger, 1990.

Newtown, George. "From St. Augustine to Paul Monette: Sex and Salvation in the Age of AIDS." In *True Relations: Essays on Autobiography and the Postmodern* Ed. G. Thomas Couser and Joseph Fichtelberg. Westport, Conn. Greenwood, 1997.

Osmond, Dennis. "Classification and Staging of HIV Disease," pp. 1.1-1– 1.1-15. In *The AIDS Knowledge Base: A Textbook on HIV Disease from the University of California, San Francisco, and the San Francisco General Hospital*, 2nd ed. Ed. P. T. Cohen et al. Boston: Little, Brown, 1994.

Painter, Kim. "AIDS Deaths Drop 13% in First Decline." *USA Today*, February 28–March 2, 1997, p. 1A.

Patton, Cindy. *Inventing AIDS*. New York: Routledge, 1990.

Peabody, Barbara. *The Screaming Room: A Mother's Journal of Her Son's Struggle with AIDS*. San Diego: Oak Tree Publications, 1986.

Pearson, Carol Lynn. *Good-Bye, I Love You*. New York: Random House, 1986.

Peavey, Fran. *A Shallow Pool of Time: An HIV+ Woman Grapples with the AIDS Epidemic*. Philadelphia: New Society, 1990.

Petrow, Steven. *Dancing Against the Darkness: A Journey Through America in the Age of AIDS*. Lexington, Mass.: D. C. Heath, 1990.

Preston, John *Winter's Light: Reflections of a Yankee Queer*. Hanover, N.H.: University Press of New England, 1995.

Price, Monroe E. *Shattered Mirrors: Our Search for Identity and Community in the AIDS Era*. Cambridge, Mass.: Harvard University Press, 1989.

Quam, Michael D. "The Sick Role, Stigma, and Pollution: The Case of AIDS," pp. 29–44. In *Culture and AIDS*. Ed. Feldman. New York: Praeger, 1990.

Reed, Paul. *The Q Journal: A Treatment Diary*. Berkeley, Calif.: Celestial Arts, 1991.

Rosin, Hanna. "The Homecoming." *New Republic*, June 5, 1995, pp. 21–23, 26.

Schoub, Barry D. *AIDS and HIV in Perspective: A Guide to Understanding the Virus and Its Consequences*. Cambridge, U.K.: Cambridge University Press, 1994.

Schow, H. Wayne, with journal entries by Brad Schow. *Remembering Brad: On the Loss of a Son to AIDS*. Salt Lake City, Utah: Signature Books, 1995.

Sergios, Paul. *One Boy at War: My Life in the AIDS Underground*. New York: Alfred A. Knopf, 1993.

Shilts, Randy. *And the Band Played On: Politics, People, and the AIDS Epidemic*. New York: St. Martin's, 1987.

Sontag, Susan. *AIDS and Its Metaphors*. New York: Farrar, Straus, & Giroux, 1989.

Sontag, Susan. *Illness as Metaphor*. New York: Farrar, Straus, & Giroux, 1978.

Stein, Gertrude. *The Autobiography of Alice B. Toklas*. New York: Random House, 1933.

Stribling, Thomas B., with Verne Becker. *Love Broke Through: A Husband, Father, and Minister Tells His Own Story*. Grand Rapids, Mich.: Zondervan, 1990.

Taylor, Christopher C. "AIDS and the Pathogenesis of Metaphor," pp. 55–65. In *Culture and AIDS*. Ed. Feldman. New York: Praeger, 1990.

Treichler, Paula A. "AIDS, Gender, and Biomedical Discourse: Current Contests for Meaning," pp. 190–266. In *AIDS*. Ed. Fee and Fox. Berkeley: University of California Press, 1988.

Verghese, Abraham. *My Own Country: A Doctor's Story of a Town and Its People in the Age of AIDS*. New York: Simon & Schuster, 1994.

Whitmore, George. *Someone Was Here: Profiles in the AIDS Epidemic*. New York: New American Library, 1988.

Williamson, Judith. "Every Virus Tells a Story: The Meaning of HIV and AIDS," pp. 69–80. In *Taking Liberties*. Ed. Simon Watney and Erica Carter. London: Serpent's Tail, 1989.

Wiltshire, Susan Ford. *Seasons of Grief and Grace: A Sister's Story of AIDS*. Nashville, Tenn.: Vanderbilt University Press, 1994.

5. Crossing (Out) the Border

Arlen, Michael J. *Passage to Ararat*. New York: Farrar, Straus, & Giroux, 1975.

Beisser, Arnold R. *Flying Without Wings: Personal Reflections on Being Disabled*. New York: Doubleday, 1989.

Callahan, John. *Don't Worry, He Won't Get Far on Foot*. New York: Random House, 1989.

Connors, Debra. "Disability, Sexism, and the Social Order," pp. 92–107. In *With the Power of Each Breath: A Disabled Women's Anthology*. Ed. Susan E. Browne, Debra Connors, and Nanci Sterne. Pittsburgh: Cleis, 1985.

Eakin, Paul John. *Touching the World: Reference in Autobiography*. Princeton: Princeton University Press, 1992.

Fine, Michelle, and Adrienne Asch, eds. "Introduction: Beyond Pedestals," pp. 1–37. In *Women with Disabilities: Essays in Psychology, Culture, and Politics*. Philadelphia: Temple University Press, 1988.

Fischer, Michael M. J. "Ethnicity and the Postmodern Arts of Memory," pp. 194–223. In *Writing Culture: The Poetics and Politics of Ethnography*. Ed. James Clifford and George E. Marcus. Berkeley: University of California Press, 1986.

Gabriel, Trip. "His Latest Never-ending Battle." (New London, Conn.) *Day*, April 15, 1996, pp. A4–A5.

Goffman, Erving. *Stigma: Notes on the Management of Spoiled Identity*. Englewood Cliffs, N.J.: Prentice-Hall, 1963.

Golden, Marita. *Migrations of the Heart*. 1983. Reprint, New York: Ballantine Books, 1987.

Hevey, David. *Creatures Time Forgot: Photography and Disability Imagery*. New York: Routledge, 1992.

Hockenberry, John. *Moving Violations: War Zones, Wheelchairs, and Declarations of Independence*. New York: Hyperion, 1995.

Hurston, Zora Neale. *Dust Tracks on a Road: An Autobiography*. 1942. Reprint. New York: HarperPerennial, 1991.

Jones, Edward E., et al. *Social Stigma: The Psychology of Marked Relationships*. New York: Freeman, 1984.

Kingston, Maxine Hong. *Woman Warrior: Memoir of a Childhood Among Ghosts*. New York: Vintage, 1975.

Kriegel, Leonard. *Falling into Life*. San Francisco: North Point, 1991.

Lionnet, Françoise. *Autobiographical Voices: Race, Gender, Self-Portraiture*. Ithaca, N.Y.: Cornell University Press, 1989.

Longmore, Paul K. "Screening Stereotypes: Images of Disabled People in Television and Motion Pictures," pp. 65–78. In *Images of the Disabled, Disabling Images*. Ed. Alan Gartner and Tom Joe. New York: Praeger, 1987.

Mairs, Nancy. *Plaintext*. Tuscon: University of Arizona Press, 1986.

Marshall, Paule. *Praisesong for the Widow*. New York: G. P. Putnam's, 1983.

Murphy, Robert. *The Body Silent*. New York: Henry Holt, 1987.

Oliver, Michael. *Understanding Disability: From Theory to Practice*. New York: St. Martin's, 1996.

Parsons, Talcott, with Rene Fox. "Illness and the Role of the Physician: A Sociological Perspective." *American Journal of Orthopsychiatry* 21 (1951): 452–60.

Price, Reynolds. *A Whole New Life: An Illness and a Healing*. New York: Atheneum, 1994.

Price, Reynolds. *Clear Pictures: First Loves, First Guides*. New York: Atheneum, 1989.

Sacks, Oliver. *A Leg to Stand On*. New York: Summit Books, 1984.

Shapiro, Joseph P. *No Pity: People with Disabilities Forging a New Civil Rights Movement*. New York: Times Books, 1993.

Sienkiewicz-Mercer, Ruth, and Steven B. Kaplan. *I Raise My Eyes to Say Yes*. Boston: Houghton Mifflin, 1989.

Silko, Leslie Marmon. *Ceremony*. 1977. Reprint. New York: Penguin, 1986.

Stone, Deborah A. *The Disabled State*. Philadelphia: Temple University Press, 1984.

Thomson, Rosemarie Garland. "Redrawing the Boundaries of Feminist Disability Studies." *Feminist Studies* 20 (1994): 583–95.

Thomson, Rosemarie Garland. "Speaking About the Unspeakable: The Representation of Disability as Stigma in Toni Morrison's Novels," pp. 238–51. In *Courage and Tools: The Florence Howe Award for Feminist Scholarship, 1974–1989*. Ed. Joanne Glasgow and Angela Ingram. New York: Modern Language Association, 1990.

Wendell, Susan. "Toward a Feminist Theory of Disability," pp. 63–81. In *Femi-*

nist Perspectives in Medical Ethics. Ed. Helen Bequaert Holmes and Laura M. Purdy. Bloomington: Indiana University Press, 1992.

Wilson, Daniel J. "Covenants of Work and Grace: Themes of Recovery and Redemption in Polio Narratives." *Literature and Medicine* 13.1 (Spring 1994): 22–41.

Zola, Irving Kenneth. *Missing Pieces: A Chronicle of Living with a Disability.* Philadelphia: Temple University Press, 1982.

6. Signs of Life

Adams, Timothy Dow. "Deafness and Deftness in CODA Autobiography: Ruth Sidransky's *In Silence* and Lou Ann Walker's *A Loss for Words.*" *Biography* 20.2 (spring 1997): 141–55.

Ballin, Albert. *The Deaf Mute Howls.* Los Angeles: Grafton, 1930.

Bauman, H-Dirksen L. "'Voicing' Deaf Identity: Through the 'I's' and Ears of an Other," pp. 47–62. In *Getting a Life: Everyday Uses of Autobiography.* Ed. Sidonie Smith and Julia Watson. Minneapolis: University of Minnesota Press, 1996.

Baynton, Douglas C. "'A Silent Exile on This Earth': The Metaphorical Construction of Deafness in the Nineteenth Century." *American Quarterly* 44 (1992): 216–38.

Bragg, Bernard. *Lessons in Laughter: The Autobiography of a Deaf Actor.* As signed to Eugene Bergman. Washington, D.C.: Gallaudet University Press, 1989.

Cohen, Leah Hager. *Train Go Sorry: Inside a Deaf World.* Boston: Houghton Mifflin, 1994.

Davis, Lennard J. *Enforcing Normalcy: Disability, Deafness, and the Body.* London: Verso, 1995.

Edwards, Jonathan. "Personal Narrative," pp. 81–96. In *Jonathan Edwards: Basic Writings.* Ed. Ola Elizabeth Winslow. New York: New American Library, 1966.

Higgins, Paul C. *Outsiders in a Hearing World: A Sociology of Deafness.* Newbury Park, Calif.: Sage, 1980.

Hurston, Zora Neale. *Their Eyes Were Watching God.* 1937. Reprint, New York: Harper & Row, 1990.

Keller, Helen. *The Story of My Life.* New York: Doubleday, Page, 1903.

Kisor, Henry. *What's That Pig Outdoors? A Memoir of Deafness.* New York: Hill and Wang, 1990.

Konner, Melvin. "Misreading the Signs." Review of *Mask of Benevolence,* by Harlan Lane. *New York Times Book Review,* August 2, 1992, pp. 14–15.

Krupat, Arnold. *For Those Who Come After: A Study of Native American Autobiography.* Berkeley: University of California Press, 1985.

Krupat, Arnold. "Native American Autobiography and the Synecdochic Self," pp. 171–94. In *American Autobiography: Retrospect and Prospect.* Ed. Paul John Eakin. Madison: University of Wisconsin Press, 1991.

Lane, Harlan. *The Deaf Experience: Classics in Language and Education*. Trans. Franklin Philip. Cambridge, Mass.: Harvard University Press, 1984.

Lane, Harlan. *The Mask of Benevolence: Bio-Power and the Deaf Community*. New York: Alfred A. Knopf, 1992.

Lane, Leonard G., and Ivy B. Pittle, eds. *A Handful of Stories: Thirty-Seven Stories by Deaf Storytellers*. Washington, D.C.: Gallaudet University Press, 1981.

Merker, Hannah. *Listening*. New York: HarperCollins, 1994.

Padden, Carol, and Tom Humphries. *Deaf in America: Voices from a Culture*. Cambridge, Mass.: Harvard University Press, 1988.

Preston, Paul. *Mother Father Deaf: Living Between Sound and Silence*. Cambridge, Mass.: Harvard University Press, 1994.

Rankin, Tom, ed. *"Deaf Maggie Lee Sayre": Photographs of a River Life*. Jackson: University Press of Mississippi, 1995.

Rodriguez, Richard. *Hunger of Memory: The Education of Richard Rodriguez*. Boston: Godine, 1981.

Rothman, David J. "The Sounds of Silence." Review of *Mask of Benevolence*, by Harlan Lane. *New Republic*, August 17 and 24, 1992, pp. 43–46.

Sacks, Oliver. *Seeing Voices: A Journey into the World of the Deaf*. Berkeley: University of California Press, 1989.

Schaller, Susan. *A Man Without Words*. New York: Summit Books, 1991.

Sidransky, Ruth. *In Silence: Growing Up Hearing in a Deaf World*. New York: St. Martin's, 1990.

Spradley, Thomas, and James Spradley. *Deaf Like Me*. 1978. Reprint, Washington, D.C.: Gallaudet University Press, 1985.

Stokoe, William C. *Sign Language Structure: The First Linguistic Analysis of American Sign Language*. 1960. Rev. ed., Silver Spring, Md.: Linstock, 1978.

Twain, Mark. *The Adventures of Huckleberry Finn*. New York: Charles L. Webster, 1884.

Walker, Lou Ann. *A Loss for Words: The Story of Deafness in a Family*. New York: Harper, 1986.

Warfield, Frances. *Cotton in My Ears*. New York: Viking, 1948.

Warfield, Frances. *Keep Listening*. New York: Viking, 1957.

West, Paul. *Words for a Deaf Daughter*. New York: Harper, 1970.

West, Paul. *Words for a Deaf Daughter* and *Gala*. 1970 and 1976. Reprint, Normal, Ill.: Dalkey Archive, 1993.

7. Epilogue

Brody, Howard. "My Story Is Broken: Can You Help Me Fix It? Medical Ethics and the Joint Construction of Narrative." *Literature and Medicine* 13.1 (spring 1994): 79–92.

Brookes, Tim. *Catching My Breath: An Asthmatic Explores His Illness*. New York: Vintage, 1995.

Brooks, Peter. *Body Work: Objects of Desire in Modern Narrative.* Cambridge, Mass.: Harvard University Press, 1993.

Broyard, Anatole. *Intoxicated by My Illness, and Other Writings on Life and Death.* New York: Fawcett Columbine, 1992.

Croce, Arlene. "Discussing the Undiscussable." *New Yorker*, December 26, 1994, and January 2, 1995, pp. 54–60.

Doty, Mark. *Heaven's Coast: A Memoir.* New York: HarperCollins, 1996.

Douglass, Frederick. *Narrative of the Life of Frederick Douglass, An American Slave.* 1845. Reprint, New York: New American Library, 1968.

Dubus, Andre. *Broken Vessels.* Boston: Godine, 1991.

Frank, Arthur W. *At the Will of the Body.* Boston: Houghton Mifflin, 1991.

Frank, Arthur W. *The Wounded Storyteller: Body, Illness, and Ethics.* Chicago: University of Chicago Press, 1995.

Fussell, Samuel Wilson. *Muscle: Confessions of an Unlikely Bodybuilder.* New York: Poseidon, 1991.

Grealy, Lucy. *Autobiography of a Face.* Boston: Houghton Mifflin, 1994.

Hawkins, Anne Hunsaker. *Reconstructing Illness: Studies in Pathography.* West Lafayette, Ind.: Purdue University Press, 1993.

Holleran, Andrew. *Ground Zero.* New York: Morrow, 1988.

Hull, John M. *Touching the Rock: An Experience of Blindness.* New York: Pantheon, 1991.

Klinkenborg, Verlyn. "Dangerous Diagnoses." Review of *Living in the Shadow of Death*, by Sheila M. Rothman. *New Yorker*, July 18, 1994, pp. 78–80.

Kriegel, Leonard. *Falling into Life: Essays.* San Francisco: North Point, 1991.

Mairs, Nancy. *Carnal Acts: Essays.* New York: Harper, 1990.

Mairs, Nancy. *Plain Text.* Tucson: University of Arizona Press, 1986.

Miller, Jonathan. *The Body in Question.* New York: Random House, 1978.

Murphy, Timothy. "Testimony," pp. 306–20. In *Writing AIDS: Gay Literature, Language, and Analysis.* Ed. Timothy Murphy and Susan F. Poirier. New York: Columbia University Press, 1994.

Sacks, Oliver. *The Man Who Mistook His Wife for a Hat, and Other Clinical Tales.* New York: Summit Books, 1985.

Updike, John. *Self-Consciousness: Memoirs.* New York: Alfred A. Knopf, 1989.

Index

Wisconsin Studies in American Autobiography

William L. Andrews
General Editor

Robert F. Sayre
The Examined Self: Benjamin Franklin, Henry Adams, Henry James

Daniel B. Shea
Spiritual Autobiography in Early America

Lois Mark Stalvey
The Education of a WASP

Margaret Sams
Forbidden Family: A Wartime Memoir of the Philippines, 1941–1945
Edited, with an introduction, by Lynn Z. Bloom

Journeys in New Worlds: Early American Women's Narratives
Edited by William L. Andrews

Mark Twain
*Mark Twain's Own Autobiography: The Chapters
from the* North American Review
Edited, with an introduction, by Michael J. Kiskis

American Autobiography: Retrospect and Prospect
Edited by Paul John Eakin

Charlotte Perkins Gilman
The Living of Charlotte Perkins Gilman: An Autobiography
Introduction by Ann J. Lane

Caroline Seabury
The Diary of Caroline Seabury: 1854–1863
Edited, with an introduction, by Suzanne L. Bunkers

Cornelia Peake McDonald
*A Woman's Civil War: A Diary with Reminiscences of the War,
from March 1862*
Edited, with an introduction, by Minrose C. Gwin

Marian Anderson
My Lord, What a Morning
Introduction by Nellie Y. McKay

American Women's Autobiography: Fea(s)ts of Memory
Edited, with an introduction, by Margo Culley

Frank Marshall Davis
Livin' the Blues: Memoirs of a Black Journalist and Poet
Edited, with an introduction, by John Edgar Tidwell

Joanne Jacobson
Authority and Alliance in the Letters of Henry Adams

Kamau Brathwaite
The Zea Mexican Diary
Foreword by Sandra Pouchet Paquet

Genaro M. Padilla
*My History, Not Yours: The Formation of
Mexican American Authobiography*

Frances Smith Foster
*Witnessing Slavery: The Development of Ante-bellum
Slave Narratives*

Native American Autobiography: An Anthology
Edited, with an introduction, by Arnold Krupat

American Lives: An Anthology of Autobiographical Writing
Edited, with an introduction, by Robert F. Sayre

Carol Holly
*Intensely Family: The Inheritance of Family Shame
and the Autobiographies of Henry James*

*People of the Book: Thirty Scholars Reflect on Their
Jewish Identity*
Edited, with an introduction, by Jeffrey Rubin-Dorsky
and Shelley Fisher Fishkin

G. Thomas Couser
Recovering Bodies: Illness, Disability and Life Writing